P9-DEW-121

Yoga for Health, Happiness and Liberation

By Yogi Bharat J. Gajjar

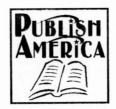

PublishAmerica
Baltimore

© 2007 by Yogi Bharat J. Gajjar.
All rights reserved. No part of this book may be reproduced, stored in a retrieval system or transmitted in any form or by any means without the prior written permission of the publishers, except by a reviewer who may quote brief passages in a review to be printed in a newspaper, magazine or journal.

First printing

At the specific preference of the author, PublishAmerica allowed this work to remain exactly as the author intended, verbatim, without editorial input.

ISBN: 1-4241-6994-1
PUBLISHED BY PUBLISHAMERICA, LLLP
www.publishamerica.com
Baltimore

Printed in the United States of America

**Dedicated
to**

my wife and inspiration

**Rupal B. Gajjar
(Anandi Narayani Ma)**

Acknowledgements

There are no words that can justly express my appreciation for the blessings and teachings of my Guru H. H. Swami Vishnu Devananda Maharaj. I'd like to thank him for introducing me to Yoga and to his Guru, Master Sivananda Saraswati. I'd like to thank my Brother Navin J. Gajjar for his help, guidance and encouragement in starting my life here in the US. I especially express my gratitude to the following:

Meeta Gajjar Parker, my daughter, who organized, typed and spent endless hours helping me to complete this book
John Akerley (Shankar), for volunteering to edit the book
Bhaskaran Krishnan, for also volunteering to edit the book
Cindy Kerr, for organizing all the images and helping organize the book
Ajay B. Gajjar, for writing the chapter on Anandi Narayani Ma (Rupal B. Gajjar)
Marc Weisburg (Arjun) for writing the Preface
Leslie Gouffray, Paul Moston and Jose A. Perez Jr. for the their art work
Manohar L. Kataria, Bharat J. Gajjar and Rupal B. Gajjar for their photography
Gregg Hill (Gopal) for proof reading

All my Yoga students, members of the Sivananda Yoga Center and the girls in the Village in the Baylor Women's Correctional Institution in New Castle, Delaware, 19720, for their contributions.

Preface

I would like to tell you how it all started. Let me explain the philosophy which has helped me a great deal in my life, and which may help you in yours.

When my father retired, a lot of people used to come see him and one day I told him, "Dad it's so nice that so many people come to see you." He replied, "I have 2 hobbies, one is astrology and the other is to know all about America. Now because I realize how important America is going to be in the world I have sent Navin (his oldest son) to study there."

It was 1949, when most Indians used to go to Great Britain to study. He believed America was the up and coming country that would grow and dominate in the future. So people used to come to find out about astrology or learn about America from my Father.

Then he told me his philosophy, "If you know one subject so well, people will need you and they will forgive all your bad habits or short comings. You should have a hobby that you love and should perfect it so well that when you retire it becomes your main business. If you want to get ahead, the way to do it is to work hard and not just sweet talk."

This advice is what I followed in my life. I was a textile engineer, majoring in knitted fabrics, and graduated from Philadelphia University. When DuPont hired me in Delaware, to do research in knitted fabrics, I made sure I knew every little detail about weft and warp knitted fabric technologies. I collected every article on this subject and did research in knitted fabrics. So, when I retired I wrote a textbook on warp knitted technologies. Because I was an expert on knitted fabrics, a lot of people within the DuPont company used to come and see me for my advise in their projects. Because I made myself very needed no one would let go of me or fire me.

During my years of work I chose Yoga as my hobby and I perfected it to my ability. Now the time has come and I realize that I can write a book on Yoga. I have taught Yoga to hundreds of people over the last 40 years.

There are many reasons why this book will benefit you. It is very practical and written in direct and simple English. This book is very authentic Yoga and covers all parts of Yoga. The book begins with goals of Yoga and following chapters help you to achieve your goals. The book will prepare you for beginning Asanas. There are hundreds of postures. In this book I've pulled out the most important Asanas that you should practice regularly. They are explained with pictures in detail.

Once you master these 28 Asanas that are recommended by H. H. Swami Vishnu Devananda Maharaj, a master of Yoga, additional advanced postures are presented. To emphasize the 3 supreme Yoga Asanas, I've written a separate chapter to concentrate on them. There is an entire chapter dedicated to the art of relaxation. Yogic breathing techniques are explained in detail with Mudra Yoga. Meditation and Mantra Yoga has been so beneficial in my life that I am excited about having the opportunity to present the basic techniques so that you can also incorporate them into your life.

During my many years of teaching Yoga I have encountered miracles of Masters through Yoga and I am able to share them with you through this book. If you want to practice Yoga, you have to do Yogic Sadhana (Practice), to achieve your goals. To make progress in spirituality Kriya Yoga (cleansing) is very essential and you will understand the depth of it's meaning.

To understand Yoga I have taken great effort to look into the Bhagavad Gita and Patanjali Yoga Sutra and included excerpts so that you can get a deeper understanding of where Yoga comes from.

For those who are struggling with health problems and trying to become vegetarian, I've included several chapters on Yogic diet, given simple vegetarian recipes and shown how this diet will improve your health. I have touched on the subjects of Brahmachara (celibacy), Hinduism and included messages from my students regarding their personal experiences with Yoga. I included a chapter dedicated to my work teaching Yoga to the women in the correctional institution in Delaware and how it has impacted their lives.

One of my dedicated Yoga students, who took a Mantra initiation from me, has written a write up for this preface that I have included here.

For 40 years, Bharat Gajjar ran a Sivananda Yoga Center in Wilmington, Delaware. The center was a large three-story house with a Yoga center and Satsang hall on the ground floor and two apartments above that helped pay the bulk of the expenses. This enabled Bharat to teach Yoga and give Satsang without concerning himself too much with money. The extra money he collected from class fees and from donations either went to the Sivananda Yoga Center or charitable organizations supporting Hindu culture and life. Bharat never personally profited from the Center. Teaching Yoga and giving Satsang is not a job or occupation for Bharat, but simply a part of his life and culture. Bharat's job until recently was at the DuPont Company working as a textile engineer. Now he is retired and devotes most of his time to studying, teaching and writing about Yoga.

Until he became a widower, Bharat's wife Rupal also helped manage the center and teach Yoga. Bharat knows what it is to lead a busy life with a wife, two children, and career responsibilities and still lead a life of Yoga. He is a Karma Yogi worshipping the Lord by serving Him through society and family.

For those forty years at the Yoga Center, Bharat showed us how to lead and teach without ego. Once a year Bharat would call all his students together at the beginning of the year and ask for advice on how to improve his Sivananda Yoga Center. Bharat would patiently listen to every suggestion without judgment, without defensiveness. Not once have I heard Bharat complain about a Yoga student. This is extraordinary since Bharat has taught Yoga to thousands of people. He is the most patient, accommodating man I have ever met.

Once a Swami came to Bharat's Satsang and gave a short lecture to his students. Afterwards the Swami said to Bharat, "I can see a few of your students are really serious." Without pause Bharat gently corrected the Swami saying, "Everybody here is really serious."

I will attempt to briefly outline my favorite teaching from Bharat's Satsang: "If you are miserable, then change your philosophy. If you are miserable, then you are following the wrong philosophy. If you are miserable and you think your philosophy is great, that is just foolishness. You have to change your angle of vision. Look at life differently. What is needed is a paradigm change. You are Spirit Soul; part of God; Divine Bliss; Joy forever."

Since about 1990, I have been very close to Bharat. I was fortunate enough for five years to serve him at the Sivananda Yoga Center and make him my Yoga teacher and mentor. Making Bharat my mentor has made my life. He gave me Mantra initiation and taught me the essentials of how to live like a Yogi, follow Hinduism (Sanatana Dharma), and lead a spiritual, joyful, moderate, family life.

Although Bharat initiated me into his Yoga lineage he advised me to go to India and find a living guru "in the flesh" as he put it and study outside his lineage. Bharat gives advice specifically suited to the person seeking that advice. He does not give generic advice. He gives advice out of his acute sense of compassion. In my experience whatever Bharat advises is spot on. If you have the sense that this book speaks to you, it is not a coincidence. Bharat is speaking to you and knows what is good for you.

Arjun (Marc Weisburg)

Table of Contents

Chapter 1

Introduction

Yog or Yoga is a Sanskrit word which means union. The mother tongue of English is Sanskrit. The English word yoke, which means joining, came from the Sanskrit word Yog. In America, the word Yoga is used instead of the Sanskrit word Yog because most of the Indian Yoga teachers in the USA came from South India where they put an "a" on the end of the word. However, Yoga is now the word used for the Science of Yoga. Yoga is not the end, but it is a way to the Supreme. In the material world, the human being feels separated from the Lord. When he or she walks toward God or the Supreme to unite with him/her, the process is called Yoga.

A great Hindu Saint from India Swami Vivekananda defines Yoga as follows, "To the worker, it is union between men and the whole of humanity; to the mystic, between his lower and higher self; to the lover, union between himself and the God of Love; and to the philosopher, it is the union of all existence. This is what is meant by Yoga."

Any person of any age and religion can practice Yoga. Yoga believes that God is one but names are many. Truth is one but Religions are many. All these types of Yoga will help one to achieve better health, happiness and liberation or Moksha. One can say it is a path to better physical, mental and spiritual health. One can say it is a technique to remove stress in a person's life and give inner peace. Yoga is not a religion but a way of living and a road to reach God Realization. You cannot separate Meditation from Yoga, they both go together. Some say that Yoga heals and purifies the mind, body and soul. In reality we have a body, mind, soul and an astral body. Yoga helps all four aspects of physiology. Yoga is harmonizing everything within oneself and all that is outside of oneself.

Who is a Yogi or Yogin? It is a person who declares himself a Yogi, who lives and practices Yoga, and believes in the Yoga Sutra of Patanjali as the Word of God. It is a person who studies, practices and teaches Yoga and spreads the good word. They have a Guru and at one point become a Guru, but it is not necessary. A Yogi or Yogin practices the Ashtanga Yoga, is disciplined and has high character as well as one who "serves, loves, gives, purifies and realizes" so says Swami Sivananda. He/she is on her way to God Realization, Self Realization and Life Realization. A Yogi does not have to believe in God, but it is beneficial if they do.

To most people in the West, Yoga means physical stretching, exercise, breathing, and a process of relieving stress or bringing peace. But, is much more complex, and there are many meanings of Yoga to many people. Some are as follows:

Yoga unites mind, body and soul. Yoga unites one to all in this material world through Om consciousness. Yoga is not a religion but a way of life. It can be practiced by anyone of any religion and of any age. You don't even have to believe in God to practice Yoga. Yoga is a path to better one's physical, mental and spiritual health. It is a road to better one's relationship with his fellow beings and nature.

Yoga is concerned with this material world and the life after this life or reincarnation. But a person does not have to believe in reincarnation to practice Yoga.

Yoga believes that by practicing Yoga, one can go beyond many physical laws (stop and start his heart, walk on water, etc). These supernatural gifts are called Siddhis.

If you ask a Yogi who gave Yoga to humanity, he will say, "God." Yoga is as old as man and as young as modern science. Yoga has been practiced in India for thousands of years, however, in the year of 2400 BC Maharishi Patanjali complied the Yoga science that was practiced in his time. He wrote a famous book in Sanskrit called Yoga Sutra. The word Sutra means a thread in the fabric of Yoga. He did not teach the whole spectrum of Yoga but gave just the essence of it. There are many interpretations and commentaries on his book, the Yoga Sutra of Patanjali. To a true Yogi, Yoga Sutra of Patanjali is the Bhagavad Gita or Bible of Yoga.

Yoga has four sources. The first is, Patanjali Yoga Sutra. The second is Vedanta, which presents Bhakti (Devotional-love) Yoga, Jnana (Knowledge and truth) Yoga, Raja (Meditation and Atman) Yoga, Karma (Service and good deeds) Yoga, Mantra (Vibrations and harmony) Yoga and Hatha (Body, discipline and energy) Yoga. The third tradition comes from the Bhagavad Gita where Lord Krishna presented Yoga and the fourth tradition is Kundalini Yoga, which is mystical Yoga.

In ancient India, most families practiced Yoga. However, after the Muslim invasions, Brahman families were the ones who mostly practiced Yoga in Ashrams, and also other religious people as well as Yogis. Swami Sivananda Saraswati of Rishikesh, India, was a great sage and a Yogi. He had many followers and disciples. He told them to go all over the world and spread the word of Yoga to the people to bring them health, happiness and liberation. One of his disciples, Swami Vishnu Devananda Maharaj came to America, practically penniless, and started teaching Yoga in New York City. Eventually he settled in Canada, opening an Ashram in Val Morin, Quebec. He was a great Yogi and also became my Guru. He was the first person to begin a Yoga teachers' training program and trained hundreds of Yoga teachers, helping make Yoga a household word in the US. Now the work of many Yogis has spread Yoga around the world.

A Yogi is a man or a woman who practices Yoga. That person lives Yoga and has declared himself or herself a "Yogi." Some people call a woman who does Yoga, a Yogini. A Yogi can be married or single. If a Yogi is initiated into Sanyasi or becomes a monk, they are called a Swami, and they are attached to an institution. If a person takes the oath of Sanyas and does not belong to an organization, he is called a Sadu, a wandering monk. A Swami or a Sadu can be, but doesn't have to be, a Yogi. They are both Hindu Monks, celibate, and take the oath of poverty. A traditional Yogi not only practices Yoga, but also has a Guru and accepts and follows faithfully the teachings of Maharishi Patanjali, and teaches Yoga, spreading the word. They are all lacto-vegetarian.

Blessed are those who are born in the family of a Yogi, who are lacto-vegetarian and are taught Yoga from an early age. Yet, children cannot truly appreciate the value of Yoga study because they are already in the Yoga discipline. Yoga comes completely natural to children and with ease. When age comes into play, then the value of Yoga is understood by all. The muscles begin to loose their natural flexibility and a person begins to feel the aches and pains of age. Yoga is not only beneficial to the individual but also to families practicing together. In this book all the postures demonstrated are by my family at different ages and my Guru H.H. Swami Vishnu Devananda Maharaj. In the postures he is demonstrating he was young.

I am a Spirit Soul (Self or Atman)

Yoga emphasizes knowing that I am a spirit soul (Self or Atman), and not this body. Yet, the body is the temple and it needs to be kept clean, strong and flexible on this journey towards God. The following Sloka emphasizes the Atma Puja—Worship of the Self. Fold hands and chant: (The Sanskrit Sloka says)

*deho devalayah proktah jivo devassanatanah
tyajedajnananirmalyam so'ham bhavena pujayet*

The English translation says:

The body is the temple. The jiva (your inner-self) is the deity of this temple since the beginning of time. May one remove wilted flowers that are looked upon as ignorance and worship the Lord with an understanding that he is not separate from oneself.

This message of Atman is greatly emphasized by Lord Krishna in the Bhagavad Gita.

The following summary of the Bhagavad Gita, by an unknown writer, is very uplifting to the spirit.

ESSENCE OF GITA
LORD KRISHNA SAYS IN THE BHAGAVAD GITA

1. Why do you worry unnecessarily! Who are you afraid of? Who can kill you? The soul neither takes birth nor does it die.

2. Whatever happened was good; whatever is happening is good; whatever will happen will also be good. Do not repent on the past. Do not worry about the future. Do your duty (Dharma), which is at hand.

3. What have you lost that you grieve for? What did you bring when you came into this world that you have lost? You came empty-handed and will go empty-handed. All your worldly possessions are simply changing hands; they belonged to someone else in the past and will be somebody else's some day. Your belief that your possessions are permanently yours is an illusion and is the only cause of your miseries.

4. Change is the law of this creation. What you think (fear) is death is only life because it frees you from the present changeable body which has become old and sick and gives you a whole new body and life. The notion this is mine, and that is yours, rich and poor, strong and weak, is born out of identification of the soul with the body. When you know the real nature of Self (Soul or Atman) you will find that all belongs to you and you belong to all.

5. You are not this body, but the soul residing in the body. This body is composed of physical matter and will disintegrate into physical matter when your Self leaves it.

6. Surrender to God (Paramatman—big self). He or she is the only refuge. Whoever experiences this becomes free from fear, worry and grief forever.

7. Whatever you do, dedicate it to God. By doing so, you will enjoy the Supreme bliss of a liberated soul.

The following story conveys the concept "I am spirit soul." There once lived a powerful King named Janaka. One night, he dreamt that he was a beggar, being persecuted by a group of villagers. They had tumbled him onto the ground, and were beating him with their fists, throwing stones and clods of dirt at him. All of a sudden, he awoke.

There he was, King Janaka, swathed in silk and jewels, being fanned by servants in his luxurious castle. Shocked by the contrast, he closed his eyes, and fell immediately back into the dream, where the villagers were still beating him, as he cowered on the ground in fear for his life. Once again, he awoke, finding himself back in the lap of luxury. This happened twice more. Janaka was fascinated and intrigued by the experience. Both states felt equally real when he was in them. How could he know which one was true and which was Maya, illusion? Was he the beggar or the king?

Back in the waking state, King Janaka called in all of his wise ministers and advisors, and asked them which state was real. None was able to answer the question to his satisfaction. The king expressed his displeasure by sending all of these so-called wise men away to be locked up indefinitely. In the meantime, a young son of a sage stepped into the courtyard. He was crippled and made quite a spectacle as he hobbled down the aisle to the throne. Many of the townsfolk had gathered, and were laughing at this ridiculous figure. The boy knelt down before the king, and with great effort stood back up saying, "Your majesty. I have come to answer your question." Now the bystanders really began to whisper and chuckle. This kid was asking for trouble.

But the king saw a light around the boy's face, and was guided by deep intuition to allow him to say his peace, even though it seemed unlikely that this boy would ever be able to answer the question. "Fine," said the King. "Tell me which state is real, the waking state or the dream state?"

The young boy smiled softly through his disfigured body, and replied. "O King. Neither the waking state nor the dream state is real. Only the Self is real, the Self that is beyond all Maya."

Lord Buddha said, *"The phenomena of life can be compared to a dream, a ghost, an air bubble, a shadow, glittering dew, the flash of lightning— and must be contemplated as such."*

There are 6 types of Yogis. They are Jnana Yogi, Bhakti Yogi, Raja Yogi, Karma Yogi, Mantra Yogi and Hatha Yogi. All Yogis practice Hatha Yoga, Pranayama and Meditation, however each one emphasizes one of the basic 6 types of Yoga.

Chapter 2

Goals of Yoga

Every philosophy, every technique has goals and Yoga is not an exception. When a person wants to take Yoga, usually that person has basic goals. The first is to achieve more flexibility. The second is to get peace of mind. Most people now believe that you can obtain these goals by practicing Hatha Yoga, which is a branch of Yoga. There are three distinct philosophies of Yoga, they are: 1) Yoga Sutra of Maharishi Patanjali (Ashtanga Yoga—8 limbs), 2) Vedanta Yoga (Intellectual, Physical and Social—Six types), and 3) Kundalini Yoga (mystical) and they all originate from Ancient India (Fig. 1.1).

In all of my teaching, I summarize the goals of Yoga as follows: Yoga leads to health, happiness, and liberation. These three words give the essence of the Yoga Sutra of Patanjali. The first and most important thing is to have good health. Practicing Yoga will also give you good health plus peace of mind and that leads to happiness. The whole Yoga tradition is designed to lead you to obtain Moksha. That means complete inner freedom and freedom after you die (outer freedom) so that you do not come back to this material world. Instead, you will join with God.

ASHTANGA YOGA—Yoga Sutra of Patanjali

The Yoga Sutra of Maharishi Patanjali is also known as Ashtanga Yoga (8 limbs of Yoga) because it describes Yoga as an 8-step process. The 8 limbs (steps) are Yama, Niyama, Asana, Pranayama, Pratyahara, Dharan, Dhyan, and Samadhi. His basic objectives are to offer good health and peace of mind. The first 5 steps not only prepare a person for good health and peace of mind, but also prepare a person for Meditation. The last 3 steps involve Meditation. The 6th step is contemplation, the first part of Meditation, which prepares one for deeper Meditation (step 7). Deep Meditation will lead you to Samadhi (step

8), which is the result of Meditation and is liberation (final step) See the 8 limbs (steps) of Ashtanga Yoga in Fig. 1.2).

1.   Yama—you and others

There are four Yamas, Ahimsa—non-violence, Satya—truth, Parigraha—non-possession, and Brahmacharya—continence. Lord Buddha says something similar in the following passage from the "Daily Readings of Buddha" by Swami Venkatesananda in his December 17th message.

"The Lord Said:

You have heard me teach the three decisive steps, which are: control of mind, known as Sila, which leads to contemplation or Dhyana, and then to wisdom or Prajna.

If living beings abstain from sexual desire they will not be subject to the round of birth and death. On the other hand, their practice of Meditation will not successfully eradicate defilements if lust is not completely eliminated. Hence, teach worldly men to get rid of lust. If this is not done, the practice of Dhyana will be futile, even as cooking gravel for food.

Again, if people do not abstain from killing they will continue to be subject to the round of birth and death. They who eat meat are but demons that will sink into the bitter ocean of birth and death and they cannot be my disciples. Therefore, you should teach people who wish to practice Meditation not to kill. This is the second decisive deed. If one does not stop killing and yet pretends to practice Samadhi, it is like one who is crying aloud while shutting his own ears and thinking that no one can hear him. Bhiksu (monks) should not wear garments made of silk, or shoes of leather or fur; they should not consume milk or dairy products. Then they will not transmigrate in this cycle of birth and death.

Again, if people cease to steal, they will not be subject to birth and death. Hence I teach that monks should not cook for themselves but live on alms. They should live here as travelers live in an inn. If they do not refrain from stealing from keeping more garments than are absolutely essential, if they do not give away food which may be in excess of their own requirements, if they are not ready to give away their own body in the service of the community, their practice of Dhyana is like pouring water into a vessel which has no bottom.

Again, people should, after being established in the above three, refrain from falsehood. If they lie, they will lose the Tathagata seed and begin to search for name and fame. Therefore, you should teach all the people not to lie. If they lie, their practice of Dhyana will be like making an image with excrement (instead of sandalwood) and expecting it to be fragrant as a statue made of sandalwood.

If the monk practices all these virtues, I will seal his realization of the bodhisattva's supreme Bodhi."

2. Niyama—You and your body

There are 5 Niyamas. They are, Sanca that means cleanliness and purity, Santosa that is contentment, Tapah that is religious fervor, Stadhyaya which is self study, and Isvarapranidhanami which means to surrender to God (or self).

Sanca—Cleanliness and Purity

Cleanliness has 2 aspects, one is your body and the other is the surroundings or your home. Purity is what is internal such as your mind and your spirit. Your Soul is pure but it is covered with impurities that have to be removed. Keep your mind with good, pure, happy thoughts and keep negativity out, live a good, pure, Dharmic life, pray and Meditate for purification.

Sansota—Contentment

We all seek a better life. At some point you are trying to fulfill your desires but you have to bring a balance to be happy. We should make our life simple and beautiful. We should not make it so complex and so busy that we have no time to enjoy and have no time to read good books and practice Yoga. Whether you are a monk or not, you should be very thankful for all that God has given you.

The Tao-Te-King of Lao Tzu says:
"There is no greater crime than seeking what men desire,
There is no greater misery than having no content,
There is no greater calamity than indulging in greed.
Therefore the contentment of knowing content will ever be contented."

Tapah—Religious Fervor

Tapah means intense desire for self and God realization. It also means austerity, penance, asceticism, self-participation (your full involvement) and strong desire to know God. Here one gives the greatest effort and moves at the highest speed.

Stadhyaya—Self Study

To make progress in spirituality or God and Self-Realization one must study scriptures and also practice introspection. To know oneself, one must sit silently and do some creative thinking. When you read a book like the Bhagavad Gita you should study it, take a topic and think about it, and try to understand its deeper meaning. Make that thought yours and allow it to grow within you. Continuous learning, improving yourself and getting to know who you are is essential in spirituality.

Isvarapranidhanami—Surrender to God

A Sanskrit name for God *Is* Isvara. There are two words here, is and Vara. *Is*—means changeless reality or God, and *Vara*-means master or a person in charge. So surrender to God means to surrender to the master. Let go of your ego, stop trying to be in control and surrender to God.

3. Asana—postures (See Chapter 6)

4. Pranayama—breath control (See Chapters 10 & 11)

5. Pratyahara—withdrawal of senses. Prepare the mind and detach from desire.

6. Dharana—mind control (contemplation)

When the mind is going in many directions, focus on one object or one thought and steady the mind. Prepare it to go into Meditation. In contemplation you are three—you, God and the object.

7. Dhyan—Meditation

When you surrender to God at this stage, you drop the object, and you and God are all that remains.

8. Samadhi—oneness

This means you have merged with God and two has become one, which is called "Om Consciousness." There is no duality left, this is Advithya (advaita).

Please note that Ashtanga Yoga says the 7 steps will lead you to reach Samadhi, the 8th step. Samadhi is the final stage of enlightenment. Hindus say it is Moksha or complete liberation. Christians say it is Christ Consciousness. Some Hindus say it is Om Consciousness. The word used by Buddhists, Nirvana, has the same meaning. Buddhism says Lord Gautama reached Nirvana or enlightenment and that is the reason he was called Buddha.

Summary of Ashtanga Yoga -

The first step of the goals of Maharaji Patanjali is self-discipline. You cannot go into a higher Yoga until you discipline yourself. The second step is observance. You can call both of these steps part of the "10 Commandments." The third step, Asana, means postures. Maharishi Patanjali says postures are very important and they will lead you to higher consciousness. I have observed many people come to learn Hatha Yoga. Once someone experiences Asanas with deep breathing they seek more advanced Yoga. The fourth step is Pranayama—Yogic breathing (deep breathing or full breathing). Pranayama is very important in Hatha Yoga. The fifth step is Pratyahara. That is when a person has to withdrawal his or her senses. This detachment will lead one to Dharana, which is mind control. Once a person reaches Dharana, he or she is ready for Dhyan or Meditation. Once a person does deep Meditation, he or she will be reaching enlightenment and Samadhi.

I have created a pyramid (Fig. 1.1) called "Yoga is a Way to Samadhi (Om)" to help in explain Ashtanga Yoga.

KUNDALINI

The Sanskrit word "Kundalini" means "Coiled up like a snake." Kundalini refers to the mothering intelligence, which awakens a person's spirituality. It is usually associated with an altered state of consciousness brought about through the practice of Yoga, Meditation or a near-death experience. When Kundalini Yoga is practiced it is generally associated with mysticism. According to the Yogic tradition, Kundalini is curled up in the back part of the root Chakra in three and one-half turns around the sacrum bone.

Kundalini Yoga also has 8 Chakras, which are really steps that lead you to Samadhi. The 8 steps or Chakras are as follows: 1. Mooladhara, 2. Swadhishatana, 3. Manipura, 4. Anahata, 5. Vishudha, 6. Ajna, 7. Sahasrara, 8. Samadhi (Om) (Fig. 9.3).

VEDANTA YOGA

The Vedas are the Old Testament of Hindus. The Vedanta philosophy came after and at an even later time Bhakti Yoga was introduced. Vedanta philosophy teaches that to reach Om Consciousness, Nirvana, or Samadhi one must practice one or more of the 6 types of Yoga, which are: Jnana Yoga (Knowledge), Bhakti Yoga (Devotion), Raja Yoga (Meditation), Karma Yoga (Service), Mantra Yoga (Loving Vibration) and Hatha Yoga (Discipline). Japa

Yoga is part Mantra Yoga and part Bhakti Yoga. (Table 2.1) Vedanta says any one of these 7 methods will take you to final Samadhi.

Vedanta also says that there are 6 basic types of human beings or Yogis. For example, if a man is a Hatha Yogi, he is basically inclined to do Hatha Yoga only. However, he may have another type of Yoga less prominent in him, such as Bhakti Yoga. But a Hatha Yogi can reach enlightenment or Samadhi just by practicing Hatha Yoga.

HATHA YOGA

In Sanskrit, the HA in Hatha Yoga means sun and the THA means moon. In Yogic philosophy it is said that there is a universe inside the human body. It goes further to say that that the right side of the human body is the sun side and that the left side of the body is the moon side. Both sides of the body are on opposite poles. Modern science has proven and accepted that humans have two sides of their brain, the right and left side. The right side controls the creative side and the left side controls the analytical side (Fig. 1.3).

	Right Side of Body	Left Side of Body
In the physical body	Ha = Sun	Tha = Moon
	Hot	Cold
	Male	Female
	Siva	Shakti
In the astral body	Pingala Naadi	Ida Naadi

Hatha Yoga is the physical side of Yoga practice. There are several types of Hatha Yoga. They are: Asana—Yoga of posture, Pranayama—Yoga of breathing, Kriyas—Yoga of cleansing, SavAsana—Yoga of relaxation, Laya—Yoga of rhythm, Naada—Yoga of sound, Kundalini—energy center, Bandhas—stoppage of energies, Siddhi—Yoga of power or going out of the body, Tratak—Yoga of gazing, Mudra—Yoga of body language, and Tantra—Yoga of sex energy.

We humans have three bodies: the Gross body which we can see; the Astral body which includes the mind and records everything experienced in this life and subconscious memories from past lives; and the Subtle body, which is a "non-material" vessel for your soul. The Astral body cannot be seen, but it came with our soul when we came into this world. It keeps memories of all our past lives when the soul leaves the body. It goes with the soul and enters into the Astral plane. There are three planes in the material universe, (1) Material (2) Astral and (3) Celestial plane. Brahman or the Spiritual World is not a part of the three planes of the universe. The material plane is what we can observe with our physical senses. The Celestial world has many different worlds, one of which is "Heaven," the world inhabited by the gods and goddesses who regulate the universe. The Celestial plane is also a part of the material world. Hindu philosophy says one cannot come out of this circle of life and death from the Astral or Celestial planes. One has to come to the material world to attain Mookti or freedom. This is the reason to be in the material world. It is a grace from God. Swami Sivananda says, "Do not waste any time in this world."

In the Astral body, there are three Pranic channels: on the right side, is the Pingala Naadi or Surya Naadi or Sun Channel; on the left side is the Ida Naadi or Chanda Naadi or Moon Channel; in the middle, there is a Shushumna Naadi. There are 101 Naadis in the astral body. Every two hours Pranic forces switch from Ida to Pingala Naadi and after two hours they switch again. At the same time, nostril breathing also changes. Every two hours one of the nostrils predominates by being more open than the other (Fig. 10.9).

There is a great connection between a person's breathing and his mental and emotional health. Balanced breathing is linked with a peaceful mind and good emotional health in the same way that unbalanced breathing is linked with a disturbed mind and emotional instability. A person experiencing anxiety or anger will have certain breathing patterns. By breathing in a manner associated with a peaceful mind, a person in fear or anger can bring the mind back to a peaceful state. The objective of Pranayama is to balance the breathing and healing the mind and emotions through proper breathing techniques.

The ultimate goal of Yoga is to balance through the practice of Pranayama and Mudra Yoga and Meditation and enter into higher consciousness. Entering into the Shushumna Naadi through Pranayama, one may subsequently awaken the Kundalini Shakti, the Divine Mother, to attain enlightenment, Samadhi and subsequently reach the goal of Mookti (freedom or liberation) and go into the Spiritual World; that is to merge with Brahman.

Ordinary people have three types of minds. One is balanced; a little happy, a little sad, a little frustrated, but overall it is balanced. We will call this the first type of mind. The second is disturbed with anxiety and over-activity. The third is depressed.

During Pranayama practice for the first type of mind, which is basically balanced and normal, one should practice alternate breathing or what is called

Analoma Veloma or Visanya Virti Pranayama (See chapter on Pranayama). For the second type of mind one should breathe from left to right only, because the left side is the moon side or cool side. Inhale through the left nostril and exhale through the right nostril. This will create a calm mind and bring the mind into balance. The breathing will also become balanced.

During Pranayama practice for the depressed type of mind, one should practice inhaling from the right nostril and exhaling from the left nostril only. This will uplift the mind, as the right side of the body is the sun or the hot side.

If one cannot or does not want to practice alternate nostril breathing, one can use one-sided breathing. That means, for the overactive type of mind, inhale from the left nostril and also exhale from left. It will have the same type of impact as alternate nostril breathing.

The goal of Yoga is to unite into oneness with Brahman and achieve Mookti, or liberation, and come out of this circle of life and death.

Types of Hatha Yoga and Their Goals
There are 14 types of Hatha Yoga. They are:
1) Asana—Postures which lead to better flexibility, strength, peace, spinal health, balance, toning, improved blood circulation, inner and outer harmony and realignment.

2) Pranayama—Deep breathing, which leads to body cleansing and healing, allows you to control and gain energy, increases life force and improves blood circulation, and brings mental peace.

3) Nindra Yoga or (Savasana)—Relaxation which leads to body and mind relaxation, heals the body and emotions, and improves health.

4) Bhandas—Locking energy that promotes better blood circulation and faster healing.

5) Mudras—Talking to God and your subconscious using body and hand postures to communicate with the astral body and subconscious mind and promote healing, cleansing, and higher consciousness.

6) Mind Control—Blocking useless thoughts and allowing only positive and creative thoughts leads to making you a more loving and compassionate being, brings peace and harmony, and allows you to live a dynamic, positive life.

7) Fasting—Controlling of your diet leads you to weight control, cleans the body, and teaches the mind discipline by working on controlling desires.

8) Tantra—Achieving higher consciousness through letting go, using sex to achieve God-realization. It is exactly the opposite of typical Yoga philosophy. Yoga means self-discipline and Tantra means indulge in all your desires to obtain enlightenment.

9) Diet—Vegetarianism leads to longevity. Fresh, healthy food in your system will provide proper weight and nourishment as well as a more disciplined lifestyle (free from drugs and alcohol).

10) Tratak—Gazing at candlelight helps you to control your mind and leads you to higher consciousness and allows you to go into a higher dimension.

11) Kriya—Cleansing of the body, mind, soul and astral body through ancient Yogic techniques removes diseases leads to better health.

12) Kundalini—Mysticism awakens the energy charkas for mystic experiences. Some people say that Kundalini is part of Hatha Yoga. It is part of Yoga, but not part of Hatha Yoga.

13) Laya—Yoga of rhythm. The goal is to attain higher consciousness through rhythm.

14) Naada—Yoga of sound. The goal is to attain higher consciousness through singing.

Bhakti Yoga and Raja Yoga relate to the soul:
Bhakti Yoga is devotional Yoga. This is practiced by surrendering to God, by singing devotional songs, going to Satsang or group activities, and through prayer or reading scriptures.

Raja Yoga is Meditation. This is practiced by meditating, opening up your third eye, seeking a Guru, and practicing Kundalini Yoga, which is mystical Yoga.

Jnana Yoga and Mantra Yoga relate to the mind:

Jnana Yoga is enlightenment through knowledge. This is practiced by reading scriptures, seeking truth and knowing yourself by witnessing yourself.

Mantra Yoga is loving God through vibrations and music. It is practiced by repeating chants and singing Mantras.

Japa Yoga is remembering God through Mantra Yoga (singing) and chanting with a Mala (rosary beads). See Chapter 14.

Karma Yoga and Hatha Yoga relates to the body and the material world.

Karma Yoga is selfless service. This is practiced by working without seeking the fruit of your action.

Hatha Yoga is self-discipline. This is practiced by doing Asanas, Pranayama, and Kriyas.

Summary

There are 3 primary goals of Yoga. I have derived them from reading the Yoga Sutra of Patanjali. They are: 1. God realization means liberation (love). 2. Self realization means enlightenment and truth. 3. Life realization means health and service. To me, these three are the primary goals of Yoga. I have made a chart (Illustration 2.1), to explain these three basic types of Yoga. To understand this chart, you have to understand the basic Hindu philosophy that in this universe there are only three forces. These are in reality the same three forces that Christians talk about. Hindus call these three forces the Father, the Mother, and the Guru. The Father is Siva, the Mother is Shakti, and the Guru is teacher. Christians say the same thing but use different words, "The Father, Son and Holy Ghost." Father is God, Son is the Only son, Jesus (Guru), and Holy Ghost or Holy Spirit, which Hindus call Divine Mother. Starting with Number 3, life realization is obtained by surrendering to Shakti, which is The Mother. This leads you to health and a dynamic life. Number 2 is self-realization, which is Guru, where you receive truth. This leads you to enlightenment. Number 1 is God realization, which is received by loving God (Siva) and surrendering to God. Opposite to life realization is laziness, pleasure-consciousness, no Dharma, and violence. Opposite to self-realization is darkness, ego, no Guru. Opposite to God realization is bondage, lack of trust, no Karma realization. For God realization one must do Bhakti and Mantra Yoga. For Self-realization one must do Jnana and Raja Yoga and for Life realization one must do Hatha and Karma Yoga.

Figure 1

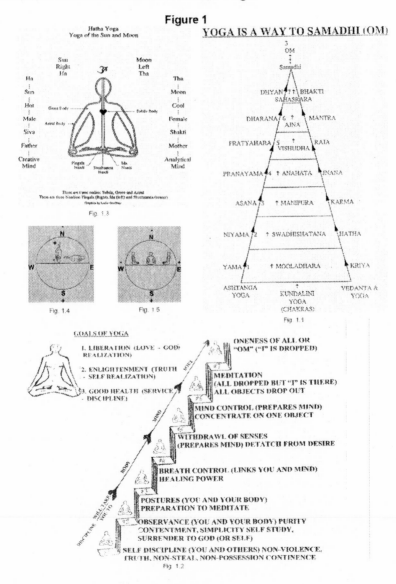

Illustration 2.1

Goals of a Yogi

1. *God Realization*

(do – Bhakti and Mantra Yoga)

Siva
Surrender; Love

OM
Liberation

↑

Problem
Bondage
No Trust
No Karma Realization

2. *Self-Realization*

(do – Jnana and Raja Yoga)

Guru
Receive; Truth

Enlightenment

↑

Problem
Darkness
Ego
No Guru

3. *Life Realization*

(do – Hatha and Karma Yoga)

Shakli
Open or Relax,
Discipline

*Health and
Dynamic
Life*

Problem
Laziness
Pleasure conscious
No Dharma
Violence

Table 2.1

Yoga Explanations

	Type	Pertaining To	Meaning	What One Should Do	Will Eliminate	Will Lead One To
1	Jnana	Mind	Knowledge	Study Scripture	Darkness	God Realization
2	Mantra	Mind	Vibration of Love	Japa or Rosary	Ego	God Realization
3	Bhakti	Soul	Devotion	Surrender to God and Guru	Bondage	God Realization
4	Raja	Soul	Third Eye	Meditate	Emptiness	Self Realization
5	Karma	Body	Service	Serve All	Pure Action	Liberation or Karma Free
6	Hatha	Body	Discipline	Build Health & Life	Negative ness	Life Realization

Chapter 3

Directions for Sleep and for Meditation

Hindu scriptures and proverbs tell you the best positions for sleeping and for Meditation. Vedic wisdom advises you to always sleep with your head in the southern or eastern direction, to always Meditate facing the north, east or west, but never facing the south, and do Japa, prayer or get married facing the south.

Thermal electricity generated by the sun travels across the earth, from the east to the west. The North Pole is a negative thermoelectric magnet, and the South Pole a positive thermoelectric magnet. Our head is negative and our feet are positive thermoelectric magnets. Like poles repel, while opposite poles attract and bring harmony.

In India, when a person dies, his head is placed towards the north and he is taken in the southward direction. It is believed that the God of death lives in the south.

The Shri Guru Gita, A Hindu scripture, says:

222. Japa done facing north-west ensures one will have no enemies, facing north-east one will acquire knowledge, facing south-east one gets one powers to attract others, and facing south-west vision (of God).

223. Japa done facing north will bring peace, facing east will attract others, facing south will cause or lead to death, and facing west will bring plenty of wealth.

224. This Guru Mantra has the power to attract all, to destroy all bonds and cause freedom. It makes Indra (king of heaven) favorable to you and can bring even kings under your control."

At weddings I would say the following:

	Sanskrit	English
(1)	Purve indraya namaha	Lord Indra resides in the East
(2)	Agne agnaya namaha	
(3)	Daksine yamaya namaha	Lord Yama (death) resides in the South
(4)	Nairtyam nairrtaye namaha	and so on.
	And so on	

I did not understand the deeper meaning of the above until I came across the following article by Swami Bua Maharaj. Here is a section of it:

"Vishnu Purana (Hindu scripture) says,

'O King! It is beneficial to lie down with the head placed eastward or southward. The man who lies down with his head placed in contrary directions becomes diseased.' The Varshaadi Nool says 'Sleeping eastward is good; sleeping southward prolongs life; sleeping westward and northward brings ruin.'

The Mahabharata says: 'Men become wise by sleeping eastward and southward.'

Two Tamil proverbs run thus: 'Vaaraatha vashvu vanthaahum dakkae thalai yaikkakkuudathu,' meaning, 'Even in the heyday of sudden fortune, one should not lie down with their head to the north' and 'Vidakketyayinum Vadakkaakaathu', meaning; 'Even the head of a dried fish should not be placed northward.'

An Ayurvedic physician seats his patients facing east before diagnosing the disease or administering his medicine. Brides and bridegrooms are always seated facing eastward on their wedding day. For effective Meditation, face east and north. Only corpses are placed with the head southward."

Healthy Method of Sleeping

To have a good night's sleep, you must not only sleep in the correct direction, but also cease tossing and turning. Poor sleeping is a health problem. Human beings are expected to spend a third of their life sleeping (about 8 hours a day). Deep sleep will help heal your body. So it is very important to know how to sleep. In this Chapter I will discuss the Yogic way of sleeping.

The first requirement is a good bed. The mattress should be nice and firm. Some Yogis like to sleep on a rug on the floor. If you have a soft bed, put a piece of plywood underneath the mattress to make it firm.

Recently one of my Indian friends living here in America, frequently had leg cramps. He tried several medicines, but had little relief. Then he went to India for a month, and his cramps almost disappeared on their own. The only thing he did differently was to switch to a firm bed. Upon returning to America, he changed his mattress to a firm one and he continued to enjoy relief from the leg cramps.

The second important thing in sleeping is to make sure your head is facing the right direction when you sleep. If your bed is facing north-south, make sure your head is facing south. If your bed is facing east-west, make sure your head is facing east. In India, the only time the head is placed northward is when a person dies/is dead. This is because your head is a negative magnet and your feet are positive. The north pole is negative and the south pole is positive. The same polarities repel whereas opposites attract and are in harmony (Fig. 1.4).

One of my Yoga students complained that she has a headache every morning. I asked her in which direction she had her head when she slept. She said she slept with her head to the north. Then I told her to switch direction and sleep with her head to the south. She was amazed that her headaches went away. When I go out of town, I take a compass with me to make sure my head is facing the south or the east when I sleep.

The medical recommendation is that children do not sleep on their stomach. In fact, no one should sleep on his or her stomach. You can sleep on your back, or on either side. If you want to burn body fat or if you feel down and want to uplift your emotions, sleep on your left side so that your right side is up. If you are hyper-tense, sleep on right side so that your left side is up, and you will experience peace. Remember, in Hatha Yoga (sun and moon Yoga), Ha— means sun (right side of your body) and -tha means moon (left side of your body). (For details see Fig. 1.3.)

People find it difficult to fall asleep at bedtime; they toss and turn or count sheep. They fall asleep once the body gets tired, but they have lost two or three hours of sleep. This is more likely to happen when you have something special planned and need sleep most. People find it even harder to sleep under these circumstances. Some people go to bed and get up in the middle of the night to go to the bathroom. On returning to bed, they are unable to go back to sleep.

I follow the Yogic way of going to bed. I fall asleep as soon as my head hits the pillow. I understand that sleep is not something I can make happen. Sleeping is involuntary, not voluntary.

A disturbed mind causes disturbed sleep. That means you have to stop your mind from thinking. Those who practice Meditation can sleep readily because they know how to control their mind. If you are not practicing Meditation, then you should do the following: Ten minutes before you go to sleep request your spouse not to talk to you, and tell yourself, "I'm going to sleep now, and I'm going to detach from the material world, the family and my projects. I will continue serving you when I wake up."

Tell the Lord, "I have worked hard and now I'm going to bed. I surrender to you, please help me out." If you have a Guru Mantra or any good Mantra like "Om," "Hari Om," or "Om Namah Shivaya," you can chant your Mantra. If you do not have a Mantra (see Chapter 14), you can use an English Mantra, "I am thine, you are mine."

If you do not like Mantras, just stop thinking. You are on the right path. Brush your teeth and get ready to sleep, and when your head hits the pillow you also will fall asleep quickly.

Suppose you still can't sleep and continue having thoughts. Then watch your breath go in and out with the Mantra Om and you will fall asleep in a very short time, because the mind cannot do two things at the same time.

If you get up at night, I recommend you go to the restroom and come back to your bed, but don't start thinking about anything, especially your next day's agenda, because if you do you may have a problem sleeping again. Just clear your mind of thoughts and fall sleep again. I taught this technique in my Yoga classes, and it has helped many of my students a great deal.

I read a very nice message in Bhagawan Ragneesh's book. He recommends that you continue your Meditation techniques before going to bed so you will spend the whole night meditating, and when you wake up you'll be absolutely blissed out. I'd like to extend this to say, remain very prayerful and very loving to God before you go to sleep so your prayers will continue during the whole night, and when you get up you will be full of love.

Some people like to take some medicine, or wine or other things to assist their sleeping. If you have to do it, it is ok, but you should make a goal to eventually stop taking sleeping pills or any other aid to go to sleep.

Everyone has some kind of dream; no one minds having good dreams, but nightmares are undesirable. Some people watch very violent movies, or TV shows before going to bed, and then have a nightmare for which they blame God. I suggest that while you prepare to go to sleep, don't watch violent programs and also pray to God, "Please don't give me any bad dreams." Bad dreams sometimes are part of past life tragedies. I'm sure that prayer can eliminate these bad dreams. Sometimes your unfulfilled desires crop up in your dreams. You can ask the Lord to remove them too. One of the ways to eliminate all this subconscious pollution is to learn and practice Meditation.

I wish you deep sleep and happy dreams every night.

Hindu Press International reports on April 1st, 2006
Study Shows Yoga Improves Quality of Sleep

"NEW DELHI, INDIA, March 29, 2006: A first-of-its-kind sleep lab now has empirical evidence that those who practice Yoga and Meditation improve their quality of sleep, says this article. Brain research also shows Yoga improving the quality of life for severe cases of epilepsy. "There is an increase in high amplitude waves in the sleep of people who practice Yoga and sudarshan kriya. The natural sleep pattern of middle-aged persons actually reverses age-related sleep degradation," said Dr. T.R. Raju, head of neurophysiology at Bangalore-based National Institute of Mental Health and Neurosciences (NIMHANS). The yet-to-be published study found that EEG of Yoga practitioners not only shows reversal of age-related degeneration of sleep but also displays a sleep pattern seen in younger people. This is the first scientific evidence on the effect of Yoga and Pranayama on the physiology of the brain. Yoga is also coming to the rescue of severe cases of epilepsy, where even drugs are proving to be less useful. "About 15 percent of epileptic patients are unmanageable by any methods of treatment. To this group, Yoga has been found to be very effective," Dr. T.N. Sathyaprabha at the department of Neurophysiology, NIMHANS, said. The team studied cardiovascular autonomic functions in epileptic patients who underwent eight weeks of Yoga therapy. The results were very encouraging: 68 percent had significant improvement of their autonomic functions (including heart rate and blood pressure) compared with pre-Yoga stage."

Conclusion

Sleep keeping your head south or east, Meditate and pray facing north, east or west but not sitting facing south (Fig. 1.5). During weddings, the priest should face the north while the bride and groom should face the east.

Chapter 4

Preparation Prior to Yoga Asana

Before you start, make sure that you are mentally ready to do a good Asana workout. Now, if you come home from outside, don't start Asanas practice immediately. First allow yourself to relax, and then start your practice. Now if you are doing Asanas in the morning, then you do not have to prepare yourself, however, to get greater flexibility it is good to take a hot shower before starting your Asana workout.

When you do Asanas properly, with single-minded awareness you can benefit greatly by the postures being done. If Asanas are done with awareness, they can be experienced as deeply meditative. The secret of awareness is that whenever you move your attention to a particular part of the body, the consciousness in that part of the body gets awakened and energized. So does the flow of Prana Shakti in that area. If one does postures, focusing their attention on each part, part by part, the whole body will come alive, cells become nourished and healing takes place. The deeper your awareness, the greater the affect and benefit you will have.

Significance of Om

Before Asanas, it is very important that you sit in Siddhasan or the Easy Posture with Jnana Mudra (Fig. 10.3). If you sit in this way you are creating a pyramid with your body and scientist say that in a pyramid all the energy flows into the center. Once you are in this position, take a deep breath and chant Om three times and say Shanti three times. Chanting Om itself is a most powerful Mantra in Hindu Dharma. I feel that many many years ago the Yogi's were meditating on the Himalayas Mountains and the wind came through the mountains the sound of Om was heard. Yogi's thought God was chanting Om and they started chanting along. You may wonder why Om and Shanti are chanted three times, the answer is that the first one is chanted for you and your inner peace, the 2nd one is chanted for all other living beings and the 3rd one is chanted for the Universe. You can even have your own 3 reasons or trinity.

Pain and Yoga Asana Practice

H.H. Swami Vishnu Devananda Maharaj used to say, "No pain no gain." In my Yoga classes, I showed Figures 2.1-2.13, charts that explain why one has to go into marginal pain to receive the maximum benefit of the Yoga practice you are doing. The chart in Illustration 4.1 shows the flexibility of a young child. Children have the maximum flexibility. The bar shows three levels A—B shows relaxed muscles of a child, B—C shows muscles being extended without pain. From C—D is the area of the margin of pain. At the point where D is shown is the breaking point of the muscle. One should not go to that point.

The 2nd bar shows the flexibility of a Forty year old that has never done Yoga. It shows minimum flexibility, and the muscles have lost its flexibility. I used to ask my students at this time, "When is a body it's stiffest? Then I would tell them, when a person is dead." But a person not doing Yoga gets stiffer as he/she gets older. I used to show them the Charlie Chaplin Walk, where all the muscles are very stiff and the legs do not bend.

The 3rd and 4th bar shows how one can come into the margin of pain during Asanas without breaking their muscles. The 4th part shows that by practicing Yoga Asanas and coming into the margin of pain, you will gradually increase your flexibility. This chart shows that if you do not come into your margin of pain your Asanas will not help you in increasing your flexibility.

The Science says everyday your body looses some parts and gains some parts through eating, breathing and through bowl movements. And every three years your body is completely replaced, so if you start Yoga at a later age, you can regain some amount of flexibility, however one cannot reach the same level of flexibility as that of a child. God has given us pain so we can live a healthy, happy and long life. I heard about a person, who had no pain; he had the greatest health problem. Pain can be your friend and it can be your enemy. You decide by how you deal with your pain. Pain is your warning signal, your red light, do not ignore it. At the same time some people take heavy medications, which is not good. One should try to solve the problem by listening to your body. Remember Safety is very important when doing your Asanas. Do not compete or showoff and get hurt.

Here's an interesting story about pain that I came across, "A man found a butterfly cocoon. One day a small opening appeared and the man watched the butterfly as it struggled to force its body through the small hole. It appeared that it had gotten as far as it could and could go no father. The man decided to help the butterfly, so he got a pair of scissors and snipped off the remaining bit of the cocoon. The butterfly then emerged easily, but with a swollen body and tiny, shriveled wings. The man continued to watch the butterfly, expecting that at any moment the wings would enlarge and expand to be able to support the body, which would contract in time.

Neither happened. In fact, the butterfly spent the rest of its life crawling around with a swollen body and shriveled wings, never able to fly.

What the man had not understood was that the restricting cocoon and the struggle required for the butterfly to get through the tiny opening were natures way of forcing fluid from the body of the butterfly into its wings so that it would be ready for flight once it achieved freedom from the cocoon.

Sometimes struggles are exactly what we need in our life. If nature allowed us to go through life without any obstacles, it would cripple us. We would not be as strong as we might otherwise be. And we could never fly." Source unknown

I have a story of my own from when I was a first year college student. I was taking a class with an Indian friend of mine. One of our assignments was to draw a picture. I had spent many years of my life studying art, and my friend watched me finish the drawing assignment in 5 minutes. So he asked me if I would help him on the assignment and draw the picture for him because it was taking him and hour to do the same drawing. So I did it. This continued for a couple of months, then the assignments started getting more and more complex, and I realized that what I was doing was actually hurting my friend because he needed to be able to do this work and he wasn't learning anything. I was crippling him. You have to go through certain pain to get the benefit in life.

There are three types of pain, mental, emotional and physical. The body pain is experienced by the mind, and different people have a different level of tolerance. Sources of pains are psychological, fear, chemical imbalance, disease, temporary or permanent bodily injury, self-inflicted, etc. Prevention is better. For that, practice Yoga, eat good balanced vegetarian food and maintain your weight. Always keep safety in mind and act accordingly. If you want to fight pain, Meditation and Pranayama are great alternative medicine. I'm sure a serious illness such as cancer etc. does require heavy medication and you should listen to your Physician.

What to Remember During Asanas

Relax your body before starting Asanas.

Wait at least 2 hours after eating before starting Asanas.

Before starting Asanas, sit in Sukhasan or Easy Posture with Jnan Mudra and chant Om and Shanti (3 times each).

Say a prayer or Yoga prayer (Om Asata Ma Sat Gamaya....)

It is good to do the practice of Pranayama or Yogic breathing before starting Asana and during your practice.

I like to start Asanas with the Swan Asana and the Sun prayer.

If you do not have much time to do Asanas, at least do the Sun Prayer (Soorya Namaskar) 3 times a day.

Do each Asana at least 3 times and hold each Asana as long as you can. Hold the Asana a minimum of 3 deep breaths—e.g. go into the cobra, inhale deeply, hold and exhale deeply. Do this 3 times and then come out of the cobra.

During Asanas, chant "Om" silently with breathing or chant your Guru Mantra, or focus on the part of the body you are working on.

Do Asanas slowly, evenly and without jerky motions.

Do Asanas meditatively and mindfully.

Work with mild pain and stay within your limits.

Do not compete with anyone. Practice Asanas at your own pace.

Keep safety in mind and avoid sharp pain.

Rest frequently.

Always stretch 3 times. Once you stretch, stay in the stretched position. The second time, stretch a little further and the third time come into the margin of pain. Always hold during inhalation and stretch during exhalation.

If possible, do Asanas religiously, daily and at the same time, place, and on the same carpet and make sure you remove your shoes before doing Asanas.

Develop your routine: some Asanas you might do once a day, some others once a week and some others once a month.

As a general rule, during most of the Asanas, when the stomach folds or contracts—you should exhale. When the stomach unfolds or expands—inhale.

Always do opposite Asanas—e.g. if you do a forward bend, then do a backward bend.

Never breathe through your mouth.

Remember Asanas are prayers to God with your body. Keep that feeling.

When you do Asanas, you are working with Prana Shakti, a living force that heals your mind, body, soul, and your astral body.

Hatha Yoga is a game of energy. Balance it and control it for better health and happiness.

If you have a cold or high blood pressure, do not do inverted postures such as the headstand or the shoulder stand.

Happy Asanas!

Asana in Raja Yoga Sutra

It is very important to know what Maharishi Patanjali says in his book "Yoga Sutra" about Asanas/Yoga postures. The following three important verses are taken from the Swami Vishnu Devananda's book entitled "Meditation and Mantras."

"Sthira-sukham Asanam

Asanas should be steady (aware) and comfortable.

Having thoroughly explained the yamas and niyamas, Patanjali now moves on to the next limb of Raja Yoga, the Asanas, or postures. This is the whole subdivision of Raja Yoga known as Hatha Yoga, which works directly with the Prana and Kundalini, the more subtle energy currents of the body. Hatha Yoga postures, always done in a specific order, massage the endocrine glands and release energy blockages in the system so that a meditative state is brought about physically rather than through sitting and watching the mind. Hatha Yoga is best practiced in conjunction with Meditation for the Asanas are a vital aid, but not the end, on the path to Samadhi.

It is said that the Asana should be steady and comfortable. Whether the posture is a simple cross-legged Meditation position or part of a set of Hatha Yoga exercises, it is important that the practitioner not be strained. He should be able to relax in the position—yet hold it perfectly still for a given amount of time. Fidgeting and loss of concentration only waste energy. Just as in Meditation, the mind and body must remain one-pointed.

Prayatna-saithilyananta-samapattbhyam

Posture is mastered by releasing tension and Meditation on the Unlimited.

There should be no strain, but only a firm and relaxed maintaining of the position. Then with the mind focused on the Infinite, one's limitations are more easily extended, and the Asana is mastered.

Tato dvandvanabhighatah

From that (mastery of Asana), no assaults come from the pairs of opposites. (likes and dislikes).

When Asanas are mastered the Yogi is not touched by the play of duality. His will and concentration are developed to such an extent that heat and cold, pleasure and pain, good and bad, and all other worldly influences do not touch him (V.46)."

MEASURE YOUR FLEXABILITY

It is important to know your flexibility. In research scientists say before you solve the problem please know your problem. An Irish proverb say's, "If you know the right road you are half way there." Youth means flexibility. Old age means stiffness only if you are not practicing Hatha Yoga.

In my Yoga classes I used to say children are the most flexible and the most like real Yogis, then I used to ask my students if they know when a human being is the stiffest. Then after they would give me several different answers, I would tell them that a human being is stiffest when they die. They are like wood.

The following is a test that measures a person's flexibility. Please measure your flexibility, it will help you to know which postures you need to concentrate on when you are practicing Hatha Yoga.

If you are a little stiff do not worry, just start your practice. Flexibility will come through practicing regularly. I am sure you will not be as flexible as a child, but you will get better because every 3 years you get a completely new body.

Then do this test, do the 14 Yoga Asanas shown in Figures 2.1—2.13. You can either do this yourself or do it with someone who knows Yoga. Rate yourself, using Table 4.1. For example Table 4.1, Number 1 is Vajarasan. Sit in Vajarasan and you decide how many points you should give yourself, 10 out of 10 of any number between 1-10. After doing all 14 Yoga Asanas, add all 14 points and see how many points you get.

Fig. 2.1 is showing a posture which is part of the Sun Prayer is Bharat J. Gajjar at age 38, Fig. 2.2 is showing the Bow Posture which is demonstrated by Ajay B. Gajjar at the age of 5, Fig. 2.3 is showing the Cobra Posture which is demonstrated by Meeta B. Gajjar at the age of 4, Fig. 2.4 is showing the Cow Posture which is demonstrated by Rupal B. Gajjar at the age of 34. Fig. 2.5 is showing a variation of the Plough Posture that is demonstrated by Meeta B. Gajjar at the age of 4, Fig. 2.7 is showing the Full Locust Posture that is demonstrated by H. H. Swami Vishnu Devananda* when he was in his twenties. In Fig. 2.6 Meeta B. Gajjar Parker (AKA MBG) demonstrating the Head Knee Posture the age of 40. In Fig. 2.8

Bharat J. Gajjar is demonstrating the Head Knee Posture. In Fig. 2.9 Meeta B. Gajjar Parker demonstrating the Yoga Mudra Posture. In Fig. 2.10 Meeta B. Gajjar Parker demonstrating the Natraj Posture. In Fig. 2.11 Meeta B. Gajjar Parker is demonstrating the Pranayama Posture. In Fig. 2.12 Meeta B. Gajjar Parker is demonstrating the Shoulder Stand Posture at the age of 20. In Fig. 2.13 Bharat J. Gajjar demonstrating the Triangle Posture.

*Picture from "The Complete Illustrated Book of Yoga" written by H. H. Swami Vishnu Devananda.

Illustration 4.1

No Pain, No Gain

(1) Young child's flexibility

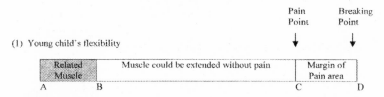

(2) 40 Years old person who does not do Yoga Asana or any stretching exercise, muscle will lose its stretch ability.

If the muscle is stretched

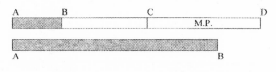

(3) For a year during Asana, come into the margin of pain

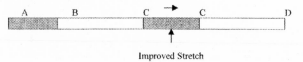

(4) After one year of Yoga Asana practice pain point "C" will shift

Improved Stretch

- To improve your health and flexibility, come into the Margin of Pain
  Be safe and make sure you do not get too close to the breaking point or sharp pain

43

Table 4.1

MEASURE YOUR FLEXIBILITY

	Yoga Asana	Yoga Posture	Plate #	Total Points	Your Points
1	VAJRASANAJ	SIT ON YOUR KNEES	1	10	
2	YOGA MUDRA	LOTUS POSTURE	2	10	
3	PASCHIMOTHANASAN	HEAD KNEE POSTURE	3	10	
4	SARVANGASAN	SHOULDER STAND	4	10	
5	HALASAN	PLOUGH POSTURE	5	10	
6	BHUJANGASAN	COBRA POSTURE	6	10	
7	DHANURASAN	BOW POSTURE	7	5	
8	SALABHASAN	FULL LOCUST	8	5	
9	SURYA NAMA SKAR #4	SUN PRAYER STEP #1	9	5	
10	----------	SQUATTING POSE	10	5	
11	----------	SQUATTING & STAND UP	11	5	
12	TRIKONASAN	TRIANGLE POSTURE	12	5	
13	NATARAJASAN	LORD NATARAJA	13	5	
14	GOMUKHASANA	COW HEAD POSE	14	5	
			TOTAL	100	

Chapter 5

Warm Up Asanas

Cross Leg Jumping

Begin by standing up. Place your left foot forward and your right foot back, and your hands on your hips. Each time you jump you switch the positions of your feet. Every time your right foot comes forward count one. Try to do at least 50 repetitions, gradually work up to 100. Inhale and exhale every time you jump. This is one of the best warm up exercises and it is good to teach this Asana in your Yoga classes. This is also a good cardiovascular exercise.

Rocking of the Back Asana

This particular Asana will massage your back. Begin by sitting on the floor with both knees pulled in. Then wrap your arms around your thighs. Now roll back, and stretch your legs out until they are straight. Then roll forward. Inhale when you roll back and exhale when you roll forward.

On the second or third round roll slightly to your right side, and on the next roll go slightly to your left. This massaging of the back will strengthen your spine and also relieve any tension around the neck. Do not roll back too forcefully as that could hurt your neck.

Wood Chopping Asana

Start by standing up. Keep your feet about three feet apart. Clasp your hands together and bend down. Inhale as you move up with your arms above your head and then bring down your hands forcefully as though you are chopping wood. A forceful downward swing is important, so make sure you remember to add force. Count one each time you go up and down. It's good to do the posture about 12 times. This Wood Chopping Asana (Figures 3.1 and

3.2) is a breathing technique that will gradually reduce back pain if you suffer from that.

Rolling of the Joints Asana

The movement and rotation lubricates the joints. The stretching, tensing and relaxing of all the associated tissues, ligaments and muscles promotes healthy blood flow.

Part 1 A

This particular Asana in Hatha Yoga is very important as it makes your joints supple. First roll your shoulders clockwise three times and then counter clockwise three times. Then continue.

Take your right hand. Begin by holding your arm straight out, away from your body. Put your left hand under your arm. Roll your arm clockwise, three times. Then roll your arm counterclockwise, three times.

Part 1 B

Now hold your right arm with your left hand, just above your elbow, and roll the lower part of your arm three times clockwise and three times counterclockwise.

Part 1 C

Now hold your right hand above your wrist with your left hand, and roll your wrist three times clockwise, and three times counterclockwise.

Part 1 D

Then open and close the fingers on your right hand.

Part 1 E

Roll each finger, three times clockwise, and three times counterclockwise.

Part 2—repeat all the steps in part 1 on your left hand.

Part 3 A

Then lie down on your left side, cradling your head with your left hand. Extend your right leg out and make large circles, three times clockwise, and three times counterclockwise.

Part 3 B

Sit up and grab your right thigh with both hands and roll your lower leg around in 3 large circles in both directions.

Part 3 C

Next, grab your ankle with both hands and roll your foot around, three times clockwise, and counterclockwise three times.

Part 4
Repeat all the steps of part 3 on your left leg.
Part 5
Roll your neck three times clockwise, and three times counterclockwise.
Part 6
Roll your eyes three times clockwise, and three times counterclockwise.
Part 7
Stand up, put your hands on your hips and roll your hips around three times clockwise, and three times counterclockwise.

Stretching of the Joints Asanas
Padanguli Naman (Toe Bending)
While sitting on the floor with your legs out in front of you, keep your feet straight and still. Become aware of the toes and bend them backward while exhaling. Hold each position for a few seconds. Practice 10 rounds. Integrate the breath with the action while placing your full awareness and consciousness on your toes. Try to become aware of the movement of "prana."

It is very important to activate the toes and feet, as the region is full of nerve endings and meridian points. Stimulating the feet activates the "pranic" flow.

Goolf Naman (Ankle Bending)
Remain sitting with your feet out in front of you, and legs straight. Point the feet backwards while inhaling, bending from the ankle joint. Point them forward while exhaling. Hold each position for a few seconds. Feel the stretch in the calves and leg muscles. Practice 10 rounds.

Goolf Chakra (Ankle Rotation)
Keep the heels in contact with the floor. Point the toes and rotate the feet at the ankle joint in a clockwise motion, as though painting a large circle with the big toe. Coordinate one rotation with one slow breath. Practice 10 rounds. Now do this exercise in a counterclockwise direction for 10 rounds.

Janu Naman (Knee Bending)
Exhale while bending the right leg at the knee, with hands clasped under the right thigh. Inhale while straightening the right leg without allowing the leg to

touch the ground. The hands remain under the thigh with the arms straightening and bending along with the leg. Practice 10 times with each leg.

Ardha Titali Asana (Half Butterfly)

Bend the right leg, placing the right foot over the left thigh. Hold the toes of the right foot with the left hand and place the right hand on the bent right knee. As you inhale gently, raise the right knee up toward the chest and, as you exhale, lower the knee to touch the floor. Slowly practice 10 rounds with each leg. This is excellent for loosening up the knee and hip joints.

Poorna Titali Asana (Full Butterfly)

Bend your knees, bringing the soles of your feet together. Clasp the feet with both hands and try to pull the feet as close to the body as possible. Relax the inner thigh muscles. Gently bounce the knees up and down, using the elbows as levers to press the legs down. Practice 30 to 50 rounds. Breathe normally.

Fingers, Wrist and Neck

For the following practices, you can sit with crossed legs in the Easy Posture or Indian style. The back must remain straight.

Mushtika Bandhana (Hand Clenching)

Hold both arms stretched straight in front of the body at shoulder level, palms down.

Then stretch the fingers wide apart while inhaling. Clench the fingers around the thumb to make a tight fist while exhaling. Practice 10 rounds.

Manibandha Naman (Wrist Bending)

Hold both arms stretched straight in front of your body at shoulder level. Keep your palms open and your fingers and elbows straight throughout the practice. Inhale while bending your hands backwards, with the fingers pointed up and towards you. Exhale while bending your hands forwards, fingers pointing down and towards you. Practice 10 times.

Skandha Chakra (Shoulder-socket Rotation)

Place your right fingers on your right shoulder and your left fingers on your left shoulder. Fully rotate both elbows at the same time in large circles. Try to touch the elbows in front of the chest on the forward movement and touch the ears while moving up. Stretch your arms back in the backward movement and touch the sides of the trunk while coming down. Inhale on the downward stroke. Practice 10 rounds clockwise and 10 rounds counterclockwise.

Both Shoulder Rotation

Roll both shoulders together clockwise three times and then roll both shoulders together counterclockwise three times.

This "Asana" helps open the shoulders and chest. It relieves strain and helps in cervical spondylitis and frozen shoulders.

Greeva Sanchalana (Neck Movements)

Slowly move the head forward, while exhaling, and try to touch the chest with the chin. While inhaling slowly, drop the head back as far as possible. Feel the stretch in the neck. Practice 10 rounds.

Slowly rotate the head in a relaxed, smooth, rhythmic manner, coordinating one complete circular movement with one slow breath. Practice 10 rounds clockwise and 10 rounds counter clockwise.

These "Asanas" relieve tension and stiffness in the head, neck and shoulder regions.

(Stretching of the Joints was developed by Paramahamsa Satyananda Saraswati and was written by Sarvath Khan, courtesy of Femina magazine, 2001.)

Hold Tight and Stretch with Breathing

"In this posture you inhale, hold, exhale and stretch during each repetition of the Asana. Sit in the Easy Posture (SukAsanan), and put your hands on your lap. Inhale deeply, and bring both your hands in front with your palms facing out, fingers locked. Now take a deep breath and hold firmly and stretch as you exhale deeply. Stay in the posture, don't relax the tension in your arms and inhale, hold and stretch again. Repeat one more time. Next take a deep breath, and during the exhalation, pull your arms straight up. Keeping your fingers locked, take a deep breath and during the exhalation, stretch your arms upward. Do not let your arms relax, maintain the stretched position and stretch again during the exhalation and repeat once more. Then take a deep breath and lower your arms behind your head, keeping your fingers clasped and inhale, hold, exhale, stretch, and pull your elbows back. Do this three times. Next, inhale, hold, and exhale, stretching your arms upward with your palms facing out, fingers clasped straight up. Then inhale, hold, and exhale bringing your arms forward, palms out and fingers clasped, and repeat this three times. Then inhale bringing your arms back up above your head straight up, exhale, stretch, and repeat three times. The last step is separating your hands and lowering your arms down next to your body and relax."

Chapter 6

Recommended Daily Asanas

It is said that there are 480,000 Asanas (postures). Out of these, the key postures, about 28, are discussed in this chapter. When I started teaching Yoga my students would ask me, "What is a good routine to practice?" When I went to the Sivananda Ashram to see my Guru, H. H. Swami Vishnu Devananda Maharaj (Fig. 14.3), I asked him this question and he gave me the following routine that I use in teaching my Yoga classes as well as in my own Yoga practice. They are given below in the order they should be practiced:

Before starting your Asana practice, chant Om, Om, Om, Shanti, Shanti, Shanti. Next Recite "Trayambakam" and sing the "Jaya Ganesha" Mantra that can be found in chapter 14. You may also recite the Yoga Prayer (see Chapter 14) or any other prayer you choose. Then do a 7 to 21 minute Meditation (if time permits), and do Pranayama as follows: first do Kapalabhati (Cleansing Breath: Three rounds, three times—One round = 12 times.) second do Visma Virtti Pranayama (Alternate Nostril Breathing or Healing Breath; three rounds). Then begin your Asanas.

Do the following as your recommended daily Asanas:
1. Swan Posture (Prostration to God and Guru)
2. Mountain Pose (PARVATASAN)
3. Sun Prayer or Sun Salutation (SURYA NAMASKAR) 3 times
4. Eye and Neck Exercises
5. Raised Leg Posture (Right & Left)
6. Body Raised Posture (Right & Left) (EKA—PADA—SIRSHASAN)
7. Shoulder stand (SARVANGASAN) &/or Headstand (SIRSHASAN)
8. Plough Posture (HALASAN)
9. Bridge Posture

10. Fish Posture (MATSYASAN)
11. Yoga Mudra
12. Head to Knees Posture (PASCHIMOTHANSAN)
13. Leg—Head Posture (EKA—PADA—SIRSHASAN)
14. Triangle Posture (HASTHA PADSAN)
15. Ankle—knee Posture (BANDRASAN)
16. Head—knee Posture (JANU—SIRSHASAN)
17. Inclined Plane (VASISTHANSAN)
18. Wheel Posture (CHAKRASAN)
19. Cobra Posture (BHUJANGASAN)
20. Half Locust (Right & Left) (SALABHASAN)
21. Full Locust (SALABHASAN)
22. Bow Posture (DHANURASAN) and rock forward and backward
23. Triangle Posture (UTTHITA & PARNKTTA & TRIKONASAN)
24. Tree Posture (EK PAD ASAN)
25. Squatting Posture
26. Twist (ARDHA—MATSYEN DRASAN)
27. Relaxed Pose (SAVASAN)
28. Wind Relieving Posture (VATAYANASAN) (Right & Left and both legs together)
(Pictures of Asanas can be found on pages 64-72.)

There are 3 supreme Yoga Asanas: the first is Yoga Asana, the second is the Headstand or Shoulder Stand, and the third is the Sun Prayer or Surya Namaskar. These three are described separately in Chapter 8 called "Three Supreme Asanas." Some people like to say that the following 14 Asanas are the key Yoga Asanas. They are, 1) Yoga Asana, 2) Headstand or Shoulder stand, 3) Sun Prayer, 4) Cobra, 5) Head to Knee, 6) Spinal Twist, 7) Plow, 8) Fish, 9) Bow, 10) Full Locust, 11) Triangle Posture, 12) Body Raise Posture, 13) Wheel Posture, 14) Savasana (Relaxation).

Swan Posture (Prostration to God and Guru)

Sit on your knees (Vajrasana) and put your hands on your knees. Take a deep breath and exhale while bending at the waist, placing your forehead on the floor with your arms stretched out. This is recommended as the first posture because it is surrendering to the Divine Lord Mudra (Fig. 3.3).

Mountain Pose (PARVATASAN)

Sit in the Lotus Posture (Padmasan) (Fig. 3.4) or in the Half Lotus (Siddhasan), or you can sit in the Easy Posture (Sukasan) and make prayerful hands. Inhale and then exhale as you bend forward and put your head on the floor. Inhale while your head is down and exhale while coming up. Put your prayerful hands on top of your head. Inhale in this position and exhale while extending your arms upward. Then take a deep breath and stretch out upward with your arms, stretching your spine upward. Staying in the stretched position, take another deep breath and try to stretch further in the upward direction. Do the last step a total of three times.

The final step is to inhale and stretch forward, bringing the head down to the floor.

This posture strengthens the spine. Your spine is your youth. This posture separates the vertebras of your spine and increases flexibility.

Sun Prayer or Sun Salutation (SURYA NAMASKAR) 3 times

Please see chapter 7 "Three Supreme Asanas" (Fig. 9.1)

Eye and Neck Exercises

Eye Exercises (Figures 3.5—3.7)

Prepare for the posture by sitting in Sukasan or Easy Posture. Put your hands on your knees. Keep your spine and neck in straight alignment. Look straight ahead, keeping your eyes open. Try to position your eyes where you can see both the ceiling and the floor at the same time. Keep the head and neck motionless while performing these exercises.

Begin the Eye Exercise by looking to your right and stretch the eyes to see further, then look left and stretch. Inhale while looking to the right and exhale while looking to the left. Perform the exercise three times

Then bring your eyes to the front. Next look up and stretch, and then down and stretch. After doing three rounds, come back to the straight-ahead position.

Next, look up at the right corner and stretch, then down at the left corner and stretch. Then come to the center. Switch corners and do the same exercise on the opposite side.

Then begin by looking down and roll your eyes all the way around clockwise three times. Then roll your eyes in the opposite direction three times.

Next, put your right hand forward with your index finger out and facing you. Keep your eyes on the tip of your finger and bring the finger towards your face until the finger touches your forehead. Then gradually take the finger back to the extended position while still gazing at the tip of your finger.

Then take the index fingers of both hands and have them facing each other while you gaze at the tip of both fingers. Pull your fingers in opposite directions slowly, then, bring the fingers slowly back together until they meet in the middle.

Neck Exercise (Fig. 3.8)

Prepare for this posture the same way as you did for the eye exercise. Then begin by inhaling and stretching your head back, open your mouth and go back further, then exhale as you bring your head forward until your chin is touching your chest. Repeat three times.

Then bring your head to the center. Turn your head to the right and stretch while inhaling. Then exhale while turning your head to the left. Do three repetitions, then come to the center.

Next, inhale while you bring your right ear down to your right shoulder. Do not raise your shoulder. It is not important that the ear touches the shoulder; just tilt the head as far as you can without pain. Repeat on the left side. Do three repetitions.

Come to the center again and roll your head clockwise three times while doing deep breathing. Then do it counter-clockwise three times.

The neck exercise will increase relaxation in your body. Some people like to do the neck exercise with their eyes closed while others like to roll their eyes with their neck. The Asana will strengthen the neck muscles.

Raised Leg Posture (Right & Left)

This posture is in preparation for the Body Raise Posture (Fig. 3.9) and leg head posture. You begin by lying on your back. If you find this difficult, you can prop yourself up on your elbows. Otherwise, your arms go next to your body with your palms down. First, raise your right leg and make sure it is straight. Bring it to a 90-degree angle. Then lower it down gradually. Then raise the left leg in the same way and lower gradually. Then raise both legs together and lower gradually. Do deep breathing three times each with each posture.

The advantage of this exercise is that it strengthens, limbers and tones the abdomen, legs, and hips.

Body Raised Posture (Right & Left) (EKA—PADA—SIRSHASAN)

Lie flat on your back and raise the head and neck while raising the right leg. Try to keep your knee straight. You can reach for your right toes or ankle. Bring the right knee to your forehead while keeping the left leg straight on the floor. Then repeat with the other leg. Then repeat with both legs. Always breathe out while folding the body forward and breathe in while extending the body. Repeat three times with the posture.

The posture benefits digestion and bowel function by the squeezing of the abdomen (Fig. 3.10).

Shoulder Stand (Fig. 2.12) (SARVANGASAN) &/or Headstand (SIRSHASAN)

Lie flat on your back while keeping your arms next to your body with your palms down. Keep both of your feet together. Raise both of your legs together slowly. Then raise your hips, supporting the small of your back with your hands, keeping the thumbs and the fingers spread apart. Bring the trunk to a vertical position with your legs extended straight up. If you cannot go up slowly, you can roll up into the Shoulder Stand. The variations for the Shoulder Stand are, spread both legs out to the sides forming a triangle, or move the legs alternately forward and back, performing splits in the air.

If you are advanced, you can bring your arms around to the front towards your knees and support your body with your head and shoulders only. In this posture, you will need to tilt your legs toward your head to help your balance.

Another advanced posture is to return your hands to their supportive position on the small of your back and fold your legs into the full lotus while on your shoulders.

The Headstand Posture (Fig. 9.2) should not be done if you have any severe ailment of the neck and head including nasal, chronic sinusitis, thyroid disorders or high blood pressure.

The benefits of this posture are to strengthen the spine, tone the body and calm the nervous system.

Plough Posture (HALASAN) Fig. 2.5, for a variation Fig. 3.11 & 3.12

This posture follows the Shoulder Stand. From the Shoulder Stand, lower your legs down in front of your head, keep your legs straight and allow your toes to touch the floor if possible. Support your back with your hands, your fingers over the small of your back and the thumbs wrapped around your sides. Try to have your body as straight as possible. Then release your arms down onto the floor opposite to your head. Do deep breathing three times.

The first advanced Plough Posture is to bring your arms forward above your head and touch your toes with your legs extended out in front of you. You will look similar to when you are doing the head to knee posture only upside down. Do deep breathing three times.

The second advanced Plough Posture is to drop your knees to either side of your head and bring your arms around from the back and wrap them around your knees. Do deep breathing three times.

This posture benefits the health of your spleen, liver and reproductive organs as well as improves your circulation.

The Bridge (Fig. 3.13)

This posture is an extension of the Shoulder Stand. From the Shoulder Stand, lower one leg at a time away from your head, arching the back while supporting your back with your hands.

Once both legs are on the floor, try to straighten out your legs so that the knees are not bent. Then bring one leg up at a time and then go back to the shoulder stand. If it is too difficult to go from the Plough Posture into the Shoulder Stand, then just come out of the posture. Otherwise, slowly roll down from the Shoulder Stand one vertebra at a time.

The benefits of this posture are that the neck is strengthened and stretched and circulation is increased in the neck and thyroid gland. The spine becomes more flexible through this Asana and the abdomen is also stretched and toned.

Fish Posture (MATSYASAN)

The Fish Posture (Figures 4.1 and 4.2) is part of spine posture group. There are three levels.

Beginner level—begin by lying on your back with your arms at your side. Tuck your hands under your buttocks. Arch your back and use your elbows to carry your weight. Lower your body slightly. Bend your head back, and rest the crown of your head on the floor.

Medium level—begin by lying on the floor on your back. Fold your legs into the Easy Posture. Prop yourself up on your elbows with your back arched. Bend your head back and rest the crown of your head on the floor. Then release your elbows and reach down for your toes.

Advanced level—begin by sitting on the floor. Fold your legs into the Full Lotus Posture. Then gently lower your back down, propping yourself on your elbows until the crown of your head is set on the floor. Then release the elbows and grab your big toes with your hands. Then make prayerful hands over your chest.

Do deep inhalation and exhalation three times in all of these postures. This posture opens up the bent spine and allows fresh blood to move into the opened areas. The legs benefit from the Lotus Posture and the Easy Posture. The abdomen is stretched and decongested. This posture aids digestion and supplies blood to the brain, pituitary, pineal and thyroid glands. It improves respiratory problems and is good for diabetes.

YOGA MUDRA

Please see Chapter 8 (Figures 8.7-8.10).

Head to Knee Posture (PASCHIMOTHANSAN) (Fig. 2.6)

Sit on the floor with your feet out in front of you. Grab your left hand with your right hand. Inhale while raising both arms over your head. Hold your breath, then exhale forward, bending from your waist. Try to keep your knees straight. As you come forward let your elbows fall to the outside of your legs. You can either grasp your toes with your fingers and pull them back or bend your index fingers to make a hook and hook them around your big toes. If you cannot grab your toes, don't worry; just put your hands on your legs. Keep trying to stretch forward on the exhale and gradually you will improve. While in the posture, try to relax and breathe normally for 20 seconds. Then inhale and come up to the starting position.

This posture helps give flexibility to your spine and back muscles. It energizes the whole body, improves digestion and corrects bowl dysfunction.

Leg—Head Posture (EKA—PADA—SIRSHASAN) (Fig. 4.3)

Begin by sitting down, and extending both legs out. Then bend one knee and cradle your foot and knee. Rock your leg as if you are rocking a baby, warming up your hip. Then grab your leg with two hands and raise your foot over your head, and if you are flexible put the back of your foot behind your neck. If you cannot do this, pull your leg up as far as you can and come into the margin of pain and hold it. Do deep breathing three times. Do the same with the other leg also.

Another variation is to lie down on your back and pull your foot up with your hands under your foot and pull it up to place it behind your neck. If you cannot do this, pull your leg up as far as you can. Remember to do both legs. There are people who can pull both legs up and place their feet behind their neck.

The benefits are improved digestion, supple joints, and greater flexibility.

Triangle Posture (HASTHA PADSAN)

Sit on the floor and spread your legs out to the sides. Keep your knees straight. Inhale and raise your arms over your head and exhale down to the right, then repeat on the left side. Then bend forward, bringing your head or chest down to the floor. Breathe deeply three times in the posture (Figures 4.4 & 6.1).

You can also do this posture standing up.

This posture will tone and firm your leg muscles and stretch your back and shoulder muscles. It improves blood flow and circulation.

Ankle—Knee Posture (BANDRASAN) (Figures 4.5 & 4.6).

Start by sitting on the floor. Bring the soles of your feet together with your knees bent. Inhale once and exhale while bending forward. Using your elbows to press your knees down, grab your feet and try to bring your nose as close to your feet as possible. Inhale coming up and repeat three times.

In the advanced posture, lift your body up and balance your weight. Try to sit on your feet with your knees bent. Bring your palms together making prayerful hands.

This posture relieves constipation, improves high blood pressure and corrects spinal weakness. It also improves blood flow to the back, legs, hips and feet.

Head—Knee Posture (JANU—SIRSHASAN)

Sit on the floor and extend the right leg out. Then either place the left foot on the inside thigh or bend the ankle and place the left foot on top of the right leg allowing the left ankle to go towards the floor. Inhale, raise both arms and fold forward at the waist while exhaling. Hold the posture for as long as you are comfortable and then inhale while raising the torso. Exhale, then repeat on the opposite leg. Do three repetitions on each side.

In the advanced posture, pull your arm around your back and grab the toe on your opposite foot. Grab your toe going forward with the arm on the same side of your body. The breathing would be the same as above.

This posture can also be performed with one leg bent back at the knee while the other leg is straight. Both arms reach forward to grab the toes of the outstretched leg. Then repeat on the other side.

This posture improves flexibility to your spine and back muscles, energizes your system and improves digestion (Fig. 4.7).

Inclined Plane (VASISTHANSAN) (Fig. 4.8)

Sit on the floor with your arms behind your back, palms on the floor and elbows locked. Extend your legs out. Inhale and lift your body up. Balance your weight between your palms and your heels. Let your head tilt back. Breathe deeply. Repeat three times. Variations of the posture are lifting the right leg only, then the left leg only, then the right arm only, then the left arm only.

After that, you can lift the opposite hand and opposite leg together and then switch sides.

These postures limber the joints and help the nervous system as well as improving circulation.

Wheel Posture (CHAKRASAN)

Begin by lying on your back. Lift your arms up, bend them at the elbows and place your hands behind your shoulders with your wrists stretched back. Bend your knees and then inhale, and push up with your legs and arms while you exhale. Hold the posture. Then come down.

From the wheel posture, you can lift your right leg up and extend it out and then bring it down. Then raise the left leg up and bring it down, right arm up and down, and then left arm up and down. Then lift the opposite arm and opposite leg at the same time and then switch opposite sides. Lower you body gently to the floor.

This posture stimulates the glands and organs, strengthens your arms and legs, and helps to make the spine more flexible (Figures 4.9 & 6.3)

Cobra Posture (BHUJANGASAN)
Half Cobra

Begin by putting your hands under your chest with your palms down and leaving 2 or 3 inches between your fingers. Inhale and raise your shoulders and head half way up, stretch your neck back and do deep breathing three times. Then come down.

Next, change the position of your hands so that the palms are down and your hands are straight and placed next to your chest. Push up with your arms until they are straight and stretch your head back, bending your spine. Do this three times. Your legs are straight and shoulder width apart. Do deep breathing and then come down.

Full Cobra

The Full Cobra (Fig. 2.3) is just like the Half Cobra, only you bend your knees and try to touch the back of your head with your feet. If you can't touch your head, don't worry, just go as far as you can. Hold the posture for three rounds of deep breathing.

This posture restores the nervous system, stretches the spine and helps move circulation.

Half Locust (R & L) (SALABHASAN)

Lay down on your stomach with legs together, head resting on your chin, hands under your thighs with palms up. Or you can make a fist with your palms up next to your thighs. Inhale, hold your breath and raise your right leg for as long as you can. Then exhale while bringing your leg down slowly. Repeat with left leg (Fig. 5.1).

This posture increases flexibility and stretches the back and legs.

Full Locust (SALABHASAN)

The full locust (Fig. 2.7) is very difficult to accomplish and requires a great deal of flexibility of the spine and strength in the arms. This is an advanced posture.

Begin by lying on your stomach. Rest your head on your chin and make a fist with your hands. Turn your hands so that your thumb is on the floor. Bring both of your arms together under your thighs. Now, using the strength of your arms, push down on the floor to provide stability. Lift both of your legs together up into the air. When this posture is mastered, your legs are at a 90 Degree angle straight up in the air. But for now, just lift as far as you can. Breathe deeply in the posture.

The benefits of this posture are increased arm strength and flexibility to the spine. This posture also helps blood flow to the neck and brain.

This posture is one of the most beneficial postures for your spine and back. If you are able to lift your legs straight up, your spine is in tip-top shape.

Bow Posture (DHANURASAN) and Rock forward and backward

Lie on your stomach, bend your knees and reach back with both arms to grab your ankles. You can have your thumb on the same side as your fingers or have your thumb on the opposite side of your foot. Pull your legs and ankles up, arching your back and balancing on your stomach. Your body should resemble an archer's bow. Your head is straight. Try to hold the posture as long as you can, breathing deeply. From here, if you are able, rock back and forth on your stomach. While your head goes down, exhale and inhale as you come up.

Another way of doing the bow posture is to grab your big toe of each foot from the front by bending your arms and reaching back with your hands. You grab the toes and pull them either to your shoulders or over your head into the bow posture. This is a very advanced posture.

You can do this on just the right side with the left arm and leg lifted up, then switch sides.

This posture is very good for strengthening the back muscles as well as keeping your back stretched and flexible. It helps more blood flow to the spine (Fig. 6.2).

Triangle Posture (UTTHITA & PARNKTTA & TRIKONASAN)

Begin by standing straight up with your legs spread apart like a triangle. Inhale, then exhale, bringing your right arm down to your right ankle. Bring your left arm up straight. Turn your head to look up at your hand that is straight up in the air.

The second variation of the standing triangle posture begins in the same way, only this time, the right hand comes down to the right ankle, and then the body bends to the right. Then the left arm comes over your head and straight out to the right. Then do the same on the other side of your body.

The third variation also begins in the same way only this time, after you exhale, twist your body forward, bringing your right hand to your left foot. The left arm goes straight up and you turn your head to look up at the hand that is in the air. Then do the same on the other side of your body.

This posture is very good for increasing blood flow through the nerves in your spine and toning the waistline and legs (Fig. 2.13).

Tree Posture (EK PAD ASAN)

Begin by standing up, bend the right knee, and pull the ankle and foot so that the foot rests on top of the thigh. If you cannot do this, then put your foot up against the inside of the left thigh. Bring the palms of your hands together. Keep your balance by focusing your eyes on one spot on the wall. Balance on the left foot. Repeat on the other side.

A variation is to grab the left ankle with the right hand while in the tree posture and then bringing the left arm up, inhale, then exhale, bending forward and lowering the left hand down to the floor. Inhale while coming up. Then repeat this on the other side (Fig. 5.2).

This posture will improve your balance, tone your legs and back muscles and also improve your concentration.

Squatting Posture (Fig. 2.8)

Begin in a standing position making prayerful hands. Come up on your toes, then inhale and exhale down. Remain on your toes and come back up to a standing position. The next time you go down, stand flat on the soles of your feet. Inhale and exhale down, while keeping your feet flat on the floor. American women find this difficult because of wearing high-heeled shoes.

If you are very flexible, you can now do the advanced posture. In this posture, while you are down in the squat posture with your knees bent and the soles of your feet flat, you bring your left ankle over your right thigh and hold it for 20 seconds, then switch sides.

This posture strengthens legs, improves your balance and soothes the nervous system. It also strengthens the bowels.

Twist (ARDHA—MATSYEN DRASAN)

Begin by sitting on the floor with both legs straight out in front of you. Bend your left knee and place your left leg over the right leg. Keep your back straight. Then take your left arm and place it on the inside of your bent leg. Grab the ankle. Take the right arm and place the palm on the floor behind your back. Then twist your body to the right and turn your head to the right. Hold the posture for 20 seconds and breathe deeply. Then twist to the left keeping your feet in the same position. Bring your right arm over the left knee and grab back at the ankle. Bring your left arm behind your back and twist your body in the opposite direction. Turn your head to the left when doing the posture. Hold for 20 seconds and breathe deeply. Now, do both of these on the opposite leg. This is the easy way of doing the twist posture.

The full Twist Posture is begun by sitting on your knees. Slide over on to your right hip. Then bring the left leg over the right knee. Start by grabbing the left ankle with your right hand and twist the body to the left. The left arm comes around your body to the left. Turn your head to the left. Breathe deeply in the posture. Try to hold the posture as long as you can. Then change hands and grab the left ankle with the left hand and twist to the right, bringing the right arm around your body. Twist to the right, and turn your head to the right.

For the more advanced posture, keep your legs where they are and bring your right arm over your left knee, twisting to the left. Bring your left arm around your body and turn your head to the left. Then do the posture on the other side.

This posture improves digestion, squeezes the abdomen and tones the liver and spleen. It massages the kidney and helps prevent back pain. It also improves the flexibility and the health of your spine (Fig. 5.3).

Relaxed Pose (SAVASAN)

After you are finished practicing your Yoga Asanas, the last thing you should do is to go into Savasana (Fig. 5.4). For further details, read Savasana in Chapter 9.

Wind Relieving Posture (VATAYANASAN) (R & L and both legs)

Begin by lying on your back and keeping the right leg straight out. Grab the left knee with both hands, inhale, and then exhale bringing your head up to your knee. Breathe deeply three times, and then do the other leg.

Bend both knees and bring them up to your chest. Wrap your arms around your knees. Inhale, and then exhale lifting your head up and bringing it to your knees. Hold and inhale, exhale three times

This posture will massage the wall of the abdomen and intestinal gasses may be released during the squeeze (Figures 5.5 & 5.6).

Figure 2

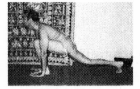
Fig. 2.1

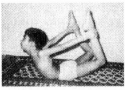
Fig. 2.2

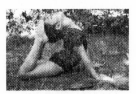
Fig. 2.3

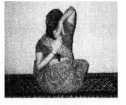
Fig. 2.4

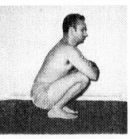
Fig. 2.5

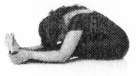
Fig. 2.6

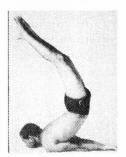
Fig. 2.7

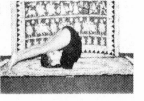
Fig. 2.8

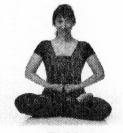
Fig. 2.9

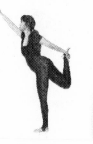
Fig. 2.10

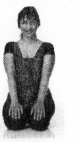
Fig. 2.11

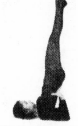
Fig. 2.12

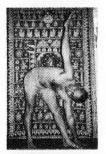
Fig. 2.13

Figure 3

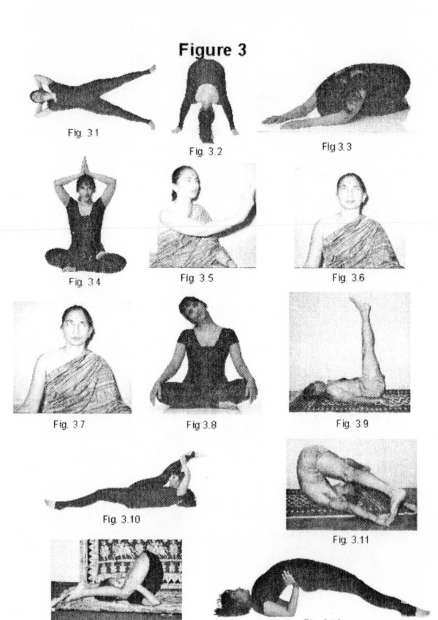

Fig. 3.1

Fig. 3.2

Fig 3.3

Fig. 3.4

Fig. 3.5

Fig. 3.6

Fig. 3.7

Fig 3.8

Fig. 3.9

Fig. 3.10

Fig. 3.11

Fig. 3.12

Fig. 3.13

Figure 4

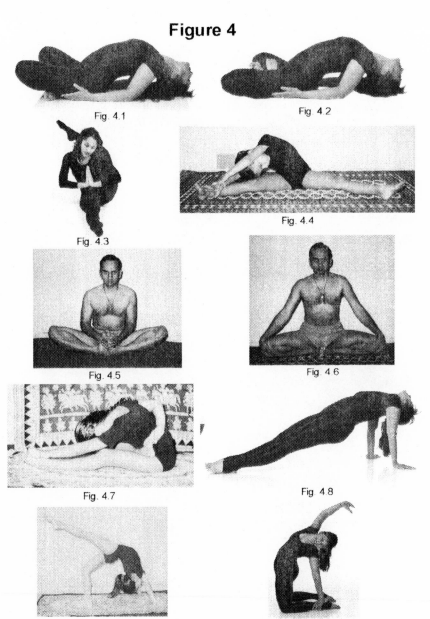

Fig. 4.1

Fig. 4.2

Fig. 4.3

Fig. 4.4

Fig. 4.5

Fig. 4.6

Fig. 4.7

Fig. 4.8

Fig. 4.9

Fig. 4.10

Figure 5

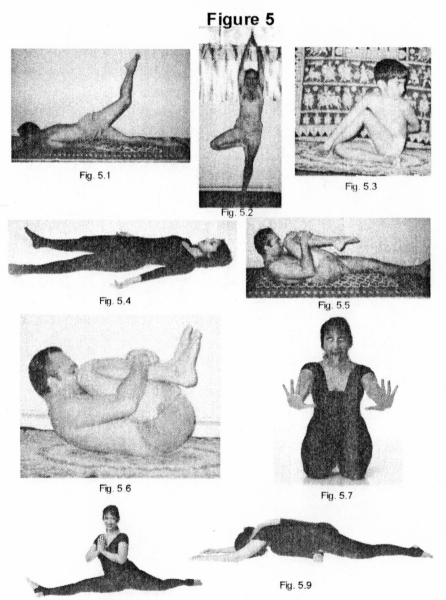

Fig. 5.1

Fig. 5.2

Fig. 5.3

Fig. 5.4

Fig. 5.5

Fig. 5.6

Fig. 5.7

Fig. 5.8

Fig. 5.9

Figure 6

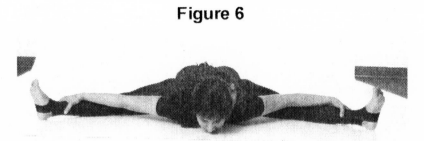

Fig. 6.1

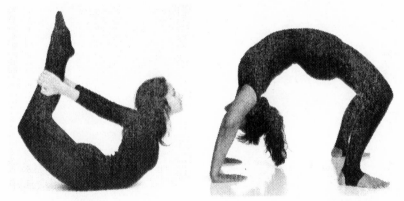

Fig. 6.2

Fig. 6.3

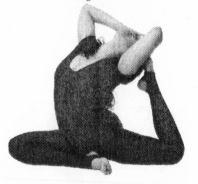

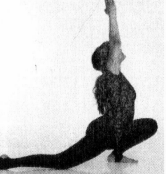

Fig. 6.4

Fig. 6.5

Figure 7

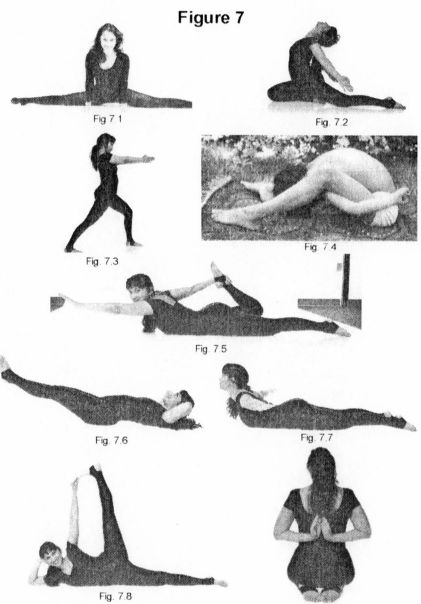

Fig 7.1

Fig. 7.2

Fig. 7.3

Fig. 7.4

Fig. 7.5

Fig. 7.6

Fig. 7.7

Fig. 7.8

Fig. 7.9

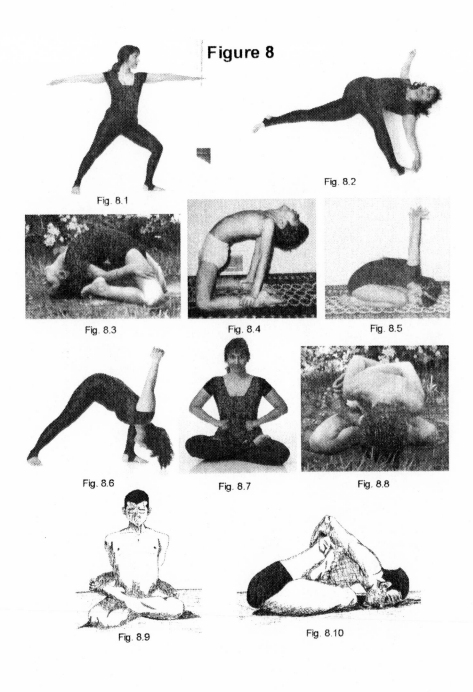

Figure 8

Fig. 8.1

Fig. 8.2

Fig. 8.3

Fig. 8.4

Fig. 8.5

Fig. 8.6

Fig. 8.7

Fig. 8.8

Fig. 8.9

Fig. 8.10

Figure 9

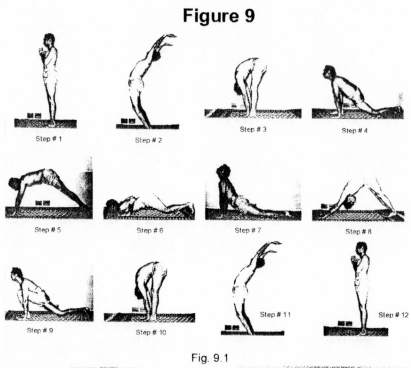

Fig. 9.1

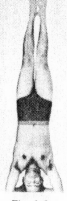

Fig. 9.2

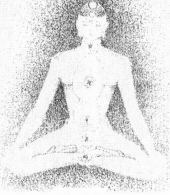

Fig. 9.3

Figure 10

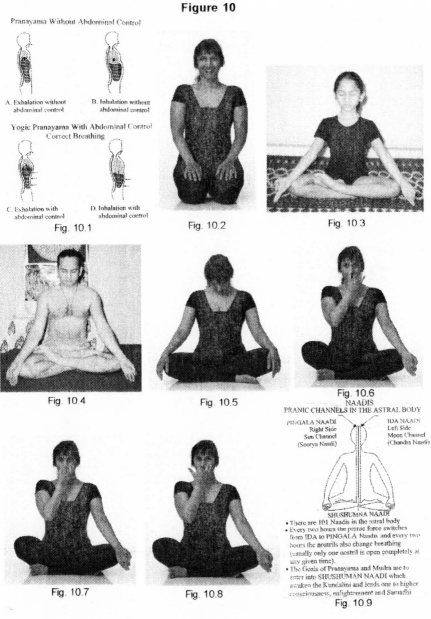

Pranayama Without Abdominal Control

A. Exhalation without abdominal control

B. Inhalation without abdominal control

Yogic Pranayama With Abdominal Control
Correct Breathing

C. Exhalation with abdominal control

D. Inhalation with abdominal control

Fig. 10.1

Fig. 10.2

Fig. 10.3

Fig. 10.4

Fig. 10.5

Fig. 10.6

Fig. 10.7

Fig. 10.8

NAADIS
PRANIC CHANNELS IN THE ASTRAL BODY

PINGALA NAADI
Right Side
Sun Channel
(Soorya Naadi)

IDA NAADI
Left Side
Moon Channel
(Chandra Naadi)

SHUSHUMNA NAADI

• There are 101 Naadis in the astral body
• Every two hours the pranic force switches from IDA to PINGALA Naadis and every two hours the nostrils also change breathing (usually only one nostril is open completely at any given time).
• The Goals of Pranayama and Mudra are to enter into SHUSHUMAN NAADI which awaken the Kundalini and leads one to higher consciousness, enlightenment and Samadhi

Fig. 10.9

71

Chapter 7

Advanced Asanas

In this Chapter, we have given 28 advanced Asanas (postures). Once you master the recommended daily Asanas, you should include in your practice these advanced Yoga Asanas. They will be easy to achieve just by looking at the pictures in the figures. As mentioned in an earlier chapter, there are 480,000 Asanas. We have selected some of them in this chapter.

Advanced Asanas

English Name	Sanskrit Name	Figure Number
1. Lion Posture	Simhasan	5.7
2. Split Posture	AnjaneyAsana	5.8 & 7.1
3. Spinal Twist Posture (Variation)	Ardha Matsendrasan	7.2
4. Yogic Sleep Posture	Yoga NidrAsana	5.9
5. VirabhadrAsana Posture I	VirabhadrAsana	7.3
6. Advanced Plough Posture	HalAsana	3.11&3.12
7. Tortoise Posture	KurmAsana	7.4
8. Tree Posture	VrkAsana	5.2
9. Side Plank Posture	VamadevAsana	
10. Bow Posture	DhanurAsana	6.2 & 7.5
11. Body Raising Posture	ArohanAsana	
Or Boat Posture	NavAsana	7.6
12. Sideways Bow Posture	Parsva DhanurAsana	7.7
13. Cow Face Posture	ComukhAsana	2.4
14. Pigeon Posture	Kapotha Asan	6.4

15. Leg Raise Posture	AnanthAsana	7.8
16. Modified Camel Posture	UstrAsana	4.10
17. Leg Split Posture	AnjaneyAsana	6.5
18. Virabhadras Posture II	VirabhadrAsana	8.1
19. Revolved Abdomen or Lying Twist Posture	Jathara ParivartanAsana	8.2
20. Angular Posture	Urdhva Mukha PaschimottanAsana	
21. Rock the Baby Posture	Not Available	
22. Diamond Posture	Supta Vajrasan	8.3
23. Camel Posture	UstrAsana	8.4
24. Anchor Posture (Part 2)	YogAsana	8.5
25. Intense Side Stretch Posture	ParsvottanAsana	8.6
26. Flying Swan Posture Hamsa		

Chapter 8

Three Supreme Asanas

Yoga tradition says there are 480,000 Asanas (postures), but out of those, three Asanas are supreme. During my 40 years of teaching Yoga, I've come to realize this truth. The three postures are, the Yoga Mudra Asana, Soorya Namaskar (Sun Prayer or sun salutations), and Sirsasana or the Headstand. If someone doesn't do any other Yoga but just does these three supreme Yoga postures, their youth will be maintained. You should sit on the floor, do three rounds of the Sun Prayer or Soorya Namaskar, and do the Headstand or the Shoulder Stand.

Yoga Mudra Asana

This is the only Asana that is called "Yoga Asana." I wondered why this is so until I realized that it is one of the most important Yoga Asanas. This Asana has the impact of Mudra Shakti on your being. There are three levels of Yoga Mudra Asana, 1) Sit in a Sukasan and make a fist with both your palms and put it under your rib cage. This is the simplest form of Yoga Mudra (Fig. 8.7). 2) Sit in a Full Lotus Posture and then make a fist with both your palms and put it under your rib cage. Inhale, and then exhale as you lower your forehead to the floor, while pushing your fists into the abdomen, creating pressure on your colon. Through the placement of your fists you send a subconscious message saying, "I will control my intake of food and I will preserve my life energy." 3) Sit in the Full Lotus, cross your arms behind your back (Fig. 8.9) and allow your right hand to grab your right big toe and allow your left hand to grab your left big toe. Now take a deep breath and touch your nose to the ground (Figures 8.8 and 8.10). Yogi B.S. Iyengar writes in Light on Yoga, "This Asana is useful in awakening Kundalini Shakti. When you do this complete Asana, please also move your head onto the right and left knees alternately with proper breathing. Crossing the hands behind the back expands the chest and increases the range of shoulder movements. Yoga Mudra Asana intensifies the peristaltic activity and pushes down the accumulated waste matter in the colon and thereby relieves constipation and increases digestive power."

If a person does Yoga Mudra Asana regularly, he/she can sit on the floor comfortably like a Yogi at the age of 80 or 90. Most people in the West cannot sit on the floor after the age of 60. This is very important for your flexibility. If somebody does not want to do this Yoga Mudra Asana, just sit on the floor and that will help a great deal.

Soorya Namaskar

Soorya Namaskar is a Sanskrit name. In English it is called Sun Prayer or Sun Salutation. Swami Vishnu Devananda (Fig. 14.2) writes about Soorya Namaskar in his book as follows:

"This exercise is called Soorya Namaskar because it is practiced in the early morning facing the sun. The sun is considered to be the deity for health and long life. In ancient days, this exercise was a daily routine in the daily spiritual practices. One should practice this at least twelve times by repeating twelve names of the Lord Sun. This exercise is a combined process of Yoga Asanas and breathing. It reduces abdominal fat, brings flexibility to the spine and limbs, and increases the breathing capacity. It is easier to practice Asanas after doing Soorya Namaskar. Before students practice the more complicated and difficult postures, the spine should acquire some flexibility."

Swami Sivananda says the following regarding the Soorya Namaskar:

"There are twelve spinal positions each stretching various ligaments and gives different movements to the vertebral column. The vertebral column is bent forward and backward alternately with deep inhalation and exhalation of breath and a little retention of breath in some cases. Whenever the body is bent forward, the contraction of the abdomen and diaphragm throws out the breath. When the body bends backward the chest expands and deep inhalation occurs automatically. In this way the body becomes flexible and the entire portion of the lungs begin to function which results in correct breathing. Moreover, it gives mild exercise to leg and arm muscles and ensures a good circulation of blood. At the same time, the sun's life-giving rays play on the man's body, sucking away the toxins along with perspiration, invigorating circulation and imparting life to the human organism-the life that the sun alone can give. For a person with stiff limbs and spine the Soorya Namaskar exercise is a boon to bring back lost flexibility.

Prayer to the Sun
Om Suryam Sundaralokanathamamritam
Vedantasaram Sivam,
Jnanam Brahmamayam Suresamamalam
Lokaikachittam Svayam;
Indradityanaradhipam Suragurum
Trailokyachudamanim,
Brahmavishnusivasvarupahridayam
Vande Sada Bhaskaram.

Translation: I always adore Soorya, the sun, the beautiful Lord of the world, the immortal, the quintessence of the Vedanta, the auspicious, the absolute knowledge, of the form of Brahman, the Lord of the Gods, ever-pure, the one true consciousness of the world itself, the Lord of the Indra, the Gods and men, the preceptor of the Gods, the crest-jewel of the three worlds, the very heart of the forms of Brahma, Vishnu and Siva, the giver of light."

After completing twelve Namaskaras lie down flat on the ground on your back and relax each and every limb one by one from toes to the crown of the head. This is called Savasana (Corpse Pose Fig. 5.4). To begin with, if one feels tired after three or four Namaskaras, he may stop with that and increase the number gradually (One everyday or every two days), all the time taking care that too much strain is not good.

The Sun Prayer has twelve steps but you have to do the twelve steps twice for balance. One time the right leg is going forward and backward and the next time the left leg is going forward and backward (Fig. 9.1). It is best to repeat the Sun Prayer twelve times. If you choose to do it less than twelve times, you should do it an even number of times, e.g. two, four, six, eight, ten. It is also very important to do the Sun Prayer exactly as it should be done and practice proper deep breathing at each step. We recommend that you do it in front of the sun with the minimum of clothing, or do it at home.

The benefits of the Sun Prayer are many. Flexibility and spinal health are major benefits. Also, if it is done in front of the Sun, you will get the proper vitamins. It is said that this is one of the perfect exercises. If you do not do any other Yoga and just do 4 Sun Prayers each day, you will maintain good health and flexibility.

Many people say the names of the Sun God at each of the twelve steps. You should recite them in Sanskrit as it creates Divine loving vibrations. These twelve names are as follows:

1. Om Mitraya Namah (Friend of All, I Bow to Thee),
2. Om Ravaya Namah (Praised by All, I Bow to Thee),
3. Om Soorya Namah (Guide of All, I Bow to Thee),
4. Om Bhanave Namah (Bestower of Beauty, I Bow to Thee),
5. Om Khagaya Namah (Stimulator of the Senses, I Bow to Thee),
6. Om Pooshne Namah (Nourisher of Life, I Bow to Thee),
7. Om Hirnaya Garbaya Namah (Promoter of Virility, I Bow to Thee),
8. Om Marichay Namah (Destroyer of Disease, I Bow to Thee),
9. Om Adityaya Namah (Inspirator of Love, I Bow to Thee),
10. Om Savitre Namah (Begetter of Life, I Bow to Thee),
11. Om Arkaya Namah (Inspirer of Awe, I Bow to Thee),
12. Om Bhaskaraya Namah (Radiant One, I Bow to Thee).

The Sun Prayer has to be practiced in a harmonious way, regularly from one step to the next with proper deep breathing. When you recite the prayer, if it is by heart, it will flow very nicely. For internal happiness and peace there are many other reasons to memorize the twelve names and meanings of the Sun God. Some of the reasons are listed below.

Sun represents your own soul.

Sun prayer is a prayer of thanks to the sun appreciating all the Lord Sun gives us for our health, our material things and happiness.

Focusing on the sun gives you a point of concentration.

Learn to reach out as a light wherever you can.

Light means knowledge.

Your soul has all the qualities of the 12 names of the Sun God.

Harmonizing your mind with the Sun can allow you to travel through the inner journey, to grow and be positive.

Teach you to be in tune with light everywhere, as the sun lights every corner of the world.

In prayer you drop your (self) attachment and try to attach yourself to wisdom and knowledge in another human being or source.

It is a good beginning—not always to see negative and be lazy and hate the whole world.

I would like to tell you the miracle of Soorya Namaskar. One of my students experienced the impact of the Soorya Namaskar in 1990. He was about 50 years old when he came into my Yoga class. He was pale and could hardly walk. He told me he had been seriously wounded in the Vietnam War, but recovered, and that after returning to the U.S. he had started drinking and using drugs. Since then he had also become a diabetic. He told me he just came out of the hospital, and while he was there he almost died and the priest came and read him his last rites, but he survived. He wanted to learn Yoga because he heard that it helps increase flexibility and strength. I told him to come to my class once a week and to become a vegetarian. I told him he could eat fish in the beginning and that he must practice about half an hour each day at home. He agreed. I taught him the Sun Prayer, which he could not even do once. I told him to start by doing 2 rounds of the Sun Prayer once a day and gradually work up to 12 rounds a day. He agreed and started doing the Sun Prayer. Guess what—within six months, he started playing tennis, and rollerblading. His numb leg became normal. This was a miracle. I took him on my public access local TV show to show people what Yoga can do. The Sun Prayer works on every muscle in your body. It should be done properly, accurately and daily. If you cannot do Yoga Asanas, just do four Sun Prayers and sit on the floor for about an hour or so. You can have greater flexibility and strength. Happy Soorya Namaskar.

Hindu Press International website reported:
World Record for Soorya Namaskar
"Gwalior, India, September 19, 2004: A unique world record was created when around 15,000 children from 180 schools gathered in Gwalior and performed Soorya Namaskar, "sun salutation," the famous hatha Yoga sequence of postures or Asanas. The children performed all the 12 Asanas of the Soorya Namaskar taking the salutation count to an astronomical 180,000.

The event was organized by Vivekananda Center and presided over by the Madhya Pradesh Chief Minister Babulal Gaur. "The most important motive behind this Sun Salutation ceremony is that there should be all-around development of personality of children and a feeling of service toward country. When they do it together it creates a sense of togetherness. And the Guinness Book of World Records was informed so that Yoga can be advertised worldwide," said Mukul Kanitkar, the organizer. "We have vowed that when we grow up we will serve our country and will stand in the face of any threat to India," said Mridul Gupta, a seven-year-old boy. Soorya Namaskar is an appreciated exercise among people of all ages and categories. It is also considered to be one of the best ways to burn calories and reduce weight. It is often recommended for obesity."

Headstand Sirshasana

Sirsasana or Headstand is one of the supreme Yoga Asanas. Beginners find it difficult to do, so they can replace it with the Shoulder Stand (Fig. 9.2) which offers 80% of the benefits of the Headstand. Swami Sivananda calls it the Topsy-turvy Pose. He says, "You have to stand on the head. This is considered to be the king of all Asanas."

Spread a fourfold blanket. Squat on the ground and prepare a finger-lock by knitting the fingers of both hands together. Make a convenient angle with the forearms. Let the finger-lock serve the purpose of a vertex. Keep the top of the head on the vertex. Slowly raise the lower part of the trunk, and then the legs. Now the whole body will stand at a right angle with the ground. Remain in this pose for 5 seconds in the beginning and slowly increase the time to half an hour. Let the breathing be normal throughout. Bring the legs again slowly down without making any sudden jerk. Relax the body. This is important.

Sirshasana is a panacea for all human ills. It is extremely useful in keeping up Brahmacharya because the seminal energy is transmuted into Ojas-Sakti and stored up in the brain. This is sex sublimation. Persons suffering from diseases of the eye, nose, head, throat, stomach, genito-urinary system, liver, spleen, lungs, renal colic, deafness, plies, asthma, consumption, pyorrhea, constipation, and many other troubles will find great relief by its practice. Grey hairs and wrinkles will disappear. It augments the digestive fire and increases appetite. Ladies also can do this Asana. Sterility vanishes. Many uterine and ovarian diseases are cured. Indeed, Sirshasana is a blessing and a gift to humanity. During the practice of this Asana the brain draws plenty of blood and energy. Memory increases wonderfully. Pt. Jawaharlal Nehru, the Prime Minister of India, was an ardent votary of Sirshasana. He managed to practice this pose daily."

Chapter 9

Relaxation (Savasana)

Prana Massage

This Prana massage can be done between two people, or in a classroom with many students. When teaching this in a classroom, I try to prevent pairing of people of the opposite sex because energies are exchanged in this technique. But it is alright when husbands and wives can be paired together. I demonstrate Prana massage on one student for all the other students to watch and learn and then I request the students to pair up in groups of two. The first person does Prana massage on the other person and then they switch.

Please do not use this technique at parties, because it is not intended to be used in that way. I developed this technique to assist in further relaxation only. The following is the technique:

Part 1

The person receiving the massage lies down on his stomach in the "Frontal Corpse Posture." This means he makes a pillow with his hands, palms down, with his cheek resting on the back of his hands, his toes touching and heels falling outward. The one receiving the Prana massage should inhale deeply through the nose. Then, during his exhalation through the nose, the massager uses his hands to exert pressure with the whole weight of their body. The massager chants "Om" each time when he applies pressure each time it is applied. The massage giver sits on his knees at the head of the person lying down and starts the Prana massage.

Part 2

Begin by applying medium pressure applied directly on the spinal column from the middle to the top. The left palm goes up the spine and the right palm presses down the spine.

Part 3

With both hands, fingers facing out, apply pressure is on both sides of the lowest part of the back, then move up a little and repeat, until you reach the upper arms. Move up the back to the shoulders, and down to the arms and then work your way back down to the low back, the starting point. The massager should ensure that the pressure is applied only during exhalation by the person receiving the massage, and that he uses his whole body weight.

Part 4

Next use both hands to massage the neck and shoulders.

Part 5

Now do hand patting all over the back.

Part 6

The massager should stand up and move to the right side of the feet of the person lying down. He should sit on his knees again and then softly place his hands on the thighs of the person lying down (right hand on right thigh and left hand on left thigh) and repeat the breathing explained in step 1. Step by step, slowly he should move his hands and weight down the legs to the ankles.

Part 7

Then the massager stands up and applies pressure with his feet onto the massage receiver's feet.

This completes the whole Prana massage, and the massage receiver should now sit up and take a deep breath.

Instant Savasana

Lie down on your back and bring both legs together. Join your heels and toes together and place the palms by the side of the body. Make sure your face is relaxed and try to be happy. Start by tightening your toes, and then tighten your ankles, and calf muscles, and knees. Now shift your attention onto your thigh muscles and tighten them and subsequently squeeze your buttocks. The next step is to breathe out and pull your abdomen in forcefully. Now tighten your fists and take a deep breath. At this point tighten your shoulders, neck muscles and tighten your face muscles. Now tighten the whole body. Then suddenly let go completely so that the whole body collapses. See how relaxed you are.

Deep Savasana

This is a deep relaxation technique. You can use this technique on yourself. A Yoga teacher can use it at the very end of class. I am explaining this technique as I would in my own Yoga class.

First, turn down the lights and ask all the students to lie down on their backs in a relaxed state (Fig. 5.4). Tell them to keep their legs slightly apart and keep both of their hands close to their body with their palms up. Now let both feet fall outward. During the wintertime, if the room is not warm enough, ask the students to bring a blanket with them. I begin by telling them to try to relax. In the beginning just watch your breath going in and out. Do not force the breath, allow it to be natural. Then I usually chant "Om" three times ending with shanti, shanti, shanti. Then I chant the "Trayambakam Mantra" for their welfare, it can be found in Chapter 14. Sometimes I chant my Guru's Mantra "Om Namo Bhagavate Sivanandaya" a few times. You can chant any Mantra. Then I ask the students to shift their attention onto their big toe. I tell them to relax their toes. I say, "Relax your toes. Relax your toes. Relax your toes." I say it three times. Then I ask them to shift their attention onto their ankles and tell them to relax their ankles. Then I tell them to think about their calf, (I say it three times). Then I tell them to point their attention to their knees, then on their thighs. Then I say both of your legs are relaxing, relaxing, relaxing. Then I ask them to shift their attention to their stomach and I tell them, "tell your stomach muscles to relax" (three times). Then I tell them to go into all the organs of the body, and tell them to be healthy and strong and to relax. Then I tell them to come to the chest area and tell them to relax all the chest muscles (three times). Then I tell them to put their attention on their heart and tell it to be strong and healthy and slow down. Then I tell them to shift their attention to their right hand, first the fingers, then the palm, then the wrist, then the upper arms, elbows and shoulders. At the end say your entire right arm is relaxing (three times). Then I repeat this for the left arm. Now I tell the students to point their attention on their lower back and tell them that the lower back is relaxing (three times), then I tell them to come to the middle back and repeat, then the upper back (three times), then I tell them to go to the bottom of their spine and start upward. As they relax their spine, gradually they come to the neck area and tell their neck muscles to relax (three times). Then I request them to come to the forehead and to tell the forehead to relax. I tell them to relax their head, their cheeks, their chin, their lips, their nose and their eyes. Then I tell them, "The

YOGI BHARAT J. GAJJAR

whole body has relaxed" (three times). I tell them, "the body is feeling heavy and it is sinking into the carpet. Now start drifting inward toward your inner self to the center of their being. They are trying to reach the atman or their true self. Now they have come to their being, their true self, which is part of God. They are divine selves, and now all their problems have disappeared and they have become transcendental and very happy and contended. Now they have gone down and down and are very relaxed." I let them stay there for 5 or 10 minutes.

Coming Out of Relaxation

First I tell them to come back (three times). Then I tell them to raise their right hand slowly and drop it, then raise the left hand and drop it. Then raise the right leg about six inches off the floor and drop it, then the left leg. Then I request them to raise their buttocks and drop it. I tell them to raise their chest and drop it. I tell them to roll their head back and forth, and take a deep breath while rolling their head from side to side. Next I tell them to raise their arms over their head and stretch their whole body. Then I tell them to bend their right leg and grab it with both arms and ask them to touch their nose to their knee, and then repeat this with the left leg. Then raise both legs with both arms and touch their nose to both knees, before lying down on their right side like a baby. I sing my Mantras: "Shri Ma, Jaya Ma, Jaya Jaya Ma," and "Shri Ram, Jaya Ram, Jaya Jaya Ram." And I think of them as my children relaxing. At the end I tell them to go into any posture they want to and stretch in any direction they please. Then I tell them to be very aware of their bodies and tell them to learn to listen to their body. Then I tell them to sit up gradually and turn on the lights.

Chapter 10

Fundamentals of Pranayama

Introduction

Yogic breathing is called Pranayama. This word is made out of three Sanskrit words; PRA = basic unit of energy, NA = energy and YAMA = control or destroyer.

Pranayama is a technique to control Prana, to capture the Prana or vital force. It strengthens the mind, and body, besides destroying the impurities within. In other words, it purifies mind body and soul.

Swami Vishnu Devananda, the great Yoga master, says, "Prana (vital air) is the body of the individual and part of the Universal breath. Regulation of breath helps the Yogi regulate and steady the mind. By controlling the mind, Prana is also controlled.

Prana is not related to breath alone. Breathing is a manifestation of a vitalizing force called Prana. By regulating the physical breathing, the Prana is controlled, and this process of controlling the subtle Prana is called Pranayama."[1]

"This vital energy is found in all forms of life from mineral to man. Prana is found in all things having life. This Prana is not the consciousness or spirit but is merely a form of energy (shakti) used by the soul in its material and astral manifestations."[1]

"Heart and lungs of a human work as long as there is Prana with the soul. Once Prana leaves the body, the soul will also leave the body."

Different people have different amounts of Prana in them. Spiritual people and people living positively have more Prana Shakti or vital force than ordinary people. Yogis who practice Pranayama have an abundance of Prana.

People unknowingly receive and lose Prana (energy). Let us look into how humans lose some amount of Prana. When one gets angry, becomes stressed out, fearful, comes in contact with negative or sick people, etc.. One will lose some Prana. But once one becomes aware of Prana one can prevent the loss of Prana Shakti or energy.

Let's focus on how one can gain Prana. It is an involved subject. One gains Prana through positive thinking and living, and by surrendering to the higher forces (God the Father) and/or Prana Shakti (God the Mother or Holy Spirit) and/or light (Guru) and of course doing Pranayama regularly.

Swami Sivananda said, "Prana is the sum total of all the energy in the universe." Yogis store Prana and direct it at will to heal their body."

"Prana can be stored in the nervous system, more particularly in the solar plexus. Furthermore, Yogi's emphasize this cardinal and essential idea that some Yoga can give us the power, through thought, or directing the current of Prana at will. Yoga, thus gives us conscious and voluntary access to the very source of life by controlling Prana. Some Yogis can even stop their heart from beating."[1] Asana with Pranayama bandhas and Mudras are done to control and direct the pranic energy. Prana is a vital force for cleansing and healing the body."

"The Chinese call the positive energy yang and attribute its origin to the sun and the stars. The negative energy is called yin and they attribute its origin to the earth. A 16th century Chinese book offers these explanations. Yang is what is light and pure. It is energy that floats up high and of which the sky is made. Yin is thick and heavy. It is that which has taken shape to form the earth. Then energy of the blue sky is up above, but the vegetables feed on it."[1]

There Are Five Basic Types of Pranayama

They are Prana, Apana, Samana, Udana and Vyana. They are explained in greater detail below:

1. *Prana*—It deals with respiration and body energy (shakti). Prana Shakti is mother power, it is Godly power that controls one's body and mind.

2. *Apana*—It has to do with excretion. It is the force that helps clean the body. The bowel movement comes from Apana, which helps purify blood and the body.

3. *Samana*—It has to do with digestion and providing body heat. With this energy Yogis can live with very little food.

4. *Udana*—It has to do with one's siddhis or powers. With Udana Shakti a Yogi can become a hypnotic speaker or singer, levitate, walk on water, fire, etc.

5. *Vyana*—It has to do with coordination and integration. When vyana leaves the body, the man dies. With Vyana Shakti Yogis can stop their heart. If one knows Vyana, one will know God.

DURING BREATHING REMEMBER THESE POINTS

1. Keep your mind on your breathing and on chanting "Om."

2. Keep track of your count.

3. Always breathe in and out through your nostrils, and keep your mouth closed, except when a technique specifically tells you to breathe through your mouth.

4. During Pranayama breathe deeply, evenly (jerkless), slowly and maintain control.

5. Chant mentally your preferred Mantra.

6. Anytime you feel dizzy, discontinue the exercise.

7. How long to hold each breath: Puraka or inhalation—2 to 4 seconds, Kumbhaka or retention—7 to 9 seconds, Rechaka or exhalation—4 to 5 seconds, Bahya Kumbhaka or Sunyaka or retention after exhalation—2 to 3 seconds.

8. Beginners should not practice Bahya Kumbhaka.

9. During Pranayama keep the body motionless, and the mind on Prana or Om or Mantra.

10. Do Pranayama 1, 2 or 3 rounds (one round = 12 times).

11. During Pranayama if one feels cool, it is good but if you feel a burning sensation, then understand that internal correction is taking place.

12. Sometimes one starts rocking or moving in a circular motion. It might be good because Kundalini might be awakening.

13. A student needs a qualified teacher to (as a) guide.

14. Pranayama becomes effective when practiced regularly. Do it, if possible, at the same time each day.

15. Before starting Pranayama, if one or both the nostrils are blocked, sprinkle some warm water on your face. It should open up the nostrils. Do not use nose spray.

16. Before starting Pranayama, wait 2 1/2 to 3 hours after eating and empty the bowels and bladder.

17. Keep your attitude positive and have faith in Pranayama.

18. During Pranayama use a chin lock or Jalandhara Bandha that is, hanging your head down from the nape of the neck.

19. Keep your eyes closed throughout, otherwise the mind will wander.

20. Expand your lungs fully, and make sure you are using your diaphragm.

21. After completing the Pranayama practice, rest in the corpse pose (Savasana) at least for a few minutes.

ABDOMINAL BREATHING

Proper breathing is abdominal breathing. It uses the diaphragm. At the outset a Yoga teacher should check the breathing of all students. The following is my method:

Lie down on your back. Put your right hand on your stomach and left hand on your chest. Now inhale deep and observe what happens. Do a few inhalations and exhalations then stop. Now ask your students what went up and down. The breathing is poor if the chest went up. If only the stomach went up, the breathing is good. In good breathing, only the stomach should go up and down. But if your chest and stomach went up, that too is alright. But breathing through the chest alone is shallow breathing. Watch a little baby breathe and you will see its stomach rises and falls as it breathes with its diaphragm.

In his book, Pranayama the Yoga of Breathing, by Andre Van Lysebth he states:

"Let us take a close look at the diaphragm and try to assess its activity in relation to the various functions of our organism. In a healthy body the diaphragm moves up and down 18 times per minute; it travels 4 centimeters up and 4 centimeters down. The amplitude of these movements is approximately 8 centimeters. 19 movements per minute or 1,000 an hour and 24,000 in 24 hours! Just think for a moment about the amount of work produced by this muscle whose surface area is considerable. It is the most powerful muscle in our body; it acts like a perfect force-pump, compressing the liver, the spleen, the intestines, and stimulating the whole abdominal and portal circulation.

By compressing all the lymphatic and blood vessels of the abdomen, the diaphragm aids the veinous circulations from the abdomen towards the thorax.

By improving the function of the diaphragm we shall always improve the functions of the liver, even if the tests are catastrophic.

Clearly, the diaphragm can play its full role only if diaphragmatic breathing includes control of the abdominal muscles. Let us first examine what happens during the diaphragmatic phase with relaxed abdominal muscles, and then compare that with what occurs when they are controlled.

The three phases of complete Yogic breathing can only be achieved successfully if they are performed with constant abdominal control. This is the only way of breathing which gives Pranayama all its good effects and all its significance. Diaphragmatic inhalation with abdominal control keeps the abdominal and thoracic phases balanced."

There are two types of breathing. The first is *abdominal breathing*, which is done without the control of the abdomen (Fig. 10.1). It shows inhalation and exhalation without abdominal control. In the exhalation the stomach remains relaxed, (Fig. 10.1) but in the inhalation, the stomach goes out. Practicing this type of breathing, according to some, causes deep stretching and eventually a big stomach, a permanent deformation of the abdominal wall and belly.

So practice Yogic Pranayama, which is the *abdominal control* breathing Pranayama. It is done in two ways. The first is exhalation with abdominal control (Fig. 10.1). The technique is to hold the stomach in and pull the abdomen in and exhale slowly, deeply and evenly.

The second technique is shown in Fig. 10.1. Hold the stomach in and then inhale slowly, evenly and deeply. The compressed air will improve the blood circulation and make the liver function better. Please note both these techniques are used.

Benefits of Pranayama
Regular practice of Pranayama will benefit a student in the following ways:
1. It will relax the mind and body. Anger is associated with heavy breathing. This is a common example of the connection of the mind and the body with the breath. If the mind affects the breath, then breath can affect the mind and also the body. Pranayama always benefits the mind and body.

2. It eliminates uneven and shallow breathing.

3. This Sadhana or spiritual practice will control the Prana, the vital force within the body and also capture Prana Shakti or force from nature, and result in more mental, physical and spiritual energy being available to help Asana as well as Meditation.

4. There are three principal Naadis (Fig. 10.9). They are Ida, Pingala and Shushumna. The Shushumna Naadi is located in the middle of the spinal column, whereas the left nostril is the path of the Ida Naadi and the right nostril of the Pingala. Pranayama practice aims to withdraw Prana from Ida and Pingala Naadis and take it to the Shushumna, which will become active subsequently. "When the Ida and Pingala Naadis are devitalized by the

operation of Shushumna Naadi, there is no night or day for the Yogi. When the Shushumna is in operation, the Yogi can transcend the limitations of time and space."[2]

5. Pranayama is done before and during Asana as well as Dhyana or Meditation to support and enhance their impact on a person's mind, body and soul.

Practice of Pranayama removes stale air from lungs, cleans and strengthens the respiratory organs and revitalizes the body. Many students of mine and I feel that as we practice Yogic breathing we have fewer "colds."

Effects of Poor Breathing

If you breathe poorly, you will have very little energy and will tire very easily. With practice of Pranayama this problem will disappear.

Blockage of Prana in one's body creates many complications. Bhagwan Rajneesh, in his book titled "Yoga" book chapter #8, page 235, writes, "Freud stumbled upon 'libido'; it is Prana ill. When Prana is not vital, when somehow the energy of Prana has become dammed up, blocked, that's what Freud has come to know and that's explainable because he was working only with ill people, neurotics and working on ill, mentally disturbed people he came to know that their bodies are carrying some blocked energy and unless that energy is released, they will not be healthy again. Yogis say, "libido is Prana gone wrong."

PREPARATION FOR PRANAYAMA

Sit in one of the following positions. During the practice of Pranayama, the preferred sitting positions are reported in the order of their preference.

1. Vajaraasan or Knee Posture (Fig. 10.2)
2. Padmaasan or Lotus Posture (Fig. 10.4)
3. Siddhaasan or Half Lotus (Fig. 10.3)
4. Sukhaasan or Easy Posture (Fig. 10.5)

Keep your spine, neck and head erect. Keep your chest out. If you sit on your knees in the Vajaraasan posture, make sure your big toes are touching. Always sit facing north, east or west, but do not face south. It helps to keep your eyes closed, to look within. Keep your mouth closed and breathe through your nostrils (there are only one or two exceptions). Breathe slow, even, long, deep breaths. Keep your mind on Prana and/or Aum (Om). Use only your right hand (in Mudras one can use both hands). Do not wear tights during exercise. Do this on an empty stomach or wait for two hours after eating. Do not do it after taking drugs or drinking alcohol. Make sure you sit with a chinlock or your chin a little bit down and controlling your air passage.

Use of Mantra

The proper way of doing Pranayama is to do it with a Mantra. There are many Mantras you could use during Pranayama, but traditionally one of the following Mantras are used:

During Pranayama

Inhalation	A	OM	O	*
Retention	U	OM	M	*
Exhalation	M	OM	Shanti	*
			(Peace)	

* Traditionally the Gayatri Mantra is repeated which is "OM Bhur Bhuvah Svah Tat Savitur Varenyam Bhargo Devashya Dheemahi Dhiyo Yo Naha Prochodayat."

Chanting a Mantra brings you closer to the Prana and helps you reach your goal quicker. The Gayatri Mantra means the following: "We Meditate on the effulgent glory of the Divine Spirit who illumines and pervades everything. Thou, O Supreme Lord, the center of this Universe, may we prove worthy of thy choice and acceptance, and may thou guide our intellects and may we follow thy lead into righteousness."

Types of Breathing

There are many types of breathing. In this chapter I will discuss two basic ones: cleansing and healing breaths. See below:

Every day practice at least one type of each kind of breathing

Sanskrit Name

Cleansing Breaths	*English Name*
1. Kapalabhati	Kapalabhati
2. Bhastrika	Bellows
Healing Breaths	
1. Vjjaya	Om Breathing
2. Visama Virtti	Analoma Veloma or Alternative nostril Breathing or 1-4-2 Technique

Kapalabhati

Kapalabhati is abdominal and diaphragmatic breathing. It is a cleansing breath that cleanses the respiratory system and the nasal passages. Swami Vishnu Devananda says, "In Sanskrit, Kapala means skull and Bhakti means shines." Therefore the term Kapalabhati means an exercise that makes the skull shine. Here the skull is the nasal passage through which the air passes in and out.

Though this is a breathing exercise, it is considered a cleansing exercise and comes under one of the Kriyas or six purification exercises. (The remaining five cleansing exercises are explained elsewhere). This is done before starting the practice of Pranayama to clean the nasal passages and to remove bronchial congestion.

In this exercise, exhalation plays a prominent part. Inhalation is mild, slow and longer than the exhalation. Except for Bhastrika, in most other breathing exercises, exhalation is longer than inhalation.

The exhalation should be done quickly and forcefully by contracting the abdominal muscles with a backward push. This sudden contraction of the abdominal muscles acts upon the diaphragm, which then recedes into the thoracic cavity, and gives a vigorous push to the lungs expelling the air from the lungs.

This is instantly followed by the relaxation of the abdominal muscles allowing the diaphragm to descend to the abdominal cavity and pull with it the lungs. This allows the air to rush in Kapalabhati. Inhalation and exhalation are performed in quick succession by a sudden and vigorous contraction and relaxation of the abdominal muscles. Exhalation takes about one fourth of the time that inhalation does. Here exhalation is quick, strong, and short, while inhalation is passive, slow, and longer. Passive inhalation and sudden expulsion of breath follow continuously, one another, until a round is completed.

One should do three rounds of Kapalabhatis. A round is 12 in and out cycles. Three rounds means 36 times. Do Kapalabhati 36 times, stop, do another 36 times, stop and rest, then do an additional 36 times. During the performance of the Kapalabhati mentally count 1,2,3… up to 36. This way you can keep an accurate count.

Bhastrika, the Bellows

"Bhastrika has taken its name from these bellows. It is a classical exercise but often misunderstood. Even the Gheranda Samhita (verses 75-6) is not very explicit: As the blacksmith's bellows dilate and contract continuously, so he (the Yogi) inhales slowly through both nostrils while distending the abdomen; he then expels the air rapidly (when it makes the same noise as bellows). Having inhaled and exhaled twenty times, he must perform Kumbhaka (breath retention) and expel the air in the same way. The wise man will practice this Bhastrika-Kumbhaka three times. He will never suffer from illness but will always be in good health."[1]

Start with the following Bhastrika technique. The preferred way of sitting is Vajarajan, Padmasan or Sukhasan. Now make a fist, bend both your hands and keep them close to your body and slowly exhale deeply. Now throw your arms up while opening your fists. While inhaling, forcefully and mentally chant "Om," and then while immediately exhaling, forcefully count one as you pull your hands down and close your fists.

At this time you have done the first count. Now repeat and count while inhaling and chanting "Om," and exhaling on count two. Do this 12 times to make one round. Rest for a few minutes and do a total of three rounds.

Bhastrika can be done without raising and lowering the arms but this technique helps concentration and creates deep and forceful Bhastrika. "Bhastrika may also be practiced as described above but with alternate breathing. Inhale through the left nostril (Ida), exhale through the right nostril (Pingala), re-inhale through Pingala, exhale through Ida, re-inhale through Ida and so on. At first go slowly in order to synchronize the movements of the hand that directs the alternation with the Bhastrika respiration. This variation is more powerful than ordinary Bhastrika, but it should not be attempted before normal Bhastrika has become spontaneous and comfortable. The respiration rate should not exceed 50 breaths per minute."[1] Bhastrika cleans the whole body.

Ujjayi Pranayama

Ujjayi is a simple healing technique and also one of the most important breathing techniques. Ujjaya means, "loud". During its practice one makes a sound during inhalation and exhalation by tilting down the head a little and partially blocking the glottis so as to stop incoming and outgoing air, contract the muscles at the base of the neck near the collarbone. You can sit in your preferred way, but keep your spine straight, keep your arms straight against the knees, your palms up, holding Jnan Mudra.

The technique requires inhaling slowly, deeply and evenly, while chanting "Om" mentally and then holding your breath as long as you can. Then one exhales slowly and evenly. During inhalation count by saying mentally, "Om," exhale one, then inhale "Om," exhale two and so on until you count up to 12, which is one round. Do at least three rounds of Ujjayi Pranayama. Note: Do not hold your breath after the exhalation.

In practicing Ujjayi Pranayama you can do abdominal breathing or abdominal control breathing.

Analoma Viloma

It is also called Alternate Nostril breathing. This is a healing breath. You can also call this technique the "1:4:2" technique. It means if you decide to use count 5, you multiply all parts of 1:4:2 by 5, which gives a count of 5:20:10. In this technique inhale counting to 5, and then hold the breath counting to 20 and then exhale counting to 10. But always say Om before every number you count. For example, during inhalation, while counting to 5, mentally say Om one, Om two, Om three, etc.

Once you master unit count 5 (5:20:10), go to count 6, then count 7, but you need not go beyond unit count 8 (8:32:16). In reality, unit count 8 is 16:64:32 seconds, as you say Om before a number.

The alternate nostril breathing exercise is as follows. Sit on the floor (if you are uncomfortable sitting on the floor, you may sit in a chair, but the floor is preferable). Take your right hand and make the palm face you. Now make the Vishnu Mudra using only the right hand by tucking the index and middle fingers into your palm. Now practice a minimum of three rounds of Anuloma Viloma Pranayama (one round means 12 times). One time Anuloma Viloma is shown in the following six steps using 5:20:10 unit counts.

(1) Close the right nostril with your thumb and breathe in through the left nostril (deep and evenly) and count 5 (say Om one, Om two, etc) (Fig. 10.6).

(2) Close both nostrils. Right nostril with thumb and left nostril with your ring and little fingers. Now hold your breath counting to 20 (say Om one, Om two, etc) (Fig. 10.7).

(3) Now take the little finger and ring finger and close the left nostril and exhale through the right nostril counting 10 (Om one,...Om ten) (Fig. 10.8).

(4) Now breathe in through the right nostril keeping your left nostril closed (count 5).

(5) Hold your breath keeping both nostrils closed (counting 20).

(6) And the last step is to exhale through the left nostril keeping the right nostril closed (reverse the finger movement).

The above six steps makes one time. Twelve of them will be one round. One should do a minimum of three rounds but not less than one round. Why one round? Because Yogis believe that there is a Universe outside as well as inside a human being and there are 12 months in a year and the number 12 represents inner harmony to the Yogi.

While practicing Anuloma Viloma, the left hand should be kept straight, resting on the knees with palms facing up, making a Jnana Mudra. In this Jnana Mudra, the thumb and the index fingers touch and form "O" and the other three fingers remain straight. This Mudra does not allow the energy to go out of the body.

Serious students of Yoga should study the "Hatha Yoga Pradipika" written by Yogi Swatmarama of the 17th or XVII century and of course the "Yoga Sutra" of Maharishi Patanjali.

References

1. "Pranayama, the Yoga of Breathing," by Andre Van Lysebeth—Unwin Paperback—London 1983, page 158, published by George Allen & Unwin Ltd.

2. The Complete Illustrated Book of Yoga by H. H. Swami Vishnu Devananda.

3. "Light on Yoga" by B. K. S. Iyengar.

4. The Sivananda Companion to Yoga, written by Lucy Lidell, Narayani and Giris Rabinovitch.

5. "Hatha Yoga Pradipika" by students of Swami Vishnu Devananda, Published by Lotus Publishing Company, Sivananda Yoga Vedanta Center, 243 West 24th Street, New York, NY 10011.

Chapter 11

Pranayama with Mudra Yoga

INTRODUCTION

Pranayama, or Yogic breathing, has been practiced for thousands of years in India. It is practiced even more now, in this fast modern world. Energy is wasted today through high tension and improper breathing, or shallow breathing, which weakens and tires people and which makes it necessary for more sleep and relaxation. Pranayama, a method to control pranic energy, offers good health and more energy to work and feel good. It may impart Prana Shakti, or Divine Mother's power, and lead one to higher spiritual consciousness.

Pranayama removes toxins. Prana or living forces is understood by gati or movement. It is not static but it is dynamic. This higher energy can be gained only by removing mental and physical disorders. It helps a great deal to understand the five basic tatwas or earthly elements. The elements are: Jamin (earth), Pani (water), Agni (fire), Vaayu (air), and Akash (ether). Everyone has to work with these five elements.

I received this divine knowledge from a great Yogi: Swami Poornananda of India (See his photo in Fig. 12.6). Swamiji was a very spiritual person and captivated the whole audience at his seminar in Wilmington, Delaware, on Pranayama, with his personality and dedication to Yoga. You could tell he practiced and believed every word he taught us. Swamji has made a great impact on my life. These teachings have helped me and I am sure it will help many more. These were his messages:

IMPORTANCE OF YOGIC BEATHING

Pranayama or Yogic breathing is very important, not only for good physical and mental health, and happiness but also for spiritual progress. With age the spine stiffens, legs weaken, joints do not bend easily, and diaphragm and abdominal muscles get weak. It has been proven that Pranayama makes old people stronger and more flexible. Pranayama is the only internal exercise that provides stamina and energy. It offers Prana, a living force. For proper breathing, lung expansion is very vital. Some feel that full chest expansion is full lung expansion, which is not true. For full lung expansion the lung has to go down to push the diaphragm out. Regular breathing brings toxins and poisons. The removal of these can only be done by Kapalabhati Pranayama (which is called cleansing breath-deflation of the lung). Jyeshtha Pranayama (which is a true healing breath, this type of breathing fully expands the lungs). (Page 71)

PRANAYAMA EXPLAINED

Pranayama is a Yogic breathing technique. It is conscious breathing which cleans and heals the body, bringing more energy and leading one to higher consciousness. Before we talk about Yogic breathing we must talk about our lungs. The human lung is divided into three parts or lobes. Most people use only the lower and middle lobes. Breathing should be conscious, slow, even and deep and cover all three lobes. The human body has a chest, diaphragm and abdomen. In Yogic breathing, the diaphragm moves downward and the abdomen expands outward. The abdomen rather than the chest should expand outward.

Prana is energy needed by the body and mind. Prana is not oxygen. Prana is circulated through our astral bodies by a network of special channels, which are called Naadis. In Sanskrit "Naadi" means movement. Naadis do not exist in the physical body but they exist in the astral body. Naadis are Pranic channels (Fig. 10.9). There are three basic channels. They are Ida, Pingaala and Shushumna. Ida Naadi is on the left side of our body. It is our female side. It is the moon channel and is also called Chandra Naadi. The Pingaala Naadi is on the right side of our body. It is the male side. It is the sun channel and it is also called Soorya Naadi. There are 101 Naadis in our astral body. Every two hours, force switches from Ida to Pingaala, or vice versa. The nostril also changes breathing unusually. Humans favor either the left or right nostril. Both nostrils are not fully used at the same time. The practice of Pranayama opens up the Naadis which heal our body, offers increased energy and imparts Prana Shakti, which means Divine Mother's power or living force. This leads to the awakening of Kundalini Shakti. At this point it is very important to understand the basics of this complex subject of Kundalini Yoga. In our astral bodies, there are seven major centers of cosmic energy situated in a line along the Shushumna Naadi which are located along the spinal cord.

These seven centers are called Chakras, (wheels) or Padmas (lotuses). In the lowest Chakra, the Muladhara Chakra, which is situated at the bottom of the spine there resides a dormant energy called Kundalini, the Divine Mother, who is symbolized by a coiled snake. At the top of the spine, in the head, the seventh and highest Chakra is called Sahasrara Chakra there resides the Divine Father, Lord Shiva. The objective of Pranayama is to awaken the Kundalini Shakti and guide her upward to meet Lord Shiva. When that occurs the highest experience happens. When you meet God it is an experience that cannot be described but must be experienced.

BENEFITS OF PRANAYAMA

Pranayama offers many benefits to the mind, physical body, astral body, and can help in spiritual life. These breathing techniques bring mental peace. They help control anger and help control the mind.

Breathing is the bridge between the mind and body. Therefore Pranayama with the help of the mind reduces bodily stress. This technique slows the pulse by teaching the heart to take more oxygen in a shorter time. The ideal pulse is 60 beats per minute. Pranayama also cleans the air sacks and thus makes the lungs more efficient and helps avoid lung cancer. Pranayama is the only way one can massage the heart and lungs. This technique with Prana Shakti energizes the body and mind and heals them without any medicine. This energy also tones the nerves of the body. Proper Yogic breathing could increase body temperature. Many Yogi's say that proper Pranayama controls one's sexual energy.

Spiritually, Pranic energy with the help of Pranayama directs Pranic energy and helps one go to the Naadis, which exist in our astral bodies. Pranayama, with the help of Mudras or Mudra Yoga (Yogic body language) which opens our inner channels, we can then enter into the Shushumna Naadi and awaken our Kundalini and go into higher consciousness. Pranayama deepens our Meditation, helps us reach enlightenment and subsequently Samadhi or Mookti (freedom). Yoga Vashistha says: Prana is a living force. Life leads to movement and movement leads to Prana, which gives us better health, happiness and leads us to Mookti.

DURING PRANAYAMA

Complete one or two or more rounds because we have a complete universe within ourselves. There is an internal cosmic rhythm. Beginners should make the sound by pressing within the throat at the beginning only. Once you have mastered the art of breathing, you do not have to make any sounds. Please note:

Puraka means Inhalation—4 to 5 seconds
Kumbhaka means Retention—7 to 9 seconds
Sunyaka means Empty lungs 2 to 3 seconds
Bandha means contract and control a certain part of the body

Beginners should not try Sunyaka (holding lungs empty) as it requires mastery, without which it is dangerous. Practice 20 minutes but 50 minutes is better. During Pranayama one should not move. During Pranayama a cooling sensation is a good effect but during the sensation know that improvement is taking place. Sometimes you start rocking and moving in a circle. That is good, maybe your Kundalini is awakening. Morning is the best time for the practice of Pranayama.

PRANAYAMA TECHNIQUES

Swami Poonananda divides Pranayama into three basic categories and they are listed below, in the order one should practice them. One should do Pranayama with selected Mudra to achieve their benefits.
  1. Kapalabhati
  2. Deerghaswasa Sharira Mudra
  3. Pranopasana
        A. Kanishta—lower lobe
        B. Madhyama—middle lobe
        C. Jyeshta—upper lobe
        D. Purna—full
        E. Merudanda—spinal
        F. Prana Kriya Mudras

Always sit with spine erect, head balanced and shoulders out and be relaxed.
  1. Kapalabhati (See Kapalabhati in the chapter 10)
  2. Deerghaswasa Sharira Mudra (Fig. 11.1)

After sitting properly for breathing exercise, interlace the fingers and extend the middle fingers out straight and keep the thumbs also straight. The heels (base) of the palms press lightly together, palms must touch (Fig. 11.1). Now touch the tips of the thumbs to the middle of the sternum while placing the tips of the middle fingers in the base of the throat. While keeping the elbows raised and parallel to the ground and now start deep breathing. One should do at least three rounds of breathing (one round is 12 times). Deergha Swasa Sharira Mudra expands the lungs and also brings the lungs to their full functions.

3. Pranopasana

A. *Kanishtha:* (Lower lobe) (Fig. 11.2)

To do Kanishta Mudra Pranayama, keep all your fingers together and straight; but keep the thumbs away from all the fingers. Now keep the elbows forward, palms facing down and parallel to the ground and keep the palm touching the body keeping them one inch below the last rib. In this Mudra air goes to the lower lobe.

B. *Madhyama* (Middle lobe) (Fig. 11.3)

To do Madhyama Sharia Mudra Pranayama keep the fingers, thumb and palms to the same way as kanishta except the thumbs are into armpits while the forefingers remain straight and on the sidewalls of the upper ribs and breastbone. Keep the elbows forward and parallel to the ground and start Pranayama Kriya or exercise. In this Mudra air goes to the middle lobe.

C. *Jyeshta Pranayama* (Upper lobe) (Fig. 11.4)

To do Jyeshtha Pranayama keep all the fingers straight. Put both the palms together and onto the shoulder blades. Keep the spine straight, head up, shoulders away from the ears, and elbows raised up keep little pressure on the hands on the shoulder blades and arms touching the head. Now start Pranayama. In this Jyeshtha Pranayama, air goes to the upper lobe and it gives relaxation as energy goes to the head.

Alternatives to those techniques shown above

The above three Kanishta, Madhyama, and Jyeshtha Pranayama are all basic exercises but they are done in the following three ways, to reach Sushumna Naadi for ultimate experience Naadi Mudra and Mookti or liberation.

a. *Kanishta Prana Naadi Mudra* (Fig. 11.5) Join the tip of the thumbs and forefingers, keep little, ring and middle fingers straight. Keep palms downward and rest on the knees or thighs. Now start Pranayama. This Mudra not only takes the Prana Shakti to lower lobe of the lung but it controls the Naadis.

b. *Madhyama Prana Naadi Mudra* (Fig. 11.6)

In this Mudra keep the hand Mudra the same as Kanishtha except all three little, ring and middle fingers bent and touching the palms. Now do Pranayama. This guides Prana to the middle lobe and it also controls the Naadis.

c. *Jyeshta Prana Naadi Mudra* (Fig. 11.7)

In this Mudra keep the hand Mudra the same as Kanishtha except thumb inside the palm and all the fingers over the thumb, palms down, keeping them on your knees or thighs (Fig. 11.7) and start Pranayama. This Mudra leads the Prana to the upper lobe and controls the Naadis.

D. *Purna Pranayama* (Fig. 11.8) Some Yogis do this Poorna Prana Mudra with their thumbs tucked inside the palms and fingers on top of the thumbs and keeping the fists up, and keeping the little fingers tucked against the abdomen just below the navel. After holding the Mudra properly start the Pranayama. This is one of the most important breathing exercises. The word poorna in Sanskrit means perfect or complete. This Mudra opens the Shushumna Naadi.

E. *Merudanda Mudra*—Meru means mount Meru, the spine and Danda means staff in Sanskrit. This Mudra with Pranayama begins the Prana Shakti, the living force penetrates into the deep area of the central nervous system. These Mudras are separate from other Mudras. They are a class by themselves.

Merudanda Mudra are three types. To do them put your fists on the thighs. In these three Mudras the positions of the thumbs decide the following three Merudanda Mudras.

a. *Merudanda Mudra* (Fig. 11.9) Keep your thumbs straight up and palms facing each other.

b. *Adho Merudanda* (Fig. 12.1) Keep your thumbs facing each other and palms down.

c. *Vrdhra Merudanda* (Fig. 12.2) Keep your thumbs away from each other and palms up. After holding the proper Mudra start Pranayama.

F. *Prana Kriya Mudra*—These Mudras are Kriyas or cleansing processes. It cleanses the gross body, astral body and subtle body. This Mudra is also called Jnana Mudra. If you want to remember anything, just hold this

Mudra to remember anything you want to remember. This Mudra is one of the Kriyas, or purifying exercises. Put your palms upon your knees or thighs. There are three parts of Pranayama. They are as follows:

a. *Shraddha Purna Prana Mudra* (means wisdom) (Fig. 12.3) Index finger touching the base of thumbs for the Prajna Poorna Prana Mudra.

b. *Medhya Purna Prana Mudra* (means higher wisdom) (Fig. 12.4) Index finger touching middle joint of thumbs for Medhya Poorna Prana Mudra.

c. *Prajna Purna Prana Mudra* (Means intuitive awareness) (Fig. 12.5) Index finger touching tip of the thumbs for the Shraddha Poorna Prana Mudra.

Once correct Pranayama is learned practicing the above Kriyas leads one to higher consciousness, and may awaken Kundalini or Shushumna Naadi or activate one of the Granthis.

Granthis

Swami Poornananda said to activate the Granthis is a science of Raja Pranayama. Granthis are glands (Fig. 12.7). Humans have 108 Granthis plus one that is the highest. When a Granthi is activated one gets power of the Granthi. For example, when a boxer activates his elbow power he gets incredible power in his elbow. Pranayama awakens one or more Granthis. There are three types of Granthis; they are:

1. Prithvi or earth (below navel)
2. Antariksha or space (in the middle between neck and navel)
3. Dyau or heaven (neck and above—Fig. 12.7)

The Prithvi or earth part of our body which is below our navel, is where there are 33 Granthis and they control sex, lust, base emotions, etc. The Antariksha or space area is the part of our body between the neck and the navel. It has 33 Granthis. It represents love, goodness, digestion etc. The Dyau or heaven part of our body is above the neck. It represents light, memory, enlightenment, high consciousness, freedom, etc. It is important to note that the three lobes of the lung affect the three types of Granthis. The lower lobe affects the Prithvi, the middle lobe affects the Antariksha, and upper lobe affects the Dyau. However, it is a known fact that most of the humans use only the middle and lower lobes. With the help of Raja Pranayama one can reach the upper lobe and subsequently activate the Granthis in the Dyau part of our body, and reach the highest state.

In conclusion Pranayama improves physical health, mental health, purifies the astral body, awakens powers, that lay within, deepens mediation, awakens Kundalini Shakti and takes one to a higher consciousness and ultimately to the attainment of Mookti or liberation.

Figure 11

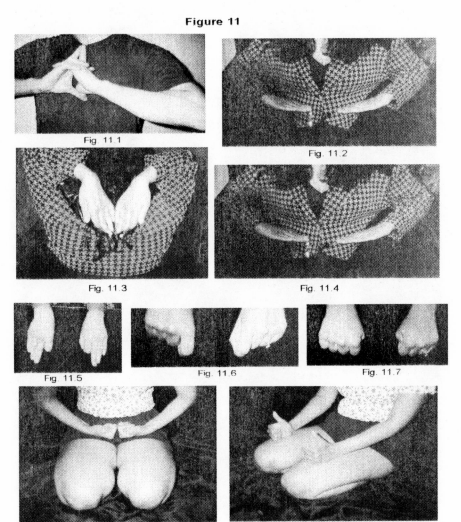

Fig. 11.1

Fig. 11.2

Fig. 11.3

Fig. 11.4

Fig. 11.5

Fig. 11.6

Fig. 11.7

Fig. 11.8

Fig. 11.9

Figure 12

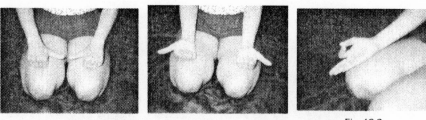

Fig. 12.1   Fig. 12.2   Fig. 12.3

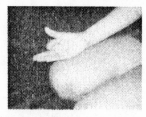

Fig. 12.4 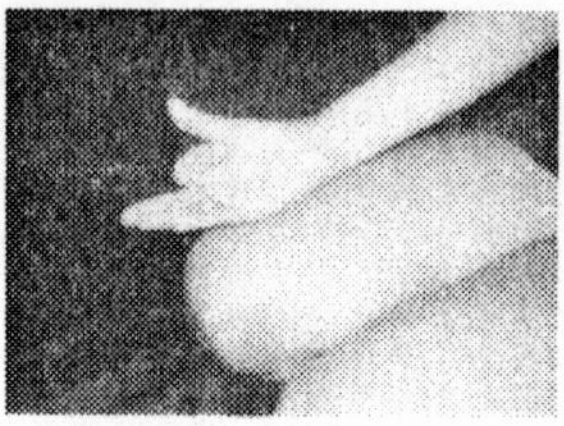   Fig. 12.5

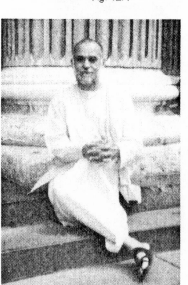

Fig. 12.6

RAJA PRANAYAMA

There are three types of Pranayamas:

1. DAYU or Heaven (neck and above)
2. ANTARIKSHA or Space (in the middle)
3. PRITHIV or Earth (below the navel)

(Total: 108 + 1 GRANTHIS or Glands)

          OM (Mookti or Liberation)

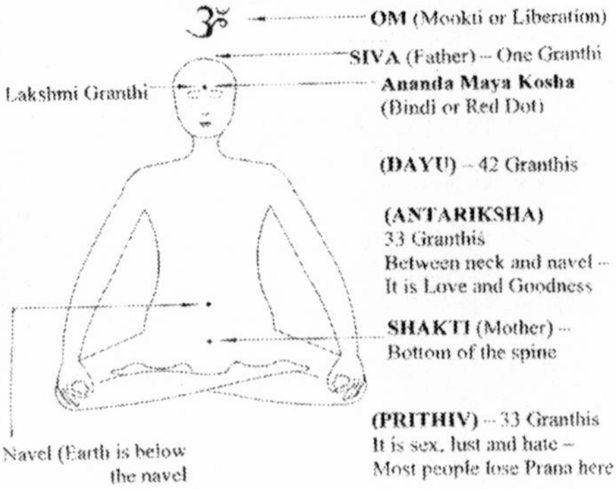

SIVA (Father) – One Granthi

Lakshmi Granthi   **Ananda Maya Kosha**
(Bindi or Red Dot)

(DAYU) – 42 Granthis

(ANTARIKSHA)
33 Granthis
Between neck and navel –
It is Love and Goodness

SHAKTI (Mother) –
Bottom of the spine

(PRITHIV) – 33 Granthis
It is sex, lust and hate –
Most people lose Prana here

Navel (Earth is below
the navel)

Fig. 12.7

Chapter 12

Mudra Yoga

Introduction

Mudra could be translated as body language. In English, body language is used to communicate with others, but in Yoga Mudra or Mudra Yoga it is used in communicating with one's self or healing one's mind, body and/or one's astral body. One could say Mudra Yoga communicates with divine self or God. There are four types of Mudra Yoga. They are:

1. Yog or Yoga Tatva Mudra Vigyan used in breathing
2. Yog Pranayama Mudra used in breathing
3. Yog Dhyan Mudra used in Meditation
4. Yog Asan Mudra used in Asana

Yog Tatva Mudra Vigyan (vigyn means science)

The ancient Shastras explain the various sciences for investigation and treatment of the human body. One of these is the Yog Tatva Mudra Vigyan or the science of finger postures related to the elements.

These Shastras base themselves on two important facts:

1. That the human body is made from five distinct elements. They are: Fire, Wind, Ether, Earth, and Water. Medical knowledge available from the Indian sciences of Ayurveda and metaphysics affirm that distortion or impairment of the five elements create outer disturbance and inner sickness in the body. To calm the disturbances and cure the inner sickness it is necessary to bring back to normal the five elements in the entire body. For this, Nature, Yoga, Ayurveda, Mental Strength, Power of Mantras and many other tools may have to be used. The five fingers of the hand represent these five elements and are

YOGI BHARAT J. GAJJAR

instrumental in achieving desired results when used as per the laws of Mudra Vigyan.

2. There are 10 types of Vayus (winds) that circulate in the nerves of the human body. Five of these are the 'Mukhya Vayus (Main Winds) and the other five the 'Upvayus' (Secondary Winds).

The above Vayus, whether working independently or in conjunction with other Vayus, help keep the body Nirmal (Pure) and in perfect working order. Any imbalance leads to malfunctioning in one or more systems of the body. Mudras in this case help in cleaning the physical and astral bodies and help the mind to be concentrated and peaceful.

Because this science specifies how postures formed with the fingers help in balancing of the elements and the winds, it is correctly called Tatva Yoga Mudra Vigyan or Mudra Vigyan for short.

In Mudra Vigyan the fingers are folded in specific postures to provide the necessary tension on the nerves and achieve curative effects. Thus, Mudra Vigyan is a neural science that works on the nervous system and helps to keep the body fit.[1]

Every human being consists of five natural elements, in the same way that in this world there are only five basic Tatva elements. They are 1) Pani (water), 2) Prithvi (earth), 3) Akash (space), 4) Vayu (air), and 5) Agni (fire). On a person's hands there are five fingers, and each finger on both hands represents an element and its energy. They are as follows:

Five Fingers	Elements
1. Little Finger	Jal (water)
2. Ring Finger	Prithvi (earth)
3. Middle Finger	Akash (space)
4. Index Finger	Vayu (air)
5. Thumb	Agni (fire)

Yogis discovered and developed the science in which the energy of any finger represented above is greatly increased when the tip of the finger is touched to the tip of the thumb. They also discovered that when the tip of any finger touches the base of the thumb the energy represented by that finger decreases. Thus the word Mudra refers to the holding of fingers in the many ways mentioned above and its impact affects the entire being.

Some Mudras are also done by holding onto both arms separately and some are done by holding both arms jointly. There are many types of Mudras but they affect the five basic parts of the human body. Each Mudra has its unique impact. It can affect one part or more than one part of the body. Areas that can be affected are the nerves, mind, and subconscious mind in Meditation, or the energy level of the body or any particular organ in the body.

The effects of Mudras are greater depending upon practice and the person's faith in the Mudra Vigyan, as well as how long a person holds the Mudra. The optimum length of time to hold a Mudra is continuously for about 45 minutes a day without a break. A good minimum amount of time would be 10 or 15 minutes for 4 or 5 times throughout a day. One can increase the length if they feel it would be more beneficial to them. Some Mudras affect a person immediately while other Mudras can take 2 to 4 months or possibly longer before a person can feel its effect.

How to Hold the Jnan or Dhyan Mudra

Jnan or Dhyan Mudra, one of the most important Mudras, is used a great deal in practicing Yoga, in practicing Meditation and also in achieving knowledge and peace. The way to do Jnan Mudra is to connect the tip of the index finger with the tip of the thumb and make sure to keep all of your other fingers are straight. This Mudra is more powerful when it is combined with Yoga Asana and Pranayama or Yogic breathing. (Fig. 13.1)

The tip of the index finger should touch the tip of the thumb, while the other fingers remain straight. This is the most important and widely used Mudras in Yoga and Meditation practice. One should sit in a Lotus Posture before starting their Yoga practice with the Jnan Mudra (Fig. 13.1). In the Jnan Mudra the index finger is Vayu (air) and the thumb is fire. When both fingers get together, energy gets moving, but when one sits in Padmasan with the Mudra, a triangle is formed where all energy starts going into the center of one's body and the mind becomes peaceful. This is the moving principle of the Mudra science.

Before you start your Yoga postures, breathing, Meditation, or teaching your Yoga class, do the following:

1. Sit in Padmasan (Lotus Posture) or Sidhasan or Sukhasan (Easy Posture) (See Fig. 10.4).

2. Keep you hands straight holding Jnan Mudra. (See Fig. 13.1)

3. Chant Om three times and then say Shanti three times before you start your Yogic breathing postures or Meditation.

It is important to do this because when you are sitting in this posture you are making a pyramid. In the pyramid, all energy goes into the center. "How is it a pyramid?" you might ask (Fig. 10.4). It is a triangle forming a pyramid. All of the energy starts flowing into the center. You are holding Jnan Mudra, which also directs energy into the center of your being. Chanting the Om Mantra also brings divine peace within the self. It is very important for you to do this posture with Mudras and chanting Mantra before you start breathing exercises, Hatha Yoga or Meditation practice.

Jnan Mudra is called Jnan Mudra because it means knowledge and it brings peace. Yogis say, if you want to remember something, hold this Mudra and you can remember everything you read and hear. In America, I've heard there is a company that gives a seminar to increase your power of memory and charges $500 for the weekend. They teach this Mudra in their seminar.

I would like to tell you another interesting thing about this Mudra. For the last 4 years, I have been teaching Yoga at the women's prison in Delaware and I showed this Mudra. The girls have told me that when a girl at the prison is hard to control, they make that girl hold this Mudra and walk around for the whole day. This makes the girl calm down and become more peaceful.

Dhyan Mudra is called Dhyan because it means Meditation. If you do this Mudra and do Meditation, your Meditation will be more concentrated, more powerful and more peaceful.

If one feels sleepy and lazy, one should practice Jnan Mudra for 45 minutes and he/she will feel full of energy. Many Yogis say that if you hold this Jnan Mudra you can remember anything you read or listen to. This Mudra has concentration power and is the reason that it was named Jnan or Mudra of knowledge. This Mudra is also called Dhyan (meaning concentration) Mudra because this Mudra is used during Meditation. Then chant Om three times. After that one should start their practice of Asanas.

Dyan or Jnan Mudra

The following section was taken from a pamphlet written by Arvind Joshi
"Vayu Mudra:—Steps: (Fig. 13.2)
1. Touch the index finger to the base of thumb.
2. Cover the index finger with the thumb.
3. Keep the other three fingers straight with ease.
Practice for 45 minutes or 15 minutes for three times in a day. "This Mudra helps reduce Vayu (gas) within the body. This gets rid of problems such as spondylitis, lumbago, knee pain, sciatica, etc. Some of these conditions require determined and regular practice of this Mudra for weeks or months until complete relief of symptoms has occurred. Sleeping under a fan can make your body feel heavy and lethargic. But if one practices Vayu Mudra while falling asleep, one does not suffer the ill effects of the fan. If one gets cramps at night, doing this Mudra will ease it. The pain caused by Vayu (gas) settling within the tendons, muscles, nerves and brain cells can be eased by using the Vayu Mudra.

Akash Mudra:—Steps: (Fig. 13.3)
1. Touch the tip of middle finger with that of thumb.
2. Keep the remaining three fingers straight with ease.
This is for strengthening the bones. Practice for 15 minutes to 45 minutes every day according to your needs. "The effect of this Mudra is to strengthen the bones. Cardiac patients benefit a lot by practicing this Mudra. Some ear problems are eased by this Mudra. Doing this Mudra during yawning or hiccups prevents locking of the jaw.

Shoonya Mudra:—Steps: (Fig. 13.4)
1. Touch the tip of middle finger to the base of the thumb.
2. Rest the thumb over the middle finger.
3. Keep the remaining three fingers straight with ease.
This Mudra is very helpful in ear problems. Practice this for 15 to 60 minutes every day per your needs. During an earache, if you hold this Mudra for 15-20 minutes, it will ease your pain. People with deafness or reduced hearing should practice this Mudra for 10 to 60 minutes a day for true benefit.

Pruthvi Mudra:—Steps: (Fig. 13.5)

1. Touch the tip of ring finger to that of thumb.
2. Keep the other three fingers straight with ease.

Practice this for 15 to 45 minutes each day and when necessary hold it longer. This Mudra will increase the Pruthvi (earth) element in the body and thus strengthen the body and other controls. Weak and underweight people can benefit by strengthening the body and increasing their weight. Energy levels increase to give you more enthusiasm, contentment, a better aura and better immunity. People find this Mudra can temporarily ease control an urency of a bowel movement, Untill you find facilities.

Surya Mudra:—Steps: (Fig. 13.6)

1. Touch the tip of the ring finger to the base of the thumb.
2. Rest the thumb over the ring finger.
3. Keep the other three fingers straight with ease.

This Mudra can assist in burning off excess fat and thus lead to slimming. Practice this for up to 60 minutes twice a day. This Mudra is recommended to be performed in Padmasana, but it can also be practiced in the cross-legged posture. This is very beneficial to heavy set and obese people. It also assists in easing of mental tension.

Varun Mudra:—Steps: (Fig. 13.7)

1. Touch the tip of little finger to the tip of the thumb.
2. Keep the other fingers straight with ease.

This is for dry skin and lack of water in the body. Practice for any amount of time and length of time as required. This Mudra assists in increasing the jal (water) element within the body. Thus it achieves lubrication where dryness exists in the body. Dryness of skin and mouth is eased. This can be very helpful in cases of gastroenteritis and also eases suffering from acidity.

Ruksha Mudra:—Steps: (Fig. 13.8)

1. Touch the tip of little finger to the base of the thumb.
2. Rest the thumb over the little finger.
3. Keep the remaining three fingers straight.

This is for excess of urination, sweat and for reducing water from the body. This Mudra reduces the Jal (water) element in the body and thus should be practiced only as needed and then stop. Do not practice in excess. This benefits patients suffering from ascitis, fluid in the lungs, etc. If one is desperate to pass urine and cannot find a suitable place, then this Mudra can help to hold it some time longer. People who sweat excessively can also benefit from this Mudra.

Apana Mudra:—Steps: (Fig. 13.9)
1. Touch the tips of middle and ring finger to the tip of the thumb.
2. Keep the remaining two fingers straight with ease.

This Mudra makes the body very purified. Excretory matter and toxins are expelled out of the body with ease. This enhances the purity of the body and mind and directs one towards Sattvic (pure and balanced) feelings. This Mudra has been found to be beneficial in cases of difficulty in urination, gases, acidity, stomachache, constipation and diabetes. People who don't sweat and thus have some discomfort can practice this Mudra and encourage the body to sweat, thus easing the problem. If there is phlegm blocked in the chest and throat area, this Mudra can ease the phlegm and one can perceive it moving lower and lower and thus ease the problem. This may help some patients suffering from cancer growths and could also be a preventive measure.

Apana Vayu Mudra:—Steps: (Fig. 13.10)
1. Bring the tip of the index finger to the base of the thumb.
2. Touch the tips of the middle finger and the ring finger to the tip of the thumb. Keep the little finger straight.

This is to pass out gases from the stomach. Practice this early morning, after meals and anytime when required for at least 15 minutes. This Mudra, when practiced after meals, is conducive to releasing gas and assists people who suffer from bloated stomach, or tightness in the chest after meals. It can also reduce and stimulate the bowel movements if practiced early in the morning. In an acute case of heart attack, this Mudra can be useful as first aid.

Pran Mudra:—Steps: (Fig. 13.11)
1. Touch the tip of the ring finger to the little finger to that of thumb.
2. Keep the remaining fingers straight.

This is an important Mudra to remain energetic. Practice this at anytime, anywhere for any length of time. True to its name, it enhances Pran Shakti (vital energy), leads to increase in immunity to disease and prevents fatigue. It will improve vision and reduce weakness of the eyes and stops deteriorating vision. Doing this Mudra 10 minutes after a meal can harmonize digestion.

Shankha Mudra:—Steps: (Fig. 13.12)
1. Enclose the thumb of the left hand in the palm of the right hand.
2. Grip the thumb in such a way that the tip of the index finger of the left hand touches the tip of the thumb of the right hand.
3. Other fingers of the left hand are folded over the right fist.

This is for any disorder of digestion and speech. Practice this for any length of time. This Mudra can also be done vice versa, by interchanging the hands. This Mudra will correct any disorders of speech, improve digestion and appetite.

Linga Mudra:—Steps: (Fig. 13.13)
1. Interlock the fingers of both hands.
2. Expose the thumb of any one hand vertically.
3. The vertical thumb must be enclosed by the other hand's thumb and index finger.

This Mudra increases the heat element within the body and thus reduces any chill within the body. Phlegm is reduced. Chronic cold is benefited. The heat from this Mudra can have an influential effect in reducing obesity. People who suffer chills and dislike cold weather find this Mudra a Godsend. Practice whenever it is needed"

Mudras for Health by Arvind Joshi[1]
Yog Tatva Mudra Vigyan by Vijay Krishna Bansal[2]

Figure 13

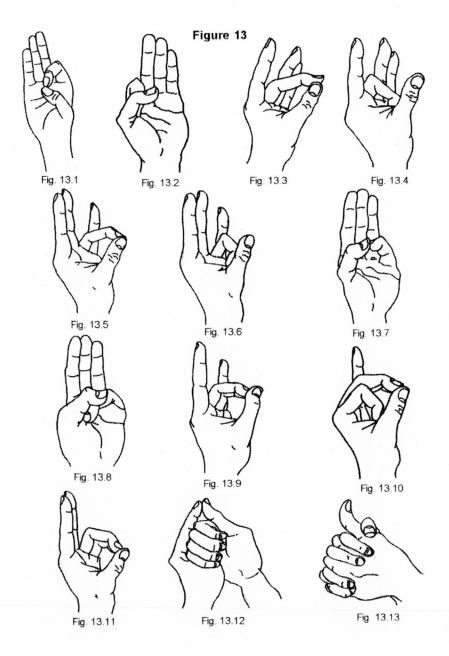

Fig. 13.1　　Fig. 13.2　　Fig. 13.3　　Fig. 13.4

Fig. 13.5　　Fig. 13.6　　Fig. 13.7

Fig. 13.8　　Fig. 13.9　　Fig. 13.10

Fig. 13.11　　Fig. 13.12　　Fig. 13.13

Chapter 13

Meditation (Dhyan)

Introduction

Meditation is as simple as this: sit down on the floor, close your eyes, stop thinking, love God, detach from all or unite with all. Meditation is also as complex as the human being. One sage said this about Meditation, "Those who know about Meditation do not talk about it, and those who do not know should not talk about it, because spiritual experiences cannot be adequately expressed by the human language." Bhagwan Shri Rajneesh (Osho) says, "Meditation cannot be taught, it can only be caught." Thus one can see that one needs a Guru or a spiritual teacher to learn mediation, or a great desire and patience to learn.

In Sanskrit, Meditation is called Dhyan. One of the benefits of Meditation is a person can control their mind which is like a wild horse. It is a game of controlling the thoughts. Meditation is very difficult because thoughts are like tennis balls, every ball comes from a different direction, different height and speed. So tennis requires you to learn and practice before you can enjoy playing. In the same way, Meditation requires you to learn it, practice it before you can enjoy it.

How to Begin Meditation

These are the recommended steps to follow when learning and practicing Meditation:

Step 1: Sit on the floor in the posture of your choice, with Jnana Mudra (see Figures 10.3 and 10.4). Soon after beginning, move your hands into your lap, palms up, one hand on top of each other with your thumbs touching. Close your eyes.

Step 2: Start marching inward, and say your favorite prayer or ask your Guru and/or God to help you Meditate.

Step 3: Focus and realize that your mind and body are not at peace, many thoughts are entering your mind.

Step 4: Try to replace all thoughts with one thought, one object, one person that you love the most, or a Mantra (your personal Mantra or the Mantra of your choice.) If you do not have one, "Om" is the most powerful Mantra. If you need a Mantra see Chapter 14, "Mantra and Japa Yoga." This is contemplation which makes many objects become one. At that point there are only three left: you, God and one object or one word.

Step 5: Repeat a Mantra, e.g. Hari Om (Hari = God, Om = Everything and everybody are one), Guru Om, Shakti Ma or any Mantra of your choice, or watch your breath go in and out. In this technique, you can focus on an object, but you do not have to. Detach and chant or watch your breath go in and out with your Mantra.

Step 6: At this stage you are entering into Meditation where your object or Mantra is dropped, and only you and God remain.

Step 7: Now drop the duality and merge into oneness or Om consciousness. You and God are one. Those who do not believe in merging with God should skip this step. This last step leads you to Samadhi or Nirvana.

Note: A Meditator does not have to believe in God or a Guru, but it helps.

Meditation Techniques
There are 108 techniques for Meditation. Eight of them are the most commonly used. Most are done sitting on the floor with eyes closed, except where indicated. Remember that prayer is talking to God, and Meditation is listening to God. These are the eight most commonly used Meditation techniques.

1) **Watch your breath technique:**—In this technique you watch the breath go in and out. One may Chant the Mantra "Om." You need to know that the mind can only do one thing at a time. If you concentrate on your breathing, your mind will stop thinking. Once the mind is quiet, the heart will open up and you will experience the love of God.

2) **Sitting thoughtlessly technique:**—Sit without any expectation, and do not allow any thoughts to enter your mind. If a thought does come, just watch

it, but do not entertain it and it will go away. The best way to continue this Meditation is to detach from the material world or merge into all with love.

3) **Mantra Meditation technique:**—In this technique, you use your Guru Mantra, or any Mantra of your choice. You replace all thoughts with the chanting of your Mantra. Mantra means the name of God. Therefore, you are loving God and focusing on the repetition of your Mantra. You are also trying to go into higher consciousness. Once you become calm and relaxed, you can drop the Mantra and sit quietly with a feeling of love.

4) **Concentrate on an object technique:**—In this technique you concentrate on an object or a thought. For example, if you love a red rose, you could focus your mind or contemplate the red rose. Often I would, in humor, tell my students, "If you have 10 boyfriends, pick out the one you like best, such as Johnny, and keep the other nine out." Some people use this technique when they are bothered by an issue. They concentrate on that one issue and listen to their higher self.

5) **Meditation on the Guru technique:**—Concentrate on your Guru or the person you love the most. For example you might select your mother, who would then be the object of your concentration. A Christian may choose to Meditate on Jesus.

6) **Know thyself technique:**—Here you focus on your own soul, or Atman, and realize that Jive Atman (you), and Param Atman (God) are the only divine reality. All others are Maya (illusion). You are concentrating on your soul, which is part of God. Your soul knows everything it needs to know, as it is part of God. Once you Meditate on the self, you go into higher consciousness and at one point you will go into Samadhi or Nirvana.

7) **Open eye Meditation technique:**—You keep your eyes partially open in this technique. You can focus on the tip of your nose or a picture of your Guru, God or a statue of God. You could sit on the bank of a river and watch the river flow. When doing this Meditation you must not entertain thoughts.

8) **Mindful walking technique:**—In this Meditation you consciously walk without thoughts but stay completely aware of everything around you.

How to Meditate

There are two important things to remember. The first is not to make yourself so comfortable as to risk falling asleep, and the second is not to be so uncomfortable as to be unable to Meditate.

The best way to Meditate is to sit on the floor, in the Easy Posture (Sukhasan). If this is not comfortable for you, then you can sit in a chair. If you sit in a chair, you could fall asleep. The traditional Yogi always sits in the Full Lotus Posture (Padmasan) or the Half Lotus (Siddhasan). However, people in the West may have difficulty sitting on the floor, because they spend most of their time sitting in chairs. You should try to keep your body upright, spine, neck and head in a straight line, keep your body totally motionless and relaxed during Meditation (see Figures 10.3 and 10.4).

Goals of Meditation
The first goal of Meditation is to become stress-free and peaceful, the second goal is to experience the love of God. The third goal is to become awakened and to become purified. The fourth is to go into higher consciousness. Through Meditation a person hopes to develop love and compassion for all as well as to lose one's ego self. Another goal is to become liberated and come out from the circle of life and death. One hopes to eventually become God Conscious.

• SUDDHI—Purification, Healing
• SIDDHI—Power, Control
• SHANTI—Peace, Full of Bliss
• BUDDHI—Knowledge, Enlightenment
• BHAKTI—Love, Compassion
• SHRADDA—Positive, Faith
• ATMA JNAN—Truth, Self-knowledge
• OM CONSCIOUS—Oneness, Feel Eternal

What is the Best Time to Meditate
Anytime is a good time to Meditate, however, Yogis recommend it be done first thing in the morning. The worst time to Meditate is right after you eat or right before going to bed. Yogis say the best time to Meditate is Brahmamurhta, which is between 3 a.m. and 6 a.m. These are called the "Godly hours," because at that time Yogis and saints Meditate. Between 6 a.m.—9 p.m., others Meditate. From 10 p.m. to 3 a.m. it is not good to Meditate, it is time to sleep.

How Long to Meditate

When you begin practicing Meditation, start with five minutes and gradually increase it to 21 minutes. True Meditation doesn't begin until after the first 21 minutes. Your goal should be to sit and Meditate for 30 minutes to an hour.

This is a summary of what Lord Buddha says in Buddha Daily Reading by Swami Venkatesananda, "There are four stages of Meditation. By reason and cause, awareness arises and ceases. By training, ideas arise and cease. The following are the ways one enters into the first, second, third, and fourth stages of Meditation:

Abandon	Train or Do **Sadhana** Do (Practice)	By Training Arises	By Training Ceases
1. Desire	Self-Restraint	Joy and	Evil
2. Ill Will	Mindfulness	Peace	
3. Laziness	(Be Aware)		
4. Worry			
5. Doubt			
(Above are hindrances to Meditation)			

By Achieving the Above State, One Enters Into the First Stage of Meditation.

Reasoning	Detachment	Subtle	Joy & Peace
Investigating	Concentration	Awareness of Joy & Peace	

One Enters into the Second Stage of Meditation

Body & Mind	Concentration	Bliss & Equilibrium	Subtle Awareness of Joy & Peace

One Enters Into the Third Stage of Meditation

World	Contemplate On 'Space is Infinite'	Absence of Pain & Pleasure	Bliss & Equlibrium

118

One Enters into the Fourth Stage of Meditation

| Self | Contemplate On 'Nothing' | Unreality of all All Objects | '0' 'No Self' |

"Now he goes beyond even that state and realizes that all his Asava (desires) have been destroyed. Mindful he emerges from that attainment. He is not attracted to anything, nor is he repelled by anything. He is free and independent. He dwells with the mind unconditionally. He knows "Thee is nothing beyond this."

Lord Buddha also said that one who has loving kindness sleeps in comfort, wakes in comfort, and dreams no evil dreams. He is dear to human beings and to non-human beings; deities guard him; fire, poison, and weapons do not affect him; his mind concentrates; his face is serene; he dies unconfused, and if he advances no higher, he will be reborn in the brahma world.

Humans Have Three Minds

"Buddhi" in Sanskrit is the "Super conscious mind," which is attached to God. The second mind is called "Mana." This is attached to the material world. The third mind is called "Chitta" which is the subconscious mind. This mind is attached or connected to all your past lives, and future lives. It is also attached to all human beings. It knows everything it needs to know. It retains the Samskaras (human tendencies) and the Vasanas (feelings). The subconscious knows the truth. When people are a nervous wreck, the doctor gives them pills to put their subconscious mind to sleep so that they can function.

The Major Types of Meditation

Hindu Meditation strives for detachment and goes from contemplation to Meditation to Samadhi (merging with the Lord). Buddhist Meditation is silent Meditation. It leads you to merge with the universe with love for all. It is a selfless Meditation, with the goal of Nirvana, where there is nothing. Christian Meditation goes from contemplation to Meditation only, in which you sit with the Lord but do not merge. Merging with God is considered by many Christians to be blasphemous. Traditional Meditation is done sitting on the floor with eyes closed. Another type of Meditation is done with your eyes open. Yogic

Meditation is active Meditation, where you try to shut your mind down etc. The Tantric Meditation is effortless. In it you let go. Transcendental Meditation is the tantric type. Some Meditation is done with Mantra, while others are done silently.

Meditation Is a Process of Detachment

This life is *Samara*, i.e. the cycle of life and death. The goal is to come out of the cycle and merge with God and be free again. We teach children to attach themselves to the material world and then our duty requires us to teach them to detach themselves from the material world and become free once again. Please know that God always grants our wishes, God gives you whatever you want. If you go on repeating to yourself, "I am no good," God will make you just that. Always remember God. That practice is called *Japa Yoga* (Rosary). Lord Krishna says in Bhagavad Gita, "And whosoever, leaving the body, goes forth remembering me alone, at the time of death, he attains my being. There is no doubt about this." (Ch #VIII-6). At the time of death whatever you think is what you become in the next birth. Lord Krishna says if you become my devotee I will make sure you remember me at the last moment of your life. The final goal of life and Meditation is to detach from all and attach to God.

Why Meditation is Difficult
Because:

• You do not see its value in your life immediately. People wonder how can something that seems so simple do so much? Can it be true?

• You have not made the resolution to practice regularly (at least 21 minutes a day.)

• You are so attached to the material world that you cannot even detach for a few minutes a day to do Meditation.

• You have too much lust. You cannot have a few minutes of silence without thinking about the opposite sex.

• You do not have a person and/or Guru who loves you unconditionally.

• You have not realized that God loves you. You believe that Meditation is harmful (such as the false belief that Meditation creates a vacuum by which the Devil might get in.)

• You do not feel the need to be purified and burn bad Karma (you feel free and saved.)

• You do not have a technique for Meditation that is right for you.

• You do not have patience to condition your mind so that Meditation can make some impact in your life.

• If you do not follow *Yama* and *Niyama* or the "Ten Commandments," without moral living, Meditation is not possible.

• If you eat too much, work too hard or sleep too little, Meditation will be difficult. Follow the middle path.

• You have not received a Mantra (initiation) from a qualified Guru.

• You do not believe that the inner self is a part of God.

You can practice Meditation without believing in God. Throughout all the years I've been practicing Yoga, and Meditating, I feel that Meditation is the real gem of Yoga. Have faith in God and/or Guru and believe that peace is love and love is God.

Focusing on the Gap

To make your Meditation stronger or more effective, focus on the gap. Bhagwan Shri Rajneesh (Osho) says in one of his books, "During Meditation, when you are watching your breath, after you inhale, right before exhalation there is a gap, if you focus on that gap your Meditation will become very powerful. Contemplating on this gap can remove mental disturbances, can bring cosmic consciousness, or God realization." Deepak Chopra says, "There is a gap between one thought and another thought and if you concentrate on that gap, it is also very beneficial."

When you are doing the eye exercise and you move your eyes from the right to the left, that junction also has a gap. Concentrating or meditating on that gap is also beneficial. Hindus pray and Meditate at the junction of when night ends and day begins and also when day finishes and night begins. Perhaps they are meditating on a gap.

Meditation is shown through drawings in Illustration 13.1.

Life Is Too Short!

Bhagwan Shri Rajneesh (Osho) writes:

"Do we really not have time or is it just a creation in our mind? You have to remember that life is not short; life is eternal, so there is no question of any hurry. By hurrying you can only miss. In existence, do you see any hurry? Seasons come in their time, flowers come in their time, and trees are not running to grow fast because life is short. It seems as if the whole existence is aware of the eternity of life. We have been here always, and we will be here always—of course not in the same forms, and not in the same bodies.

Life goes on evolving, reaching to higher stages. But there is no end anywhere, and there has been no beginning anywhere either. You exist between a beginningless life and an endless life. You are always in the middle of two eternities on both sides."

Hurry—the end is near

"Your conditioning has given you the idea of one life. The Christian idea, the Jewish idea, the Mohammedan idea—which are all rooted in the Jewish conception that there is only one life—has given the West a tremendous madness for speed. Everything has to be done in such a hurry that you cannot enjoy doing it, and you cannot do it in its entire perfection. You somehow manage to do it and rush to another thing.

The Western man has been living under a very wrong conception: It has created so much tension in people's minds that they can never be at ease anywhere; they are always on the go, and they are always worried that one never knows when the end is coming. Before the end, they want to do everything. But the result is just the opposite; they cannot even manage to do a few things gracefully, beautifully, perfectly.

Their life is so much overshadowed by death that they cannot live joyously. Everything that brings joy seems to be a waste of time. They cannot just sit silently for an hour, because their mind is saying to them, 'Why are you wasting the hour? You could have done this, you could have done that.'

It is because of this conception of one life that the idea of Meditation never arose in the West. Meditation needs a very relaxed mind, with no hurry, with no worry, with nowhere to go… just enjoying moment to moment, whatever comes." Bhagwan Shri Rajneesh (Osho)

Relaxing to eternity

"In the East, Meditation was bound to be discovered; just because of the idea of life's eternity, you can relax. You can relax without any fear. You can enjoy and play your flute, you can dance and sing your song, and you can enjoy the sunrise and the sunset. You can enjoy your whole life. Not only that, you can enjoy even dying, because death too is a great experience, perhaps the greatest experience in life. It is a crescendo. In the western concept, death is the end of life. In the eastern concept, death is only a beautiful incident in the long procession of life; there will be many, many deaths. Each death is a climax of your life, before another life begins—another form, another label, and another consciousness. You are not ending, you are simply changing the house."

When You Meditate, I Feel Love

This is a story that I feel will inspire you to Meditate. In 1959, I went to India to attend my sister's wedding, after spending seven years in the US. When I reached there, the wedding was called off. During a party while I was there, I met my wife. It was semi-arranged by a relative. We liked each other. The next day we went out together and she gave me a red rose. I knew right away that she was the right person for me. In a few days we got married. We were separated for 2 ½ years while waiting for her to obtain her green card, but eventually we began our lives together, and had two children. We had a good marriage. But now and then she used to get frustrated and say, "You don't love me." I could not understand what she meant. I would tell her, "But you want this kind of house, I got that for you, etc, I always respect you. It hurts me when you say that." I didn't know what she wanted.

In 1967, we met our Guru H. H. Swami Vishnu Devananda. We both started practicing Yoga and Meditation. As a result our happy marriage started getting even better. After that she never once said to me, "You don't love me."

I used to Meditate before going to work while she was sleeping. One day as I was Meditating, she woke up and said, "Whenever you Meditate, I feel great love." I was surprised, because while meditating I was not thinking about her, I was thinking about God. I was loving God. That reminds me that

ISKCON's Guru, His Divine Grace A. C. Bhaktivedanta Swami Prabhupada, once said, "If you love God, you love everybody." It is as if you tune into the Guru and all lights turn on automatically.

If you want to improve your capacity to love, love God, pray and Meditate on the self. Meditate on God. This will improve your relationship with your spouse or friend. It will improve your relationship with your children.

Meditation teaches you how to love, to awaken the love that is dormant within you. If you Meditate, your family and society will experience love.

At another time in my life, I had met a woman during the summer when I was visiting a Yoga camp in Canada. She told me because I practice Yoga for years that she had enjoyed Meditating for years but recently found Meditation to be very disturbing. She couldn't understand why this was happening to her. I told her, in the beginning, when you practice Meditation you experience peace but as you practice more you go into much deeper levels and all your past life negativity surfaces. It's a cleansing process. But this cleansing process doesn't work if you eat meat. So I asked her if she was still eating meat. She said, "yes." So I told her if she wanted to go deep into Meditation she had to first of all stop eating meat and at one point have a Guru. She benefited a great deal from our conversation.

Figure 14

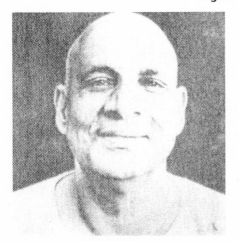

Master Sivananda
Fig. 14.1

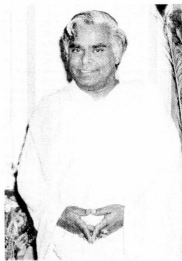

H.H. Sw ami Vishnu Devananda Maharaj
Fig. 14.2

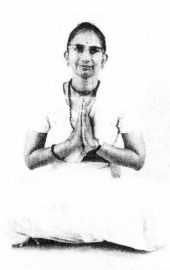

Rupal B. Gajjar
Fig. 14.3

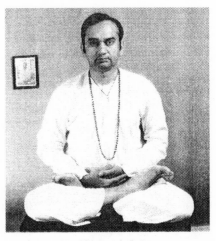

Yogi Bharat J. Gajjar
Fig. 14.4

Illustration 13.1

Removal of Mental Disturbances, Attainment of Cosmic-Consciousness and God Realization Become Reality When One Meditates on the "GAP" of Empty Space Which is Brahman or God

---

1. ▲   Night   O   Day   O   Night
Gap #1   Gap #1

2. §   O   Inhalation   O   Exhalation
Gap #2   Gap #2

3. ℜ   Thought   O   Thought
Gap #3

4.   Sleeping   O   Wake Up
Gap #4

5.   Eyes Going Right   O   Eyes Going Left
Gap #5

Hear the Silence
Or

6.   Bird Sings   O   Bird Start Singing Again
Gap #6

§   Bhagavan Rajneesh
ℜ   Deepak Chopra
▲   Hindu prays during these gaps

MEDITATION IS TO GAIN BACK OUR
FREEDOM, LOVE AND BE ENLIGHTENED

OM   OM

A Child is:
- One with God
- In Freedom and Love
- In Spirit and Self
- In OM – All is One

Freedom, Love, OM and
enlightenment (sidda)

Society conditions the Child's
Mind for his survival in the
Material world (The Child eats
the apple: or enters into Maya)

Knowledge of the Seer
(Atma Jnan)
Witness – A Seer
(A Drashta)

Soul or Self gives control to
the Mind

Discipline

Mother (Power)

Find a Guru:
A spiritual teacher
Find a Guru:
A spiritual teacher

The Mind controls the human and is fragmented.
Now humans have lost their Freedom, Love and
Self. They are robots, lost and unhappy

127

Chapter 14

Mantra and Japa Yoga

Mantra is a word that means God and it is chanted individually or in a group but when it is repeated with a mala or Rosary it is called Japa. This is a story about how I came to believe in the power of Mantras. In the summer of 1972 I visited my Guru in Val Morin, Canada. During his lecture he told us that when you are feeling afraid, if you chant "Om" or any other Mantra, your fear would disappear. I did not believe in Mantras at the time. That same year, my company, DuPont sent me on a business trip to Boston. On the way back, we boarded a small plane. During our flight to Philadelphia, we encountered a storm that caused our plane to drop about 1,000 feet. At that time, I felt that this was going to be the end of my life. I suddenly remembered my Gurus' message and I closed my eyes and started chanting "Om" within a few minutes I felt great peace enter into my heart. I opened my eyes and I noticed we were still going through the storm, but I had become a believer in Mantras. I continued to chant my Mantra until we had come out of the storm.

Mantra Yoga is an important part of Yoga. Mantra is defined as a sacred word or phrase that means God, or the quality of God, or associated with God and/or Universe. To a Yogi, Mantra is not a sacred word but it is God. This word or phrase is very powerful because it was realized by a Yogi in his or her deepest Meditation or it was given by God to a realized Saint. This word or phrase is dynamic and effective because it has been repeated by Yogis for thousands of years. Therefore, when you start repeating the Mantra, you automatically and instantly join the wavelength that has been set up through the years (like you start a T.V. or radio). The Mantra instantly starts purifying your soul, mind and sub-conscious being. Mantra is the most effective way of reaching the goals of Yoga.

Swami Vishnu-Devananda says, "Our Master Swami Sivananda emphasized the vital necessity and importance of ensuring that our Yoga practices be supported by the proper mental attitude or Bhava, by chanting Kirtans he himself strictly adhered to this principle."

When a Mantra is repeated, without singing, over and over again, it is called Japa Yoga. The repetition of Japa when carried on by verbal, whisper, or mental repetition is known respectively as Vaikhari Japa, Upamshu Japa and Manasika Japa. Also, when the Mantras are sung, it is called "Mantra chanting." Many times Mantra chanting is called Kirtan but the real meaning of Kirtan is to sing the songs of God. It is like Christian hymns. Mantras are always in Sanskrit but Kirtans can be sung in any language.

To make Mantra and Japa Yoga effective, they should be chanted with love in the heart, keeping the meaning of Mantra. However, it is not important to know the Mantra to be effective but it helps to keep love and God in the heart.

The one Mantra a Yogi repeats in Japa is the one his Guru gave him at the time of his initiation. If you are a beginner and do not know which Mantra is right for you, I would recommend that you take one of the above Mantras and repeat it for a week. Then repeat another Mantra for a week. This way you can try several of them and, during chanting, see which Mantra works on you-that means, which Mantra brings you bliss and energy. That is the right Mantra for you. Use that Mantra in your Japa. After practicing Yoga for a while, you may decide to be initiated and at that time, your Guru will give you a Mantra that is right for you. The Mantra that your Guru gives at the time of your initiation is very powerful. Again, it is important to pronounce the Mantra properly. If you are associated with our Sivananda Yoga Center, it is very simple, just come to our Sunday Satsang and we will teach you the correct pronunciation. If you are not in Delaware, go to one of the Sivananda Centers near you, and they will teach you. Otherwise, talk to someone who knows authentic Yoga or write to us, we will send you a tape. Buy a tape and learn the Mantra.

The Rudraksha Mala

Rudraksha is a favorite bead of Siva. It is highly sanctifying. It removes all sins by sight, contact and Japas.

A Mantra repeated with Rudraksha is a 100,000 times more powerful. A man wearing Rudraksha derives a hundred million times more merit.

O Goddess, as long as the Rudraksha is on the person of a living soul he is least affected by premature death.

Siva Purana: Vidyesvara Samhita Ch. 25, Verse 2.

Rudraksha means "eye of Rudra: (Rudra is the name of Lord Siva in his aspect as Transformer). It is described in the "Siva Purana" that from a desire to help the world drops of tears fall from Siva's eyes and from those tears, sprang the first Rudraksha plants. Symbolic of the renunciation of unreality, the Rudraksha bead indicates the supreme reality—Parabrahman.

In the "Siva Purana", Siva says, "If anyone wears it during the day, he is freed from sins committed during the night. If he wears it during the night, he is freed from sins committed during the day. Similar is the result with its wearing during morning, midday or evening."

Vidyesvara Samhita Ch. 25, Verse 48.

Says Mahadave, the Rudraksha as well as the person who wears it is my favorite. O Parvati, even if he has committed sins he becomes pure.

He who wears Rudraksha around the hands and arms and over the head cannot be killed by any living being. He shall roam in the world in the form of Rudra.

He shall be respected by Gods and Asuras (bad people) always. He shall be honored like Siva. He removes the sin of anyone seen by him.

If a person is not liberated after Meditation and acquisition of knowledge, he shall wear Rudraksha. He shall be freed from all sins and attain the highest goal.

Vidyesvara Samhita Ch. 25, Verses 54-59.

If one is interested in Japa, he or she should consider using Rudraksha Mala for Japa and /or wearing it. Japa-Mala could be bought at the Sivananda Yoga Center Boutique. The Rudraksha Mala can be bought at Jai Mala Company, Sister's View Park #34, 61280 Parrell Road, Bend, Oregon 97701 USA.

About JAPA, Sri Ma Anandamayi says: "Listen! Do not let your time pass idly. Either keep a rosary with you and do Japa; or if this does not suit you, at least go on repeating the name of the Lord regularly and without interruption like the ticking of a clock. There are no rules or restrictions in this: invoke Him by the name that appeals to you most, for as much time as you can, the longer the better. Even if you get tired at some auspicious moment you may discover the rosary of the mind where you will continually hear within yourself the praises of the great Master, the Lord of Creation, like the never ceasing music of the boundless ocean. You will hear the land and the sea, the air and the heavens reverberate with the song of His glory. This is called the all-pervading presence of His Name.

The world consists of Name and Form: The Name is it's beginning and the Name is its end. When the aspirant achieves perfection by concentrating on the Name, he loses himself in it. The world ceases to exist for him and his ego disappears. What then is, and what is not? Although some may realize this, it can never be expressed in words."

Sri Swami Sivananda says, "In this Kali Yoga (iron age) Japa alone is the easy way to the realization of God... Life is short. Time is fleeting. The world is full of miseries. Cut the knot of Avidya (ignorance) and drink the Nirvanic bliss. That day on which you do not perform any Japa is simply wasted."

In Sivananda Yoga Vendanta Ashram of H. H. Swami Vishnu-Devananda the following Mantras are sung before starting the Satsang (spiritual meeting). One could sing this song individually before starting one's Yoga sadhana (Yoga practice) as well.

MANTRA YOGA AND CHANTS

1. Jaya Ganesha, Jaya Ganesha, Jaya Ganesha Pahimam
Sri Ganesha, Sri Ganesha, Sri Ganesha Rakshamam

2. Saravanabhava, Saravanabhava, Saravanabhava Pahimam
Subramanya, Subramanya, Subramanya Rakshamam

3. Jaya Saraswati, Jaya Saraswati, Jaya Saraswati Pahimam
Sri Saraswati, Sri Saraswati, Sri Saraswati Rakshamam

4. Jaya Guru, Shiva Guru, Hari Guru Ram,
Jagat Guru, Parmam Guru, Sat Guru Shym

5. Om Adi Guru, Adwaita Guru, Ananda Guru Om,
ChildGuru. Chidganan Guru, Chinmaya Guru Om.

6. Hare Rama, Hare Rama, Rama Rama, Hare Hare
Hare Krishna, Hare Krishna, Krishna Krishna, Hare Hare

7. Om Namah Sivaya, Om Namah Sivaya,
Om Namah Sivaya, Om Namah Sivaya.

8. Om Namo Narayanaya, Om Namo Narayanaya,
Om Namo Narayanaya, Om Namo Narayanaya.

9. Om Namo Bhagavathe Vasudevaya, Om Namo Bhagavathe
Vasudevaya,
Om Namo Bhagavathe Vasudevaya, Om Namo Bhagavathe
Vasudevaya.

10. Om Namo Bhagavathe Vishnu-Devanandaya,
Om Namo Bhagavathe Satgurunathaya

11. Om Namo Bhagavathe Sivanandaya,
Om Namo Bhagavathe Satgurunathaya

12. Krishnam Vande Jagat Gurum Sri
Krishnam Vande Jagad Gurum

SPECIAL CHANTING MANTRAS

1. Sri Ram Jaya Ram, Jaya Jaya Ram Om
Sri Ram Jaya Ram, Jaya Jaya Ram

2. Hari Om, Hari Om, Hari Hari, Hari Om,
Hari Om, Hari Om, Hari Hari, Hari Om,

3. Guru Om, Guru Om, Guru Guru, Guru Om,
Guru Om, Guru Om, Guru Guru, Guru Om,

4. Shakti Om, Shakti Om, Shakti Shakti Shakti Om,
Shakti Om, Shakti Om, Shakti Shakti Shakti Om,

5. Shakti Ma, Shakti Ma, Shakti Shakti Shakti Ma,
Shakti Ma, Shakti Ma, Shakti Shakti Shakti Ma,

6. Siva, Siva, Siva, Siva, Sivaya Namaho
Hara Hara Hara Hara Namah Sivaya

*These are Mantras; they can be used in your Japa.

Sing the Mantras shown above at least once a day preferably with your family at the altar. These Mantras are prayers to bring love and peace into your heart, family and in the world.

There are seven most important Mantras in the Yoga Tradition, are as follows.

1. Om
Om means God, there are books written just on the Mantra Om. It is the most important Mantra in the Hindu, Buddhist, and Jain religions. It is so powerful, that when a Guru gives a Mantra initiation, they never give the Om Mantra. Rather, the Guru gives Mantras such as Hari Om, Guru Om etc.

2. MahaMantra

Hare Krishna, Hare Krishna, Krishna Krishna, Hare Hare
Hare Rama, Hare Rama, Rama Rama, Hare Hare

Maha means the greatest. This is also one of the most important Mantras available.

3. Om Namah Sivaya

This is the most important Mantra to Lord Shiva (Father).

4. Shakti Ma

This is an important Mother Mantra. It is chanted for Shakti or Mother. The mothers are Saraswati, Lakshmi, Durga and Kali.

5. Guru Om

This is an auspicious Guru Mantra.

6. Krishnam Sharanam Gachha Me

This is also a Mantra to Lord Krishna. It means, "I am surrendering to you Lord Krishna the creator of the Universe.

7. Gayatri Mantra

This is one of the most sacred Mantras. The Gayatri Mantra is called "Vedamata" "While Brahma, the Supreme Creator, was once deep in mediation, the prosody or subtle inner vibration of Gayatri revealed itself to him. This was before the Vedas, based on the same prosody, were revealed to the world's sages, Hence the Gayatri Mantra is called 'Vedamata,' the Mother of the Vedas.

The Vedic scriptures, compiled in verse, prose and song by Vyas Deva, were drawn from the Memory of the world's sages and are mankind's earliest expression of Divine Knowledge. Although compiled in India, the Vedas are not the exclusive possession of one particular religion or group but are the invisible threads forming the spiritual family of the earth into a sublime, harmonious network.

The Gayatri Mantra was revealed to the Vedic sage Vishvamitra, a preceptor of Sri Rama, and incarnation of Lord Vishnu. It is considered to be the most powerful Mantra of the Vedas.

Before chanting the Mantra one should inhale, then chant Om. Pause, inhale again, and chant the next phrase, Bhuh Bhuvah Svah. Chant the entire Mantra in this pattern, following the five conventional groupings given on the page facing.

The Mantra is divided into five steps:
1. Om
2. Bhuh Bhuvah Svah
3. Tat savituh Varenyam
4. Bhargah Devasya Dhimahi
5. Dhiyah yah nah prachodayat

The Vedamata
The Vedamata Gayatri is traditionally portrayed with five faces forming an indivisible whole. She is thereby presented as a unified manifestation of the five divine fragrances or elements of creation: kshiti (earth), ap (water), Teja (fire), Marut (air) and Vyoma (ether). With its five traditional groupings the Mantra is an undivided whole. The central break, 'Tat Savituh Varenyam,' meaning 'we adore Savituh the source of all creation' refers explicitly to the five elements.

Also symbolized in this portrayal of the Vedamata are the five stages of practice through which the sadhak (the aspirant) must pass and which open him to more and more light:

Earth - The stage in which hostile tendencies in speech and action are restrained;

Water - The stage in which hostile tendencies in the vital plane and subconscious mind are restrained;

Fire - The stage in which all of the above are harmoniously overcome;

Air - The stage in which the sadhak is centered and has reached the state of cosmic Intelligence;

Ether - The stage wherein Om is fully manifest to the realized aspirant.

With her ten hands the Vedamata protects the Sadhak from any harm that may threaten from the ten directions. The hand before her right shoulder gestures fearlessness (Abhaya Mudra). The hand on her left knee gestures reward (Barada Mudra). The lotus upon which she sits represents the principle of intellect subdued and mastered in the realization of Vedic wisdom.

The Practice of Pranayama with the Gayatri Mantra

"Stage 1. (4 Seconds)—Adjust your posture to an erect position, then breathe two or three times through both nostrils normally. Pressing the right nostril closed with the thumb, inhale to capacity through the left nostril for four seconds. While inhaling Chant mentally: Om.

Stage 2. (16 Seconds)—Closing the left nostril with the ring or middle finger while keeping the right nostril closed with the thumb, retain the air for sixteen seconds in mental silence.

Stage 3. (8 Seconds)—Free the right nostril, then exhale gradually for eight seconds. Keep the left nostril closed. While exhaling chant mentally: Bhuh Bhuvah Svah.

Stage 4. (4 Seconds)—Now inhale rhythmically through the right nostril for four seconds, canting mentally: Tat.

Stage 5. (16 Seconds)—Closing the right nostril again, retain the air in silence for sixteen seconds.

Stage 6. (8 Seconds)—Free the left nostril and breathe out for eight seconds. During this period chant mentally: Savituh Varenyam.

Rest: Now breathe two or three times through both nostrils normally."[1]

There is another technique for Chanting the Gayatri Mantra with Pranayama that is done by closing the right nostril and inhale while chanting the complete Mantra. Then close both nostrils and chant the complete Mantra one time and then close the left nostril and exhale from the right nostril while chanting the complete Gayatri Mantra. Then repeat the process on the opposite side.

The Mantra shown below is the version of the Gayatri Mantra recited along with it's meaning that was read at every Satsang at the Sivananda Yoga Center of Delaware.

Om Bhur Bhuvah Svah, Tat Savitur Varenyam,
Bhargo Devasya Dheemahi Dhiyo Yo Nah Prachodayat[1]

We Meditate on the effulgent glory of the divine Spirit who illumines and pervades everything. Thou O Supreme Lord, the center of this Universe, may we prove worthy of thy choice and acceptance and may Thou guide our intellects and may we follow thy lead into righteousness.

Please note that the Gayatri Mantra is Mother Shakti sitting in the lotus flower and has five heads and ten hands.

The following Mantras are also valuable Mantras for Japa Yoga.

Om Sri Maha Ganapataye Namah, Om Aim Saraswatyai Namah, Om Sri Maha Lakshmyai Namah, Om Sri Durgayai Namah, Om Sri Maha Kalikayai Namah, Om Namah Sivaya, Om Namo Naravanava, Om Namo Bhagavate Vasudevaya, Om Sri Ramaya Namah, Om Sri Hanumate Namah, Shanti Ma, Guru Om, Hari Om Tat Sat, and Sri Rama Rama Rameti, Rame Rame Manorame; Sahasranama Tattulyam, Rama Nama Varanane.

Everyday of a week has a Mantra that one can chant that is most auspicious for that day. These seven Mantras are as follows:

Sunday "Om Namo Narayanaya" (Ohm`nuh-mo Nah-Rai-un-Nai-uh)

Om reverence to Narayan (Vishnu) brings love, prosperity, power, and infinite glory. Wisdom, enjoyment, releases from bondage to lower consciousness. Gives the ability to dissolve obstacles resulting from egoism and ignorance. Keeps you free from calamity. Brings joy through knowledge.

Monday "Om Namah Shivaya" (OHM nuh-muh-Shi-Vai-uh)

Om reverence to Shiva. Destroys negative tendencies and effects. Gives one the power to overcome the three qualities that keep one bound to material consciousness.

Tuesday "Om Sri Subramunyaya Namah" (OHM Shree Soo-bruh-mun-Yai-uh-nuh-muh)

Om reverence to Subramunya. Gives success in any undertaking. Drives off evil influences. Gives victory both in spiritual and physical battle.

Wednesday "Om Namo Bhagavate Vasudevaya"
(OHM nuh-moh' b'hug-uh-vuh-TEY Vah-soo-day-vah-yuh)

Om reverence to the Lord of the Universe Krishna, to the divine self who is all pervading. Grants enjoyment and success in all activities. Confers divine love. Brings peace to a troubled mind.

Thursday "Om Namo Bhagavate Sivanandaya"
(OHM nuh-moh' b'hug'-uh-vuh-TEY Sivanandaya)

Thursday is guru day. By invoking the guru the great power and bliss of enlightenment, which the guru has attained, can be manifested into you.

Friday "Om Sri Maha Lakshmiyai Namah"
(OHM Shree muh-HAH luck-shmee-YAI nuh-muh)

Om reverence to the great Lakshmi, mother bestows all forms of prosperities, truthfulness, nonviolence, humility, spiritual understanding, contentment, serenity of mind, endurance, compassion, wisdom of the cosmic self. Lakshmi represents the blossoming of the consciousness.

Saturday "Om Sri Hanumate Namah" (OHM Shree huh-noo-muh-TEY nuh-muh)

Om reverence to Hanuman. Hanuman has unbounded love of Rama and his unquestioned devotion and service to Rama. This Mantra gives strength and courage. Help discover the powers of the Soul in order to triumph over all adversities and attain the highest realization. Gives control of the senses, success in devotional practices as well as worldly success.

"Everything of value lies within you. Establish contact with your inner-self. Meditation is the door to the self. Mantra helps open the door."

MANTRA INITIATION

If you want to make progress in spiritual life, you need a Guru. That Guru will give you a Mantra initiation. When my wife, Mrs. Rupal B. Gajjar (Anandi Narayani Ma 1933-1984), who was a great Yoga teacher, got initiated she wrote the following:

"Initiation is a Yoga tradition when a student learns from a Guru and serves his Guru. At one point, the student has no doubt about the Guru and at that time he/she is willing to walk on his/her path to perfection. He has developed faith. At that moment in the student's life, he or she requests an initiation. If the student is ready, the Guru gives an initiation.

The Initiation Ceremony is sacred. Through this ceremony, the student joins the Yoga path officially. He or she joins the parmpara—that means he is linked up with his Guru to all the previous Gurus and to God. Students never reveal their sacred Mantra and private ceremony to anyone.

Initiation means one-mindedness of the unlimited goal of spiritual growth. Initiation means a soul has found the source of enlightenment. Mantra given by one's teacher helps the student realize himself as a pure soul. Initiation means your fruitless wandering has reached an end. You have found peace, stability and the real path of happiness. You feel oneness with your spiritual master's lotus feet. (By this time, you realize the Guru is not this body, but is a spirit.) The student submits to his Guru's wisdom. Initiation means you love and share the spiritual path and you have found your true home. Initiation means you understand that your path is the most beautiful one, but your respect other names and ways to love God. The Initiation means a spiritual tie exist between you and your Guru's teachings and his blessings.

This article is dedicated to my Guru—Swami Vishnu Devananda and his Divine Guru, H. H. Sri Swami Sivananda, and my husband, Bharat J. Gajjar and my children—Ajay and Meeta."

HOW TO SIT IN JAPA
So Says, Sri Guru Gita

If seated on deerskin one attains Jnana, and if seated on tiger-skin one attains Moksha. If seated on Kusha-grass-seat one gets knowledge of the Self, and if seated on wellen seat one acquires all psychic powers. // 221

By doing Japa facing south-east, one gets powers to attract others, facing north-west one will have no enemies, facing south-west one will have vision (of God) and facing north-east one acquires knowledge. //222

Facing north during Japa one becomes peaceful, facing east one will attract others, facing south one meets with death and facing west one acquires plenty of wealth. //223

This Guru Mantra has the power to attract all. It destroys all bonds and causes freedom. It makes Indra favorable to you. It brings under your control even kings. //224

[1] Taken from the booklet called "The Gayatri Mantra" by Satyaan, Autumn Press 1974

Chapter 15

Yoga Prayers and Slokas

Sanskrit Yoga Prayer
Om Asato Ma Sat Gamaya
Tomaso Ma Jyotir Gamaya
Mrityor-Ma Amritam Gamaya
Om Shanti, Shanti, Shanti.

Om Lead us Thou, oh God,
From Unreal to real.
From Darkness to light.
From Death to immortality.
Om Shanti, Shanti, Shanti.
Om Peace, Peace, Peace Be unto Us All.

GAYATRI
Om, Bhur Bhuvah Svah, Tat Savitur Varenyam,
Bhargo Devasya Dheemahi, Dhiyo Yo Nah Prachodayat

We Meditate on the effulgent glory of the divine spirit who illumines and pervades everything. Thou O Supreme Lord, the center of this Universe, may we prove worthy of thy choice and acceptance and may Thou guide our intellects and may we follow thy lead into righteousness.

The Universal Prayer
O Adorable Lord of Mercy and Love.
salutations and Prostrations unto Thee.
Thou are Omnipresent, Omnipotent, and Omniscient.

Thou art Satchidananda.
Thou art Existence, Knowledge, and Bliss Absolute.
Thou art the Indweller of all beings.

Grant Us an Understanding heart, equal vision, balanced mind, faith, devotion and wisdom.
Grant us inner spiritual strength to resist temptations and to control the mind.
Free us from egoism, lust, greed, anger and hatred.
Fill our hearts with divine virtues.

Let us behold Thee in all these names and forms.
Let us serve thee in all these names and forms.
Let us ever remember Thee.
Let us ever sing Thy glories.
Let Thy name be ever on our lips.
Let us abide in Thee forever and ever.

Om Shanti, Shanti, Shanti
Hari Om Tat Sat.

Yoga Prayer
By Yogi Bharat J. Gajjar

O, Dear Lord of the Universe,
Lead us from delusion to your love,
From unhappy to happy family,
From anger to peace,
From hate to love,
From Bondage to liberation,
From hostility to harmony,
From dullness to inspiration,
From Falsehood to truth,
From injustice to justice,
From separateness to Om consciousness,
From ignorance to enlightenment,

From selfish pleasures to Dharma,
From stagnancy to creativity,
From poor health to good health,
From weakness to energy,
From chaos to discipline,
From violence to non-injury,
From poverty to riches,
From ugliness to beauty,
From unreal to real,
From darkness to light,
From death to immortality,

Om Shanti, Shanti, Shanti
Om peace, peace, peace be unto us all
Hari Om Tat Sat.

PRAYERS

Maha Mrityunjaya Mantra
Om Trayambakam

(Sanskrit)
Om Trayambakam Yajamahe
Sugandhim Pushtivardhanam
Urvarukamiva Bandhanan-
Mrityormukshiya Mamritat (rpt. 3x)

Om Sarvesham Svasti Bhavatu
Sarvesham Santir Bhavatu
Sarvesham Purnam Bhavatu
Sarvesham Mangalam Bhavatu

Sarve Bhavantu Sukinah
Sarve Santu Nirmayaah
Sarve Bhadrani Pasyantu
Ma kaschid-Dukha-Bhag-Bhavet

Om Asato Ma Sat Gamaya
Tamaso Ma Jyotir-Gamaya
Mrityor-Ma Maritam Gamaya

Om Purnamadah Purnamidam
Purnat Purnamudachyate
Purnasya Purnamadaya
Purnameva Vashishyate
Om Shanti, Shanti, Shanti

(English)
I worship the fragrant three-eyed one (Siva),
Who nourishes all beings,
And grants liberation from death as easily
As the cucumber is severed from the vine.

May everybody have prosperity,
May everybody have peace,
May everybody have perfection,
May everybody have auspiciousness.

May all be happy,
May all be free from disabilities,
May all look for the good in others,
May none suffer from sorrows.

Lead us from the unreal to the real.
Lead us from darkness (ignorance) to light.
Lead us from death to everlasting immortality.

That is perfect. This is perfect it is whole.
This perfect world arises from perfection.
If we remove the perfect world,
That which remains is indeed perfect (God).
Om Peace, Peace, Peace be unto us all.

You can bless your family, society, friends or any person by reciting this prayer. Recite this prayer everyday and it will bring liberation, love, peace and happiness.

DHYANA SLOKAS
(Gajananam)

GAJANANAM BHUTAGANADI SEVITAM
KAPITTA JAMBU PHALA SARA BHAKSHITAM
UMA SUTAM SHOKAVINASHA KARANAM
NAMAMI VIGNESHVARA PADA PANKAJAM

I prostrate myself before the lotus feet of Vigneshusara (Ganesha), the son of Uma, the cause of destruction of sorrow, who is served by the host of Bhuta-Ganas (angels), etc., who has the face of an elephant, who partakes of the essence of Kapittha and Jambu fruits.

SHADANANAM KUMKUMA RAKTAVARNAM
MAHAMATIM DIVYA MAYURA VAHANAM
RUDRASYA SUNAM SURASAINYANATHAM
GUHAM SADAHAM SHARANAM PRAPADYE

I always take refuge in Guha of six faces (Subramanya), who Is of deep red color like kumkuma, who possesses great Knowledge, who has the divine peacock to ride on, who is The son of Rudra (Siva), and who is the leader of the army Of the Devas (gods, angels).

YA KUNDENDU TUSHHARA HARA DHAVALA
YA SHUBRA VASTRAVRITA
YA VINA VARADANDA MANTITATA KARA
YA SHVETA PADMASANA
YA BRAHMA CYUTA SHANKARA PRABHRITBHIR
DEVAI SADA PUJITA
SA MAM PATU SARASWATI BHAGAVATI
NISHESHA JATYAPAHA

May that goddess Saraswati who wears a garland white
Like the kunda-flower, the moon and the snow, who is
Adorned with pure white clothes, whose hands are ornamented
With the Vina and the gesture of blessings, who is seated on
A white Lotus, who is always worshipped by Brahma, Vishnu, Siva and
other gods, who is the remover of all inertness and laziness, protect me.

OM NAMAH SIVAYA GURAVE
SAT-CHID-ANANDA MURTAYE
NISHPRAPANCHAYA SHANTAYA
SRI SIVANANDAYA TE NAMAHA
SRI VISHNUDEVANANDAYA TE NAMAHA

Salutations to Guru Siva (Sivananda) who is the embodiment. Of Existence-knowledge-Bliss Absolute, in whom worldliness does not exist, who is ever peaceful. Salutations to Sivananda, Salutations to Swami Vishnu Devananda

OM SARVA MANGALA MANGALYE
SHIVE SARVATHA SADHIKE
SHARANYE TRAYAMBAKE GAURI
NARAYANI NAMOSTU TE
NARAYANI NAMOSTU TE

I salute the three-eyed Divine Mother Narayani, who brings auspiciousness and who fulfills all the desires of the Devotee (both spiritual and material).

SHANTI MANTRAS
(Mantra For Peace)

Om Sham no mitrah sham Varunah, Sham no Bhavatvaryaman
Sham no Indro Brihaspatih, sham no Vishnururukramah
Namo Brahmane, Namaste Vayo, Twameva Pratyaksham Brahmasi,
Twaameva Prataksham Brahma Vadishyami
Ritam vadishyami Satyam Vadishyami

Tanmamavatu, Tadvaktaramavatu
Avatu Maam, Avatu Vaktaram
Om Shanti, Shanti, Shanti

May Mitra Varuna and Aryama be good to us. May Indra and Brihaspati and Vishnu of great strides be good to us. Prostrations to the Brahman. I shall proclaim thee as visible Brahman. I shall call thee the Just and the True. May he protect the teacher and me. May he protect the teacher. Om peace, peace, peace.

Om Saha naavavatu, Sahanau bhunaktu, Saha viryam karavavahsi, Tejasvi Navadhestamastu Ma Vidishavahai
Om Shanti, Shanti, Shanti

Om, May he protect us both (teacher and taught). May He cause us both to enjoy the bliss of Mookti. May he both exist to find out the true meaning of the scriptures. May our studies be fruitful. May we never quarrel with each other. Let there be threefold Peace.
Om Apyayantu Mamangani Vak Pransehakshuh Shrotramatho

Balamindriyani cha servani servam Brahmopanishadam
Maham Brahma nirakuryam; Ma ma Brahma Nirakarot
Anirakaranamastu; anirakaranam me astu
Tadatmani nirate ya upanishatsu Dharmasto
Mayi santu; Te Mayi santu
Om Shanti, Shanti, Shanti

May my limbs, speech, Prana, eye, ear and power of all my senses grow vigorous. All is the Brahman of the Upanishads. May I never deny the Brahman. May the Brahman never desert me. Let that relationship endure. Let the virtues recited in the Upanishads be rooted in me. May they repose in me, Om peace, peace, peace.

Om Bhadram Karnebhih shrunuyama devah
Bhadram pashyamakshabhiryajatrah;
Sthirairangaistushtuvamsastanubhih;

Vyasema devahitam yadayah
Swasti na Indro Vriddhashravah
Swasti nah puch vivasvavedah
Swasti nah Tarkshyo srishtanemih
Swasti no Brihaspatirdadhatu
Om Shanti, Shanti, Shanti

Om O worshipful ones, may our ears hear what is auspicious. May we see what is auspicious. May we sing your praise, live our allotted span of life in perfect health and strength. May Indra extolled in the scriptures, Pushan the all-knowing Tarkshyo and Brihaspati vouch, means safe prosperity in our study of the scriptures.

Sanskrit Prayers Hymns to the Guru

BRAHMANADAM PARAMASUKHADAM KEVALAM JNANAMURTHIM DVANDVAA-TEETAM GAGANA SADRESHAM TATVAMASY-AADI LAKSHYAM

I salute the Guru who is the incarnation of supreme bliss, who is the bestower of bliss, who is independent, who is the embodiment of the highest wisdom, who is beyond the pairs of opposites (like love and hate), who is all-pervading like space, who is the goal pointed out by secret formulas like "That Thou Art," who is without a second, who is eternal, pure and unmoving, who is the witness of all hearts, who is beyond our imagination and who is free from the play of the qualities of nature.

CHAITANYAM SHAASWATAM SHAANTAM NIRAKAARAM NIRANJANAM NAADA BINDU KALAATEETAM TASMAI SRI GURAVE NAMAH

Salutations to the Guru who is awareness itself, eternal, peaceful, formless and free from blemish, who is beyond Nada, Bindu and Kalaa.

GURUR BRAHMAA GURUR VISHNUH GURUR DEVO MAHESHWARAH GURU SAAKSHAAT PARA BRAHMA TASMAI SRI GURAVE NAMAH

Guru is the creator (of our spiritual aspirations), the Protector (of our aspirations), and the Great Lord (who destroys the evil in us): and the Guru himself is the Supreme Being. Salutations to the Guru.

AJNANA TIMIRAANDHASYA JNAANAANJANA SHALLAHKAYAA CHAKSHUR UNMEELTTAM YENA TASMAI SRI GURAVE NAMAH

Salutations to the Guru, who by wisdom removes the blinding darkness of ignorance and opens the inner eye that perceives the Truth.

DHYANA MULAM GUROR MURTHIH PUJA MULAM GUROH PADAM MANTRA MULAM GUROR VAAKHYAM MOKSHA MULAM GUROH KRIPA

The Guru's form (or image) is fit to be Meditated upon: the feet of the Guru should be worshipped, the Guru's words should be regarded as Mantra or Gospel—Truth, and the Guru's Grace will bestow liberation on us.

OM NAMAHSIVAAYA GURAVE SATCHIDANANDA MURTHAYE
NISHPRAPANCHAAYA SHAANTAAYA NIRALLAMBAAYA TEJASE

Salutations to Guru Siva (Sivananda), who is the embodiment of existence-knowledge-bliss absolute, in whom worldliness does not exist, who is ever peaceful. Salutations to Sivananda.

OM PURNAMADAH PURNAMIDAM PURNAT PURNAM UDACHYATE
PURNASYA PURNAMAADAAYA PURNAMEVAA-VASHISHYATE
OM SHANTI, SHANTI, SHANTI

Om. That is full (infinite or perfect). This is full (infinite or perfect). From that *Full*, this *Full* was born. Even after the *Full* was born of the *Full*, Fullness (Infinity or Perfect) alone remains. Om Peace, Peace, Peace.

Hare Krishna, Hare Krishna, Krishna Krishna, Hare Hare
Hare Rama, Hare Rama, Rama Rame, Hare Hare

This Mantra is called the "Maha Mantra." Maha means the greatest of all.

Yoga Practice Who Will Do?
By Bharat Gajjar

Yoga practice who will do?
We will do, we will do.
Yoga life, we sure like it.
Pranayama who will do?
We will do, we will do.
Hath Yoga, we sure like it.
Meditation who will do?
We will do, we will do.
Raj Yoga we sure like it.
Mantra Yoga who will do?
We will do, we will do.
Japa Yoga, we sure like it.
Geeta reading, who will do?
We will do, we will do.
Yoga prayer, we sure like it.
Karma Yoga, who will do?
We will do, we will do.
Satvic food we sure like it.
Service to others who will do?
We will do, we will do.
Satsang we sure like it.
Ahimsa who will do?
We will do, we will do.
Love, we sure like it.
Speaking truth, who will do?
We will do, we will do.
Yama Niyama we sure like it.
Love to God, who will do?
We will do, we will do.
Guru, we sure like him.

Figure 15

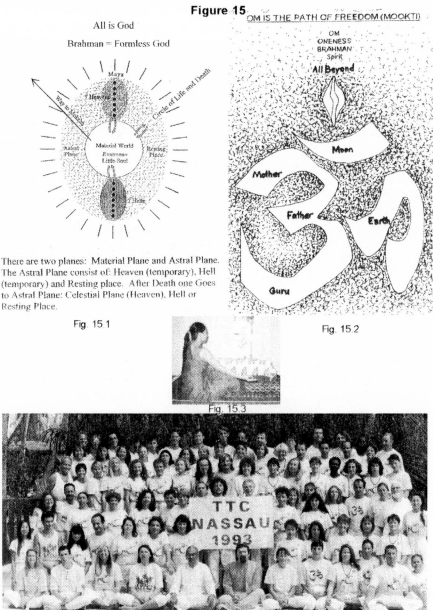

All is God

Brahman = Formless God

There are two planes: Material Plane and Astral Plane. The Astral Plane consist of: Heaven (temporary), Hell (temporary) and Resting place. After Death one Goes to Astral Plane: Celestial Plane (Heaven), Hell or Resting Place.

Fig. 15.1

OM IS THE PATH OF FREEDOM (MOOKTI)

Fig. 15.2

Fig. 15.3

Fig. 15.4

Chapter 16

Miracles of Masters

I have never met H. H. Swami Sivananda (Fig. 14.1) but I have heard about him from my Guru, H.H. Swami Vishnu Devananda Maharaj (Fig. 14.2). I'd like to tell you of the miracles that I have personally experienced with Swami Sivananda through my spiritual connection with him and through Meditation.

My first encounter with Master Swami Sivananda was before I knew who he was, but I truly believe that his spirit spoke to me. I was ten years old and at school. I heard a boy calling out to a girl, "Meeta come here!" At that very moment, a voice within me said, "That will be the name of your daughter." I was surprised how strong and clear the message was.

By the time I had finished high school and was in college, my brother was studying in America, and I heard that same voice tell me, "Go to America." So I told my father that I wanted to go to America.

He asked, "How can I send you to America when you are not getting good grades, and when you spend your time playing music, painting, writing poetry and playing sports?" Then I promised that I would not do all those things but study if he sent me to America. A year passed. Then he had a quarrel with his brother and I was getting involved in the feud, so my father turned to me and said, "Bharat, run away from India, go away from this family situation, because Pandit Nehru is a communist and anti-Hindu and he is taking India in the wrong direction." So he gave me money to buy my ticket to sail to America. I enrolled at the Philadelphia University of Textiles. My brother, Navin J. Gajjar, helped me through college financially. Later I helped my sister, Hansa N. Mehta, through college.

After graduating, I got a job at DuPont de Nemours and Co. as a research engineer. I got married and had two children. The first was Ajay and the second Meeta. When my daughter was born, my brother visited me. I told him of my interest in sending my children to India for a Hindu education. He asked, "Why do you have to run to India, why can't you bring our culture here?"

The result of that conversation led two other Indians and us to open the first Hindu Temple in Delaware. Unfortunately a feud developed in the partnership as our partners wanted to have a cultural center where we wanted a religious center. Ultimately my partners were paid off. Again I heard the voice I believed to be Swami Sivananda's who said, "This is good." I felt the Master was instrumental in the breakup of the partnership. Then one man said to me, "I'll close this temple down."

"Over my dead body," I retorted instantly and instinctively. I was taken back that I had actually said those words. I felt that the Master had spoken those words through me.

After that, every Sunday my wife, Anandi Narayani Ma, and I used to go and sit there and hold Satsang. One or two Americans would come and gradually a few more came, and their number grew gradually. Then the Master told me, "Teach Yoga here."

Now I remembered my friend, Amrit Desai, who taught Yoga fulltime in Philadelphia. I called and asked him to teach Yoga at our center. He said, "If you can get 10 students, I'll come and teach." Then I advertised and nine people committed to the class. I who had no intention of studying Yoga realized that if I didn't sign up Amritji wouldn't come.

After 10 lessons Amritji became so busy with other things that he could no longer come. This was a difficult situation and needed divine help. At the Hindu Center we had an altar with Mother Durga's picture. I sat in front of Mother Durga and prayed, "I'm going to teach Yoga even though I'm not qualified, but I know Hindu philosophy." I vowed to Mother Durga, "Whatever money comes from teaching, I will not take but I'll give all that money to the center."

I advertised and six or seven people signed up. After four or five sessions one of my students who was fascinated by the study of Yoga went to Canada and met Swami Vishnu Devananda. He came back and told me about Swami Vishnu Devananda's ashram.

Then the Master told me to go there. So our family went to the Yoga camp in Val Morin, Canada and met Swami Vishnu Devananda. We all learned so much that we kept going for a week every summer. Through Swamiji's teaching and through practice I became a better teacher. I started teaching two classes a week and conducting Satsang for the next 35 years.

Swami Vishnu Devananda initiated me. During his lecture Swamiji related an incident. The Master called him out of his tent and came in the spirit to meet him.

On returning from Canada, I thought that if Swamiji could invoke the Master's spirit, why couldn't I? So during my next Yoga class, at the time of relaxation, I invoked and prayed that the Master's spirit would come and bless the students with a peaceful, good relaxation.

After the class, one intuitive student approached me and asked who came through the door. I asked her, "Did the person look like an American, blond, and short?" She said, "No, he was tall, bald and was wearing orange drapery." I was really surprised. I asked her if she had ever seen or met an Indian Swami. She said, "No." I was amazed that Master had really come at my request.

The next incident occurred during another Yoga class, when I invoked Master's presence again during relaxation. After class, a doctor came up to me and asked, "Who touched my forehead and blessed me?" I was sitting far away from him and I had not moved from my seated position. I knew for sure that it was Master who had touched his forehead and blessed him.

I still had not become a total believer in Master Sivananda's presence. Then I had another experience at my office. My supervisor had asked me to do some important research and submit a proposal to implement this project. He only gave me four or five hours for the task. I came over to my desk and thought, let me ask the Master. If he is really there, he can help me come up with the five ideas I was seeking.

The Master spoke after two hours. He guided me to go downstairs to where the machines were running. When I got there, two ideas came to me. I went back to my desk and wrote them down. Then three more ideas came to me. I wrote them down as well. I submitted all five ideas in my proposal to my supervisor. He liked them and asked me to test them out.

Subsequently four of them became US Patents and one became a German Patent. After this, I became a believer in Master's grace and I confessed to the Master, "I will never doubt you again or ask you for any material favor."

Then one day during my Meditation at my bedroom altar, the Master came as a big, white light. I asked if it was him, but I already new, and he replied, "Yes." He also said, "You're on the right path." I was speechless. Then he left.

Later I was invited by the University of Delaware to teach Yoga. Forty-five students and five professors had signed up. I felt a lot of pressure. I wanted to prepare my lecture in advance and note down at work certain points before my two-hour class.

But I had to be out of town on business that week. Hence, I thought I'd prepare my talk at work on the day of the class. But I had gotten so busy I couldn't prepare anything. So I had to go directly from work to teach my class. On my way to the class I prayed to the Master to help me out. I started my class all excited. The lecture seemed to flow effortlessly from me and with great enthusiasm.

After class, when most people had left, one intuitive girl came over and asked me who was sitting beside me. I was taken back by the question. Then I asked her, "Did the person look like an American, blond, short?" She said, "No, he was tall, taller than you, bald and was wearing orange cloth, and after the class he left."

Another incident I remember from my early days of teaching Yoga in Wilmington. A girl who came to my class had had a car accident and the doctor had told her that her neck was permanently damaged. It hurt her all the time. I spent some time meditating on her critical condition and asked Swami Sivananda how Yoga could help her. The answer came. I repeated the message to the girl, "Inhale through your nose while chanting Om, take the Prana into the area where it hurts, surround it with the Prana and then exhale. Do this for 15 minutes every day." She did this for a month, and was completely healed.

When she went back for a checkup, her doctor was amazed by the complete healing and asked her what she had done. She told him that Yoga had healed her. She eventually became a Yoga teacher herself.

I fondly remember a man who came to another of my Yoga classes. I didn't know he was a Christian Minister, because he had never brought that to my attention. After he had had heart surgery, he called me from his hospital bed one afternoon and requested to see me. So I went to see him.

He lay in his bed, holding his cross tightly in his hand, as I entered the room and sat down next to him. He told me that during his heart surgery the previous day he saw a blue light coming towards him with the Mantra "Om Namah Shivaya" being continuously chanted and an Indian Swami. He was frightened by the vision and wanted to know what I made of it. I explained to him that it was Lord Shiva and my Guru's Guru, Swami Sivananda. He asked me if I would chant the Mantra I did during relaxation when he was in my class. So I chanted Tryambakam (see Chapter 15) and it brought great peace to him.

While working at the DuPont Company, one day one of the men from the laboratory came to me with a problem. He said he came to me because I looked spiritual. He needed help with a personal problem. His daughter had been haunted by her grandfather's ghost ever since he died a year ago. He wanted relief, or rather release, from this problem.

I gave him a picture of Swami Sivananda with the Mantra "Om Namo Bhagavate Sivanandaya" and told him to put the picture on her dresser and have her recite this Mantra every day. A month later he came back to my office and told me it was a miracle that it worked. Several years later, after he had retired and moved to Florida, I got a phone call from him. His daughter-in-law had a mental problem and he had driven back to Delaware for another copy of Master Sivananda's picture.

Just before I retired from the DuPont Company I sat down to Meditate in front of my altar as I do every morning. It was common for me to get messages from the Master during Meditation. This particular morning I got a message to go on television and spread the Master's teachings. It seemed like an odd request; I wondered if this was my ego speaking. So I ignored the message. But the message kept coming daily for the next six months. Then, one day, I answered the Master, "Ok, I'll do something about your request but I don't feel I'm qualified and don't know how to go about doing this." Then I got out the yellow pages, looked up Channel 28, which is the Delaware local cable channel and called them. I went to see the manager about a television show for the Sivananda Yoga Center of Delaware. He said a half hour show would cost $150.00. We didn't have that much money. So he suggested, "You can have a live program twice a month and run a repeat on the alternate Thursdays if you like. You can keep the last three minutes for advertisements and charge vendors $50.00 per minute."

I went to the only Indian grocery store in Wilmington at that time, and asked the owner if he would be interested in advertising his store on my TV show which would be called *Yoga For Health, Happiness and Liberation*. I was stunned and beside myself with joy when he agreed to take two minutes of advertising time per show. The Yoga Center made up the remaining $50.00, and we began the live television show twice a month in 1990. It grew into a live weekly program. In 2007, the program is still on the air. The television studio says the show is being watched by 15,000 to 20,000 people.

Amazingly, before every show, the Master tells me what I should talk about on the show, which makes my job very easy. I never imagined when I started the TV show that it would continue beyond a couple of years.

One time I had to find a book from the hundreds in my home library. I couldn't locate this one important book I needed to give a speech. Finally, I sat and Meditated, asking the Master for help. I prayed, "Please guide me, please and take me to the book." Then I got up and allowed his guidance to take me to where the book was, and I looked down, and there it was. I'm always amazed by the presence of the Master in my life.

In 1992, I was given early retirement along with many other employees. I was six months past the age of 60, and I was not prepared for retirement. Again I turned to the Master and asked him if I should start a Yoga ashram. The message he gave me was a very clear "No." Instead, he guided me to keep teaching Yoga, and write a textbook in my field of expertise.

So I began writing my textile textbook, which took me 10 years to complete. I wasn't confident about completing the book. So I decided to write every chapter as an article for a textile magazine. I sent the first two chapters to two prestigious British textile magazines. They printed both of them exactly the way I submitted them. My articles brought me to the attention of the Dean of the Philadelphia University in Philadelphia, PA. He asked if I would teach textiles in his graduate program. Thus began a new phase of my life, which lasted 10 years, until 2002. I regard this as the Master's grace.

My Encounters with My Guru H. H. Swami Vishnu Devananda

Through the grace of Master, I came to know Swami Vishnu Devananda Maharaj. The very first time I saw him I knew he was my Guru. Everything that I have learned about Yoga is through his grace. He not only taught me, but also inspired me. Every summer my family and I spent a week in Val Morin, enjoyed the beauty of the Ashram, learned more about Yoga and its benefits in a person's life. Swami Vishnu Devananda introduced the Master to me and told me about his greatness. Every time we went to the Ashram, Swami Vishnu Devananda was very happy, because he believed in families practicing Yoga together. During evening Satsang he used to invite my family onto the stage. I would bring my harmonium, and my wife and two children would sing bhajans. I used to sing with great enthusiasm. Then Swamiji commented "Emotion is not devotion." I understood what he meant, because I had a habit of singing with great enthusiasm.

Often when my family and I visited Val Moran, I asked to see Swamiji personally and he graciously invited me to his cottage in the Ashram. I presented him with my Sivananda Center of Delaware Prayer Book, which he looked over and said, "This is good, the Master wants all of us to write and spread the word."

Once I asked Swamiji if he would come to Wilmington, Delaware and conduct a Yoga workshop. He actually came and stayed with my family. At 4 am, Swamiji would get up and chant for an hour while he was in my home and then Meditate. Our seminar was over a weekend (Saturday and Sunday) from 9 am to 4 pm. On Saturday, 30 people attended the seminar. I introduced Swamiji, and he began by chanting Mother Durga's Mantra and continued for over an hour. I was sitting there worrying that all these Americans will be upset about this since they had come to learn Yoga. On the contrary, however, they all got blissed out. Spiritual vibrations are very important in learning and teaching Yoga.

After Swamiji visited Wilmington, I decided to change the name from the Hindu Center of Delaware to the Sivananda Center of Delaware, largely because I was teaching Yoga and the messages of Swami Vishnu-Devananda and the Master.

I started doing more Meditation after learning Yoga from my Guru Swami Vishnu and after a while my Meditation got much deeper. However, when you start to purify your insides a cleansing process begins. At one point I noticed the cleansing process was happening to me. I felt the hostility within me that was coming out. This frightened me so I stopped meditating and made the decision to get a Mantra initiation from Swamiji. That Summer I got initiated and I felt very peaceful and full of love. When I got home from Canada that year, I wrote the following poem.

Yoga Is A Perfect Path

Yoga is a perfect path,
    Bliss is just walking on the way.
Wake up, wake up, oh my brother,
    It is later than you think.
Walk, walk, walk with us now,
    Put an end to your suffering.

God is our supreme goal,
    Self-realization is what we seek.
Peace and energy will join us,
    Health and happiness are on the way.
Walk, walk, walk, oh my sister,
    Life is beautiful, let us make it.

Hatha, Raja and Pranayama are going with us,
    Mantra Meditation do carry with us.
Forget not to take satwick food along,
    We will need discipline to help us.
Walk, walk, walk, hand in hand,
    Forget the body and walk in the spirit.

Dark and scary is the night,
    Follow the Guru's candlelight.
Let us serve the Guru, God will liberate us,
    Time is short; far is that end.
Walk, walk, walk where we stand,
    Let us go as far as we can.

Every time I went to Yoga Camp in Val Morin, Canada, and saw Swami Vishnu Devananda I used to touch his feet and take his blessings, and every time, tears ran down my face. Once when this happened, my wife was standing a few feet away from me and couldn't hear what Swamiji was saying. From out of the blue he pointed to my wife and said, "She is your Guru." I said to myself, "She's not my Guru. I think Swamiji is mistaken." Then my wife asked me what had Swamiji said to me. I told her, "It was nothing important, forget it." But she kept asking me, again and again, for three or four days and the message was getting stronger and stronger in my heart. I couldn't ignore it. Finally, after she asked me again, I told her I would tell her when we got home. When we got home, I told her to sit on a chair and I got down on my knees. I told her that "Swamiji said, you're my Guru, and from now on you are."

She was stunned. She accepted me as her third child, which was a blessing. From then on I started calling my wife, like my children, "Mummi." It was rare, but sometimes when she got upset she would say, "You don't love me." From this day forward she never said that I did not love her. Our marriage grew stronger.

I learned one thing. In marriage, a husband and wife should play "One down," not "One up." What this means is that when you start from an equal position, when each person says, "You're the best" eventually it cannot go down any further. But when either plays "One up," saying, "I'm better than you," there is no end to arguments and quarrels, because the sky is the limit. Worse, in this game, both husband and wife lose. No one ever wins at this game. The two biggest problems on this earth are ego and seeking pleasure. They both lead to pain and destruction.

Subsequently my wife decided to get initiated from Swami Vishnu Devananda also. After her initiation she was transformed into a spiritual being. She did not want to leave the ashram, but when it was time, she did. She was upset for a couple of days, but accepted her separation from the ashram and Swamiji. I recognized the great change in her and it frightened me. She had evolved into a powerful Yogini.

I learned the Jaya Ganesha Mantra, Trayambakum Mantra, Yoga Asanas, Japa Yoga using a Mala (rosary), Pranayama and Meditation. I decided to pass on this transcendental knowledge to the Vishwa Hindu Parisad Children's Summer Camp (100 children and 50 parents) where these things were not being taught. In 1983 I asked to be allowed to teach at the camp. Eventually I taught in two camps up to 2005. I also taught Swamiji's messages and teachings in my two Yoga classes every week and Satsang every Sunday.

After receiving my Mantra initiation from Swamiji, I started giving the Mantra initiation to my students at the Sivananda Yoga Center of Delaware and promoting vegetarianism as well as giving them a spiritual name. I gave many initiations but I'd like to tell you about one particular initiation I gave.

His name was Haridas (Geesung who is from South Korea). He lived in Fort Meyers, Florida. He called up one day and asked if I'm Yogi Bharat. I replied that I was. Next he said he had heard that I give Mantra initiations. He wanted to be a Hindu and to be a Hindu Brahmin (Priest). He had studied the Vedas and the Upanishads, Jyotish (astrology) and Hindu philosophy. He was a vegetarian. He said he felt he was already a Brahmin. I told him he was qualified and initiated him in Wilmington. I prayed to the Master and asked for his name to be joined to the lineage of Sivananda. In my Meditation the name "Haridas" came to me. I have never seen anyone as happy as he was when I gave him his new spiritual name.

He would wear a Bindi and yellow cape or shawl with Mantras on it. He asked me to teach him how to perform Hindu weddings. I did, and he performed many Hindu weddings. He also learned to, and gave, Mantra initiations and gave them to many of his students in Fort Meyers, Florida, spreading the word of Master Sivananda. He taught karate, Yoga, and Indian astrology, in all of which he was proficient. He used to go to Hindu bhagans meetings and helped the Hindu community build a temple.

After his initiation, he called me once a week. He was the only one who called me Guru Ji, and always asked me, "What is the message you gave on your television show?" Then he would come see me twice a year, bringing flowers and Korean Tea. I told him not to do that, but he insisted on doing it. I used to sit on a chair. He would sit near, touch my feet and say, "Guruji, please bless me." I would always bless him.

He taught me devotion. One day he called and told me he wanted me to listen to four beautiful tapes by Bhagawan Rajneesh. He wouldn't let me pay for them so I sent him 20 Om pendants I had got from India.

Then he told me his father had just passed away, left him some money and that he desired to go to India with his children and go to the Sivananda Yoga Ashram and bathe in the Ganges. I told him that I would talk to my niece about his desire.

On September 13, 2004, I received a call from the President of the Hindu Temple of Fort Meyers, whom I had visited with Haridas. She gave me sad news. She told me that Haridas had died in a car accident in Florida. A drunk driver came into his lane and had a head-on collision with his car. Fortunately,

Haridas's mother had gone to Fort Meyers and taken charge of the children, aged 13 and 16.

On September 14, 2004, I received the four tapes that Haridas had told me he was sending me. I cried. At our Sivananda Yoga Satsang we prayed for his soul. May God bless his soul. He was one in a million.

I went to see Swami Vishnu right before he left this material world. He greeted me with love and said, "I want you to teach the Bhagavad Gita in the next Teacher's Training session at the Sivananda Ashram Yoga Retreat in the Bahamas." I was really surprised at his asking me to do that, because it was my poorest subject. However, I thanked him and consented. For the next seven months, I studied and prepared my talks for 6 or 7 hours a day making notes. I enjoyed the Bahamas and teaching the Bhagavad Gita a great deal. Eighty students from around the world attended the Teacher's Training program. On the last day, we had a group photo taken. (Fig.15.4 on page 151)

After Swami Vishnu Devananda passed away, I wrote the following article, *"Who Made Yoga Popular in the West?"* It was printed in a Yoga magazine.

"Let me ask you who made Yoga a household word in the West? I believe that Yoga is practiced now in the West as much as it is in India. Who caused this to happen? He is that great son of Bharat (India), that great saint of India H. H. Swami Vishnu Devananda Maharaj, who left his body on November 9, 1993. He was born in South India in 1927.

On the instruction of his Guru H. H. Swami Sivananda, Swami Vishnu-Devananda came to the U.S.A. in the early 1960s without money or support. He built his headquarters, Sivananda Yoga Ashram Yoga Camp, in Val Morin, Canada and was the inspiration for 25 Yoga centers around the world, including three in India. His book, "The Complete Illustrated Book of Yoga," is the Bhagavad Gita or Bible of Yoga. His most important contribution was the Teacher's Training Course (TTC) of Yoga. TTC trained hundreds of students in the West who, in turn, taught Yoga classes around the world and made Yoga a household word.

The whole world should know this truth. If not the entire world, at least Indians should know for sure.

Swami Vishnu-Devananda has initiated many able swamis in the west to continue his work. He loved everyone and inspired thousands of people to practice and preach Yoga, including me. On top of all this, he was a champion of peace. Now his spirit will guide people for generations to come. His message is, learn, practice and preach Yoga for health, happiness and liberation. His formula to be happy is 1) proper exercise, 2) proper breathing, 3) proper relaxation, 4) proper diet and 5) positive thinking and Meditation."

AUTHOR'S ENCOUNTERS WITH SPIRITUALITY

Yogi Vitaldas

I heard that a 60-year-old Indian Yogi, was teaching Yoga in New York. His name was Yogi Vitaldas. I contacted and asked him to give a weekend Yoga Seminar in January 1967. I went to the railway station to pick him up. He arrived barefoot and wearing a thin cloth (dhoti—Indian clothes) and a thin kaphani. It was snowing outside. I said, "Yogiji, don't you feel cold?" He replied, "I'm a Yogi; I don't feel cold." He stayed in my home with my family. He noticed that some of our cooking pots were made of aluminum. He also saw the oil in the kitchen as well as the large tub of Crisco, which is partially hydrogenated oil.

Yogiji told us back then that it is not healthy to eat partially hydrogenated oil and to cook in aluminum pots. After that we got rid of all our aluminum pots and bought only stainless steel pots and switched from Crisco to butter.

The Seminar of this great Hatha Yogi was excellent. During the question and answer session a lady raised her hand and asked, "Yogiji what do you think about Swami Yoganananda?" He answered that he was not a Yogi. We asked him why he said that. He said, "Yogananda got up to give a lecture and he dropped dead." So I asked, "Wasn't that a good way to die?" Yogiji answered, "No, Yogis don't die that way, a Yogi knows when he is going to die and he calls everyone and tells them, 'it is time for me to leave this material world,' and then he presses certain parts of his anatomy and his spirit leaves through the crown of his head, allowing him to attain Moksha (complete freedom)." Then I asked Yogiji if he were going to die that way. He said, "Definitely."

Yogi Shantananda

At the Sivananda Yoga Center someone brought us the news that Yogi Shantananda, a Hatha Yogi in his late twenties, had come from India. I invited him to conduct a Yoga seminar in Wilmington, Delaware. I arranged a two-day seminar over a weekend and met him prior to the seminar.

I asked him to teach Hatha Yoga, Pranayama and anything else he wanted to. At that time I asked him if he had any Siddhis. He replied, "What do you want me to do?" I said, "What would you like to do?" He said, "I can make all of them cry." I said, "That will be good."

An Indian proverb says, when people see power, they bow down. Twenty-five people attended the seminar. When it started, Yogi Shantananda took his right hand and patted his right thigh slowly and chanted the Mantra, "Shakti Ma." I watched everything very intently. Suddenly, almost everyone in the room, men and women, began crying loudly like babies. I wish I had filmed the moment. I felt like crying too, but I held back. The rest of his seminar went very well.

Swami Baba Muktananda

When Swami Muktananda first came to New York, Yogi Shantananda told me that he was a great Siddha (enlightened being). He said I should have his darshan (being in his presence and being blessed).

So I went with a few of my students from the Sivananda Yoga Center to check him out. We arrived at a small hall, and with 200 other people, waited for about 30 minutes until an older man arrived. As he entered the room, a couple of American ladies started to cry. So I asked one of them, "Why are you crying?" She said "I never felt so much love in my life." Swamiji had not even said hello to her.

I was the only Indian in the room and Baba had singled me out. When I looked in his eyes I could see the Universe through them. Then we all went and took his blessing. I decided at that moment that if he visited next year I would bring my family for his darshan.

Within a year Baba's organization had purchased a hotel and other buildings and that year more than 1,000 people came to see Baba. At that time, my daughter was about nine years old and my son was ten and a half.

My wife and I took our children to attend Baba's Satsang. At the end of Satsang Baba used to bless people individually by touching them with a peacock feather on top of their head. When Baba saw Meeta, my daughter, he was very happy to see an Indian girl. Meeta was standing next to me. As soon as he looked at her, she said, "Daddy, I feel like I have a beard like Swamiji." I assured her that she's OK. When Swamiji touched me with the peacock feather I felt like a shock ran through my body.

When Baba Muktananda passed away, his disciple Swami Gurumayi, took over. He passed on his Siddhis to her before he died. Siddhi Yogidam, their institution, has grown significantly under Gurumayi's leadership.

In 1990, a group of Indians arranged a bus trip to visit Gurumayi's ashram for a private darshan. Meeta and I went with them. Gurumayi does not touch grownups, only children. It's been said that if Gurumayi touches you, then everything in your life will work out. During the individual blessings when Meeta walked up to Gurumayi she began to cry. Gurumayi asked, "Why are you crying?" She took Meeta's hand in hers and Meeta said, "I feel your Shakti."

Yogi Amrit Desai

Yogi Amrit Desai is a personal friend. He performed my sister Hansa's marriage ceremony here in America. The Mayor signed the papers, but Amritji did the Hindu ceremony and blessed them. He was my first Yoga teacher, and introduced me to Hatha Yoga. When I began teaching Yoga, I vowed not to use any income from the Yoga Center for my personal needs. I used all that money and donations to keep the center going and to spread the message of Yoga.

I learned Meditation from my Guru, Swami Vishnu Devananda and started practicing it every day. One day, during Meditation, I got a message from Swami Sivananda that a hostile American group has gotten into Yogi Amrit Desai's organization, the Kripalu Center. I went to Kripalu to spend a few days with Amritji and his wife. I told him of the message I received that this group wants to remove him from his organization and it could be done because he gave all the power to trustees. He didn't believe me and said that everybody is really loving.

I came home and after a year or two everything I said happened and he was removed from the Kripalu Center. He came to see me and said that everything I had seen in my Meditation came to pass. I told him that it wasn't me, but the Guru who told him. I had just passed on the message.

Swami Tilak

Swami Tilak was from India and his associate from Shri Lanka. They were traveling Monks who traveled around the world, rather than from village to village. He had heard about me, and I invited them to come to our Yoga Center and give a lecture. During Satsang that Sunday, the energy in the room was so powerful. It was hard to explain, but it was felt by everyone in the room, and not me alone.

After Satsang, both Swamis came to my home. My wife cooked dinner, and Swamiji made shiro for dessert, as he really enjoyed making this sweet. While my wife was out of the kitchen, I asked Swamiji, "You have so much energy. Where does it come from?" He replied, "From pure living and from being completely celibate."

Chapter 17

Yoga Sadhana (Practice)

Learning Yoga from a qualified teacher is just the beginning. The next step is to include Yoga practice in your daily routine. This message is especially for the part-time Yoga practicer. Regular practice of Yoga Asana, Pranayama, and Meditation for 20 minutes to half an hour at least three days a week, if not for the preferable five days, is essential. A half hour of reading about Yoga or spiritual literature will be of help. Increase your Yoga knowledge and inspiration by going to a Yoga Ashram or retreat for vacation. There are many Yoga websites. You can go to Swami Sivananda's http://www.divinelifesociety.org/ and Swami Vishu Devananda's http://www.sivananda.org/teachings/teachers/swamiji/swamiji.html. If you have more time, add the following to your Yoga practice.

These are my instructions for Yoga Sadhana.

1) One does not have to drop religion or bad habits to be a Yogi. Just add Yoga and negative and undesirable habits will drop out on their own.

2) Yoga Sadhana (practices) will bring liberation (love), enlightenment (truth), good health and a good life.

3) Yoga is not dogmatic. Rather it is a way of living and a state of mind achieved with the guidance of the Guru (Spiritual Teacher).

4) Try to walk, instead of standing and go as far as you can.

For your personal sadhana:

Bhakti:—Devotion: Keep marching with faith towards God and Guru.

—Pray: Recite prayers of your choice, and be prayerful while doing it. Many Yogis recite the Yoga prayer given below.

Yoga Prayer
Om Asato Ma Sat Gamaya
Tomaso Ma Jyotir Gamaya
Mrityor-Ma Amritam Gamaya
Om Shantih, Shantih, Shantih.

Om Lead us Thou, oh God,
From unreal to real.
From darkness to light.
From death to immortality.
Om Shanti, Shanti, Shanti.
Om Peace, Peace, Peace Be unto Us All.

Surrender: To Shakti (MA-power) with Guru's love and they will take you to Siva (Father-God).
Mantra: Japa: Remember God in anyway that you can—Chant the Mantra in your heart or mind. Remember God or Self every moment available to you.
Jnana: Mala: Rosary at least three rounds a day.
Read or listen: Religious or philosophical books.
Memorize: Important verses (e.g., Gita).
Detachment: Be like a Lotus flower that rises from the mud.
Raja: Meditate: At least twenty minutes a day.
Open the third eye.
Witness the dance (accept KARMA—reincarnation).
Karma: Dharma: Serve and be dutiful to God, Guru, family, society and to yourself.
Hatha: Asana: Do a minimum of ten to twenty minutes of Yoga postures. They are prayer with your body.
Pranayama: Do two types of Yogic breathing (three rounds each).
Vegetarian: If you are not a vegetarian, first drop red meat, then fowl, fish and eggs.
Know that drugs (not medicine) are harmful to your body—Eat natural good foods. Too much salt, white sugar and spices are not good for your health. Moderation is the answer (Note: Yogi's eat milk products).
Weight: Maintain your right weight.
Kriya: Practice cleansing.

Fasting: Fast once a week or on the 11th or 13th day of the moon (lunar) calendar. Take with water alone or in combination with fruit and/or milk.

Yama and Niyama: Spiritual and positive living is the answer.

The pulls and pressures of family and job have created many part-time Yoga practicers. Time-management gurus John Robinson and Geoffrey Godbey, in their book "Time for Life," have declared Americans have more free time, not less. Their study of the daily routines of 10,000 Americans over the past 30 years reveal that people have about 40 hours of leisure per week. Usually this time is scattered in short bursts through the workweek. But Americans spend many of those hours watching TV. This was their breakdown on our time in a week: 15 hours watching TV, 6.7 hours socializing, 4.4 hours talking on the phone conversing with family members, 2.8 hours reading, 2.7 hours spent on hobbies, 2.2 hours adult education, 2.2 hours for recreation/sports/outdoors, 1.2 hours for other organizations, 9 hours cultural events, 9 hours of religion, 4 hours listening to radio or recordings. But most Americans claim that not all of this is true. This is my breakdown for an average person's time during the day.

7 hours—sleep
7 hours—work
7 hours—family, Eating, Cleaning, Fixing and Service
1 hour—fun, relax,
1 hour—hobby, reading
1 hour—walk, Yoga and Meditation

In short, a busy, married, person has about an hour a day for practicing Yoga. That isn't much time, but in a busy schedule. That is all that is available.

How many calories you burn is important, the New England Journal of Medicine claims from its study of 17,000 Harvard alumni that a person who burns 2,000 or more calories a week in moderate exercise will probably live longer than one who doesn't. A 150-pounder who irons his owns shirts will not only save money but also use up 22 calories every 10 minutes. If he cooks, he'll use up 31 calories, if he cleans the house, he will burn up 42 calories and if he shops for food, he'll burn another 42 calories. Walking a brisk 20 miles every week is the simplest way to use up the requisite 2,000 calories.

Energy Expended by a 150 Pound Person in Various Activities

Activity	Calories Per Hour
A. REST AND LIGHT ACTIVITY	
Lying down or sleeping	80
Sitting	100
Driving an automobile	120
Standing	140
Domestic Work	180
B. MODERATE ACTIVITY	
Yoga	180
Bicycling (5 ½ mph)	210
Walking (2 ½ mph)	210
Gardening	220
Bowling	270
Swimming (1/4 mph)	300
C. VIGOROUS ACTIVITY	
Wood Chopping	400
Tennis	420
Downhill Skiing (10 mph)	600
Squash and Handball	600
Running (10 mph)	900

Shaping Up: To lose a pound of fat, you need to burn 3,500 calories more than you consume, according to medical authorities. If you burn 500 calories more per day than you consume, you will lose a pound of fat per week. However, don't try to reduce your weight too quickly. Sudden weight loss, doctors say, can cause kidney stones, psychological problems and even death.

Exercise vs. calories: The table below, published by CPC North America, a food manufacturer, shows how many minutes of different exercises are required to burn up the calories acquired by eating various foods. The figures are for a person weighing 155 pounds. If you weigh less, required minutes of activity increase.

Food	Fuel Intake (calories per serving)	Minutes of Activity	
		Walking (3 ½ mph)	Running (5 ½ mph)
Apple, large	100	18	10
Beer, 8 oz.	115	21	11
Cola, 8 oz.	105	19	10
Cornflakes (with milk and sugar)	200	36	19
Cheddar cheese, (1 oz.)	110	20	10
Donut	150	27	14
Ice Cream	190	34	18
Pancake (with Syrup)	115	21	11
Hamburger (with bun, sauce)	350	64	33
Steak (10 oz. sirloin)	1,000	182	95

Source Unknown

How to Measure Your Yoga Practice

I developed the chart in Table 17.1 (page 185) for the part-time Yoga practicer. Swami Sivananda's organization, the Divine Light Society, is using the chart shown in Table 17.2 (page 186) for advanced part-time Yoga practicers. These charts will help you measure your Yoga progress.

Recommended Reading for Your Yoga Sadhana

A sadhana I recommend is reading Yoga and some spiritual books. This is the reason I'd like to recommend some books that you should look into obtaining and reading. Some books are already available online in websites such as http://www.dlshq.org/download/download.htm and http://www.divinelifesociety.org/.

1)   H. H. Swami Sivananda of Rishikesh wrote many books on Yoga as well as spirituality. I recommend the following three books on Yoga "*Practice Of Yoga*," "*Sadhana*," and "*Bhagavad Gita*."

2)   H. H. Swami Vishnu Devananda, *"The Complete Illustrated Book Of Yoga,"* is one of the most authentic books on Yoga, and his other books are *"Meditation and Mantra,"* and *"Hatha Yoga Pradipika."* The last is H. H. Swami Vishnu Devananda's translation of Hatha Yoga Pradipika written in the 17th Century from Ancient Sources by Yogi Swatmarama.

3)   B.K.S. Iyengar, *"Light On Yoga."* His books are considered to be the second most authentic books on Yoga.

4) Swami Venkatesananda, *"The Yoga Sutras of Patanjali,"* *"Daily Reading of Sivananda,"* and *"The Supreme Yoga."*

5) Sivananda Organization, *"The Sivananda Companion to Yoga,"* a very popular book on Yoga.

6) Andre Van Lysebeths, *"Pranayama."*

7) A book complied and edited by W.Y. Evans Wentz, *"The Tibetan Book of the Dead."*

Yoga in the Olympics

Since Yoga is included in the Guinness Book of World Records, why not include it in the Olympics? Some Yogis feel that hatha Yoga should not be used in competition, but if it was brought into the Olympics, it would gain world focus and more people would practice Yoga. So I propose that the International Olympic Committee include Hatha Yoga postures in the next Olympics. To excel in Hatha Yoga postures, one must practice everyday, have skill, precision, strength and grace. Yoga is taught and practiced by people everywhere for good health, flexibility and to remain beautiful. This would be an excellent way to promote Yoga, and bring good mental and physical health to the many people who need it and are unaware of its existence.

Comparison of Hatha Yoga vs. Other Exercise
(Swami Vivekananda Kendra Organization and additions by BJG)

Hatha Yoga	Other Exercise
1. At mental level	At physical level—Count numbers
—Awareness (meditative)	
2. Slow and smooth	Fast and jerky
3. Metabolism down	Metabolism up
4. Gain energy	Lose energy

5. With deep breathing	Regular breathing
6. Loose clothing	Tight clothing
7. Any age	Mostly young
8. Spiritual (uniting body, mind & soul)	Only physical
9. Harmonizing	Force
10. Stretch	Number
11. Affects nerves and glands	Affects muscles and heart
12. Static	Done many times
(did posture once, but kept it a long time)	
13. Muscle healing	Muscle building
14. Toning* down the muscles	Toning the muscles
15. Stop practice, no bad effect	Stopping will increase weight and at same time could cause heart problems
16. Improved muscle strength	Improve strength
17. Need small carpet	Machines are used
18. Yoga practice is inspiring	Some exercises are boring
19. Leads to spirituality and better health	Leads to better fitness
20. Intuitive	Competitive
21. Balanced energy (Prana)	Unbalanced energy
22. It helps play other sports better	One sport may exclude participation in other sports
23. Peaceful	Aggressive
24. Harmonizing force	Resistive force
25. Heart centered	Ego centered
26. Inexpensive	Could be expensive
27. Affects the astral and subtle body	Affects the gross body
28. Needs a Guru or teacher	Needs a teacher
29. It is a healing process	It offers better fitness
30. God given	Man given
31. It is a prayer to God with your body	It is a good exercise

* Toning means contracting the muscle; dead people's and children's muscles are long and flexible.

SPIRITUAL INSTRUCTIONS BY H.H. SWAMI SIVANANDA

These twenty instructions contain the very essence of all Yoga Sadhana. Karma, Bhakti, Jnana, and Raja Yoga will all come to one who follows them whole-heartedly. They are the unfailing keys to quick and effective development and culture of the physical, mental, moral and spiritual self of man.

1. *Brahmamuhurta*—Get up at 4 a.m. daily. This is Brahmamuhurta, which is extremely favorable for Sadhana. Do all your morning spiritual Sadhana during this period from 4 a.m. to 6:30 or 7 a.m. Such Sadhana brings quick and maximum progress.

2. *Asana*—Sit in Padmasana (lotus pose), Siddhasana (adept's pose) or Sukhasana (any pose you like) for your Japa and Meditation for half an hour, facing east or north. Increase the period gradually to three hours. Practice Sirshasana (headstand) and Sarvangasana (shoulder stand) for maintenance of health and Brahmacharya. Take light physical exercises such as walking, etc., regularly. Do twenty rounds of easy, comfortable Pranayama (breathing exercises). Do not strain while doing Pranayama.

3. *Japa*—You can repeat any Mantra (sacred syllable), such as pure *Om* or *Om Namo Narayanaya, Sri Ram, Sita Ram, Sri Ram Jaya Ram Jaya Jaya Ram, Om Namah Sivaya, Om Namo Bhagavate Vasudevaya, Om Saravanabhavaya.* Repeat the Mantra for 16 rounds of 108 (1,728 times) daily. At least one round is better than none. Devotees of Christ may repeat the name *Jesus or Hail Mary,* Mother of Jesus. Parsis, Sikhs and Muslims may select a name or Mantra from the Zend Avesta, Granth Sahib or Koran respectively.

4. *Dietetic Discipline*—Take Sattvic food. Give up chilies, tamarind, garlic, onion, sour tastes, oil, mustard, and asafetida. Observe moderation in diet (Mitahara). Do not overload the stomach. Give up those things you like very much for two weeks once or twice in a year. Eat simple food. Milk and fruits help concentration. Take food as medicine to keep life going. Eating for enjoyment is a sin. Give up salt and sugar for a week or two. You must be able to live on rice, dal and bread without any spices. Do not ask for extra salt for dal, and sugar for tea, coffee and milk. People who are normally used to a non-vegetarian diet should try their best to gradually give up flesh-eating as completely as possible. They will be immensely benefited.

5. *Meditation*—Have a separate room under lock and key. If this is not possible then a corner of a room should be set apart with a small cloth screen or curtain drawn across. Keep the room spotlessly clean.

6. *Svadhyaya*—Study systematically the *Gita, Ramayana, Bhagavatam, Vishnu-Sahasranama, Lalita-Sahasranama, Adityahridaya, Upanishads, Yoga Vasishta, the Bible, Imitation of Christ, Zend Avesta, the Quran, the Tripitakas, the Granth Sahib* and other religious books from half an hour to an hour daily, and have Suddha Vichara (pure thoughts).

7. *Elevate The Mind*—Learn by heart some prayer-slokas (prayer verses), Stotras (hymns) and repeat them as you sit in the Asana before starting Japa or Meditation. This will elevate the mind quickly.

8. *Brahmacharya*—Preserve the vital force (Veerya, seminal energy) very, very carefully. Veerya is God in motion or manifestation (Vibhuti). Veerya is all power. Veerya is all money. Veerya is the essence of life, thought and intelligence. This instruction is not for bachelors only. Householders also must follow it as far as possible. They must be extremely moderate in their martial relations with their spouse. This is very important.

9. *Charity*—Perform charity regularly, every month, or even daily according to your means. Never fail in this item. If necessary forego some personal wants but keep up this charity regularly.

10. *Have Satsang*—Give up bad company, smoking, meat and alcoholic liquors entirely. Have constant Satsang (association with holy people). Do not develop any evil habits. Deliberately exert to develop positive, virtuous qualities.

11. *Fast*—Fast on *Ekadasi* (11th day of the Hindu lunar two week period) or live on milk and fruits only. Christians must fast on alternate Sundays, Muslims on alternate Fridays, and Parsis on a suitable day every two weeks.

12. *Japa Mala*—Have a Japa Mala (rosary) around your neck or in your pocket or underneath your pillow at night. This will remind you of God. Twirl the beads during your leisure. You should repeat the Name at all times, whatever task you may be engaged in.

13. *Observe Mouna*—Observe Mouna (vow of silence) for two hours daily. Do not make gestures and inarticulate noises *during* the period of silence.

14. *Discipline of Speech*—Speak the truth at all costs. Speak a little. Speak sweetly. Always utter encouraging words. Never condemn, criticize or discourage. Do not raise your voice and shout at little children or subordinates.

15. *Be Content*—Reduce your wants. If you have four shirts, reduce the number to three or two. Lead a happy, contented life. Avoid unnecessary

worry. Be mentally detached. Have plain living and high thinking. Think of those who do not possess even one-tenth of what you have. Share with others.

16. *Practice Love*—Never hurt anybody. Ahimsa Paramo Dharmah (Non-injury is the highest virtue). Control anger by love, Kshama (forgiveness) and Daya (compassion). Serve the sick and the poor with love and affection. This is service to God.

17. *Be Self-Reliant*—Do not depend upon servants. Self-reliance is the highest of all virtues.

18. *Have Self-Analysis*—Before going to sleep think of the mistakes you have made during the day, (self-analysis). Keep a spiritual diary and self-correction register as Benjamin Franklin did. Maintain a daily routine and write down your resolution. Do not brood over past mistakes.

19. *Do Your Duty*—Remember that death is awaiting you at every moment. Never fail to fulfill your duties. Be pure in conduct (Sadachara).

20. *Remember God*—Think of God as soon as you wake up and just before you go to sleep, and at all other times whether engaged in any work or not. Repeat his name always. Surrender yourself completely to God (Saranagati).

This is the essence of all spiritual Sadhana. It will lead you to liberation. All these spiritual canons must be rigidly observed. You must not give any leniency to the mind.

SCIENCE OF 7 CULTURES

An ounce of practice is greater than tons of theory. Practice Yoga, religion and philosophy in daily life and attain self-realization.

These 32 instructions give the essence of the Eternal Religion (Sanatana Dharma) in its purest form. They are suitable for modern busy householders with fixed hours of work. Modify them to suit your convenience and increase the period gradually.

In the beginning take only a few practical resolves that form a small but definite advance over your present habits and character. In case of ill health, pressure of work or unavoidable engagements, replace your active Sadhana by frequent remembrance of God.

Health Culture

1. Eat light and simple food moderately. Offer it to God before you eat. Have a balanced diet.

2. Avoid chilies, garlic, onions, tamarind, etc. as far as possible. Give up tea, coffee, smoking, meat and wine entirely.

3. Fast on Ekadasi days. Take only milk, fruits or roots.

4. Practice Yoga Asanas or physical exercises for 15 to 30 minutes. Take a long walk or play some vigorous games daily.

Energy Culture

5. Observe silence (Mouna) for two hours daily and four to eight hours on Sunday.

6. Observe celibacy according to your age and circumstances. Restrict the indulgence to once a month. Decrease it gradually to once a year. Finally take a vow of abstinence for just whole life.

Ethical Culture

7. Speak the TRUTH. Speak little, speak kindly, and speak sweetly.

8. Do not injure anyone in thought, word or deed. Be kind to all.

9. Be sincere, straightforward, and openhearted in your talks and dealings.

10. Be honest. Earn by the sweat of your brow. Do not accept any money, things or favor unless earned lawfully. Develop nobility and integrity.

11. Control fits of anger by serenity, patience, love, mercy and tolerance. Forget and forgive. Adapt to men and events.

Will Culture

12. Live without sugar for a week or a month. Give up salt on Sundays.

13. Give up cards, novels, cinemas and clubs. Fly from evil company. Avoid discussions with materialists. Do not mix with persons who have no faith in God or who criticize your Sadhana.

14. Curtail your wants. Reduce your possessions. Have the ideals of plain living and high thinking.

Heart Culture

15. Doing good to others is the highest religion. Do some selfless service for a few hours every week, without egoism or expectations of reward. Do your worldly duties in the same spirit.

16. Give two to ten percent of your income in to charity every month. Share what you have with others. Let the world be your family. Remove selfishness.

17. Be humble and prostrate to all beings mentally. Feel the Divine presence everywhere. Give up vanity, pride and hypocrisy.

18. Have unwavering faith in God, the Gita and your Guru. Make a total self-surrender to God and pray: "Thy Will be done; I want nothing." Submit to the Divine Will in all events and happenings with equanimity.

19. See God in all beings and love them as your own self. Do not hate anyone.

20. Remember God at all times or at least on rising from bed, during a pause in work and before going to bed. Keep a Mala in your pocket.

Psychic Culture

21. Study one chapter or 10 to 25 verses of the Gita with meaning daily.

22. Memorize the whole Gita, gradually. Keep it always in your pocket.

23. Read Ramayana, Bhagavata, Upanishads, Yoga Vasishtha or other religious books daily, and on holidays.

24. Attend religious meetings, kirtans and Satsangs of saints at every opportunity. Organize such functions on Sundays or holidays.

25. Visit a temple or a place of worship at least once a week and arrange to hold kirtans or discourses there.

26. Spend holidays and leave periods, whenever possible, in the company of saints or practice Sadhana at holy places in seclusion.

Spiritual Culture

27. Go to bed early, Get up at 4 o'clock. Answer calls of nature, clean your mouth and take a bath.

28. Recite some prayer and kirtan Dhwanis. Practice Pranayama, Japa and Meditation from 5 to 6 o'clock. Sit in Padma, Siddha or Sukha Asana throughout, without movement by gradual practice.

29. Perform your daily Sandhya, Gayatri Japa, Nitya Karma and worship, if any.

30. Write your favorite Mantra or Name of God in a notebook for 10 to 30 minutes.

31. Sing the Names of God (Kirtan), Prayers, Slokas and Bhajans for half an hour to an hour at night with family and friends.

32. Regularity, tenacity and fixity are essential. Record Sadhana in a Spiritual Diary daily. Review it every month and correct your failures.

ETHICS OF YOGA

SERVE, LOVE, GIVE, PURIFY, MEDITATE, REALIZE

Serve

1. Service has elevated me. Service has purified me.

2. I ever keep myself fully occupied.

3. I never leave a work till it is finished.

4. I never procrastinate on any work.

5. I serve all.

6. I pray and do kirtan for peace in of the whole world, for the health and peace of sick people, and for the peace of the departed souls and the earth-bound spirits also.

7. I serve the poor.

8. I massage the legs of sick persons and Sadhus.

9. I attend on guests very caringly.

10. I keep my promises.

11. I give very promptly reply to all my letters.

12. I serve all sincerely selflessly.

13. I get work done through kindness, service, respect, and love.

14. I obey.

15. I am humble and simple.

16. I am frank and straightforward.

17. I am bold and cheerful.

18. I can bear insult and injury.

19. I talk a little. I think much. I Meditate much. I try to do much and serve much.

Love

20. I love all.

21. I respect elders and Sadhus (Monks).

22. I respect all saints and prophets of all religions, respect all religions, all cults, all faiths and all creeds.

23. I am ever happy and joyful. I make others happy and joyful.

24. I always speak sweetly.

25. I am perfectly tolerant and catholic (universal).

26. I am merciful and sympathetic.

27. I am child-like in my Swabhava (nature).

28. I am forgiving.

29. I am free from vindictive nature.

30. I return good for evil. I serve that man who has injured me, with joy.

Give

31. I rejoice in giving. I always give.

32. I have spontaneous and unrestrained generosity.

33. I take immense delight in feeding the poor and my students.

34. I try to be a mother to my students.

35. I do a lot for charity.

36. I do not keep anything.

Purify

37. I always serve my masters with sincerity and intense faith and devotion.

38. I wandered without food during my Parlvrajaka life. I slept on the roadside at night without clothing during the winter. I ate dried bread with water.

39. I developed many virtues.

40. I stick tenaciously to my principles and ideals.

41. I fast on Ekadashi. I do not take salt on Sundays.

42. I practice Ahimsa, Satyam and Brahmacharya.

43. I always look with introspection. I analyze and examine myself.

44. I am very regular in doing Asanas and exercises. I also do Pranayama regularly.

45. I lead a well-regulated life.

46. I lead a simple life.

47. I respect all. I do salutations to all first.

48. I do not argue much. I live in silence.

49. I study sacred books.

Meditate

50. I perform worship of Atma at all times. I work for the good of others.

51. 'Aham Brahm Asmi; Sivoham; Soham; Sat-Chitananda Swarupoham'— This is my favorite formula for Vedantic Meditation.

52. I constantly Meditate on the following: Prajnanam Brahm, Aham Brahmasmmi, Tat Twam Asi, Ayam Atma Brahm; Satyam Jnanam Anantam Brahm; Santam Sivam Adwaitam; Aham Atma Gudakesa; Aham Atma Nirakarah Sarvavyapi Swabhavatah; Brahma Satyam Jagan Mithya Jeevo Brahmaiva Na Aparah; Akartha Abhokta Asang Sakshi; Ajo Nityah Saswatoyam Purano, Jyotishamapi Tat Jyotih.

53. I never go to the mountains or seaside for a holiday. Change of work gives rest. Meditation gives abundant rest.

54. My joy is inexpressible. My treasure is immeasurable. I attained this through Sanyasa, renunciation, untiring selfless service, Japa, Kirtan and Meditation.

Realize

55. I talk to others on things that I have myself practiced.

56. I practice and advocate the Yoga of Synthesis.

57. I do not pay lip service to Vedanta. I am a practical Vedantin.

58. I mix with all. I become one with all.

59. I see the Lord in all.

60. I do mental prostrations to animals, trees, bricks, stones, and all creatures!

Extracted from the inimitable autobiography of Sri Gurudev "SIVANANDA GITA," this self-revealed Code of Sivananda-Ethics gives you the essence of all the scriptures in the world.

RAJA YOGA—MEDITATION
Swami Sivananda gives these 24 instructions on Meditation.

1. To render the mind fit for Meditation is the purpose of all Sadhana.

2. Meditation is the last rung of the ladder.

3. Immortality is the fruit of Meditation.

4. All problems will be solved by Meditation. This faith you must have.

5. Meditation is the greatest Tapasya. No other kartavya is greater than Meditation.

6. Meditation is to quiet the mind and give it a direction towards its goal.

7. Through the mind itself you realize that you have gone off the point of concentration, and the mind, through will power, brings us back to the point.

8. Empty the mind and create a condition by which it can concentrate on one object (Mind should be totally free from all activities).

9. You must use your intelligence and try to make concentration as pleasant and interesting as possible. The ultimate analysis will reveal that concentration is hampered by desire and attachment.

10. The gross mind cannot still the thoughts. It is only the fine mind that can concentrate.

11. Lust, anger and greed are the main foes of a seeker. These are the greatest obstacles to Meditation. These impurities have to be eliminated from the mind. By making the life sattvic, by filling ourselves with **Sattva**, we can annihilate these enemies.

12. Either you think of the things you do not like or of a thing you like and to which you are attracted. Therefore attachment and repulsion are at the root of the problem. It means lack of **Valragya**, dispassion.

13. Meditation is the point where all Yogas are unified.

14. The most effective way of growing into the divine nature is not so much by picking out your little weaknesses, as by filling yourself with virtues.

15. I shall give you some valuable suggestions for success on the path of Meditation. They are:

    (a) Constant recollection (fill your mind with thoughts of the supreme being).

    (b) Continuous prayerfulness.

    (c) Repetition of the Divine name.

16. Where love is, there the mind and heart are; therefore, develop love for God.

17. Meditation is the process of the total spiritualization of your entire being.

18. Meditation is the technique of living in the world of conflicts while being unaffected by them.

19. The aspirant of today starts Meditation as soon as he reads some books. But, Meditation is almost the last stage of the **Sadhana.** It is the very threshold of the kingdom of heaven or realization.

20. Meditation is one percent theory and 99 percent practice.

21. Contemplate upon the ideals into which you wish to grow.

22. The mind at first will try to jump about in a hundred different directions. It will run about most uncontrollably. But do not be perturbed. Just allow it to run. Stand apart from it. Remain alert within and observe its antics.

23. All of us who are striving for God should always remember that success in Meditation depends upon the intensity of our love for Him. The more we love God, the more our attention is attracted towards him. The more we feel this attraction, the more we enjoy our Meditation.

24. Meditation leads to that unique spiritual faculty lying deep within each human soul, the faculty of intuition, which is also called the third eye, or the eye of wisdom. That faculty alone is the rightful instrument of the soul.

The following is an excerpt from page 124 of the book "Power of Intention" in Dr. Wayne W. Dyers book by Swami Sivananda.

"The best thing to give:
to your enemy is forgiveness;
    to your opponent, tolerance;
    to your friend, your heart;
    to your child, a good example;
    to your father, deference (honor);
    to your mother, conduct that makes her proud of you;
    to your self, respect;
    to all men, charity.
        —Swami Sivananda, a sage who lived in India

Table 17.1

(Example – Make yours bigger)   Yoga Practitioners Weekly   Name:_____
                                   Record Keeping Table   _____

Day of Week	Not Less	Your	S	M	T	W	R	F	S	S	M	T	W	R	F	S
Date	Than	Goal														
	Minutes															
Daily																
1 Prayers of your choice; Sanskrit and Trayambakm	1															
2 Pranayama - Kapalabhathi - rounds	3															
Pranayama - Ujjayi - rounds	1															
3 Meditation	20															
4 Asana Postures	15															
5 Puja Kirtan and Parsad	10															
6 Read Gita - how many pages or slokas	10															
7 Malas (Rosary) - how many rounds	3															
8 Chanted Mantra during other activities (or wrote Guru, Ishta, Mantra)	-															
9 Number of meals eaten (moderate)	2															
Balanced diet (satisfied)	-															
Abstained from eating between meals	-															
Abstained from eating meat	-															
Abstained from eating fish																
Abstained from eating eggs	-															
Abstained from alcohol and other drugs	-															
Abstained from desserts	-															
Abstained from coffee	-															
10 Drank how many glasses of water	6															
11 How many hours slept	7															
12 How many minutes in company of wise	-															
13 How many minutes in selfless service	-															
14 How much TV and other reading																
15 Hours with family - in real sense	-															
WEEKLY																
1 Studied religious or philosophy book	-															
2 Walked or played musical game	-															
3 Wrote in spiritual diary	10															
4 Fasted - water or fruit and/or milk	yes															
5 Brachmachalye (celibacy)	-															
6 Observe Mouna (silence)	-															
7 Did you attend religious place or Satsung or group meeting	yes															
8 Abstained from reading, listening or participating in violence or lies	yes															

Table 17.2

Spiritual Diary

This is for your information, Master Sivananda recommends the Yoga Practitioner keeps the following diary for their Sadhana

From .... To .... 19 ....

	Mon	Tue	Wed	Thur	Fri	Sat	Sun	Total
1 How many hours did you sleep?								
2 When did you rise from bed?								
3 How many rosaries (Mantra repetition) did you say?								
4 How long did you chant Mantras?								
5 How many Mantras did you write?								
6 How long in Pranayama (breathing exercises)?								
7 How long in Asanas (yoga postures)?								
8 How long in physica exercises?								
9 How many hours in Mouna (complete silence)?								
10 How many Slokas (verses) did you read?								
11 How long in study of religious books?								
12 How many hours in useless company?								
13 How long in company of the wises?								
14 How much time in selfless service?								
15 How much given charity?								
16 How many lies told and with what self-punishment?								
17 How many times angry, how long and with what self-punishment?								
18 How many times failed in Brahmacharya (celibacy)?								
19 How many times failed in control of evil habits and what self-punishment?								
20 Fast which days								
21 How long spent in Meditation Saguna or Nirguna?								
22 Were you regular in your Meditation?								
23 What virtues are you developing?								
24 What evil qualities to eradicate?								
25 Which sense is troubling you most?								
26 Bed time?								

Chapter 18

Kriya (Cleansing) Yoga

Kriya Yoga is part of Hatha Yoga. Kriya means cleansing. It is cleansing of the body, mind and astral body. The recommended Yoga Sadhana (practice) methods of cleansing are:

A. Ashtanga Yoga

    1. Yama, 2. Niyama, 3. Asana, 4. Pranayama, 5. Pratyahara, 6. Dharana, 7. Dhyana, 8. Samadhi.

B. Vedanta & Yoga

    1. Bhakti, 2. Jnan, 3. Raja, 4. Mantra, 5. Karma, 6. Hatha, 7. Kriya

C. Kundalini Yoga (Mystic Yoga)

D. Swami Sivananda says:

    Serve, Love, Give, Purify, Meditate, Realize, Be Good, Do Good, Practice Yoga

E. Swami Vishnu-Devananda says:

    "Do five things."

    1. Proper Exercise (Yoga Asana), 2. Proper Breathing (Pranayama), 3. Proper Diet (Balanced vegetarian diet), 4. Proper Relaxation (tension free life), 5. Positive thinking.

F. Yogi Bharat's Recipe.

    Pursue these by practicing Yoga

    1. God Realization, 2. Self Realization, 3. Life Realization

One of the goals of Yoga is to attain Moksha, which means final liberation, i.e. coming out of the circle of life and death. One has to clean up and become pure to attain final liberation. But Kriya first emphasizes the cleaning of the body. So I'll focus on that. To walk on the path of Hatha Yoga the body needs to be clean and strong. Some say that Kriya means cleaning the mind, body and soul. But the soul is part and parcel of God and hence cannot be impure. Therefore it does not need cleaning. However, some Yogis say that the soul is covered with impurities, which must be removed.

There are two types of cleaning, spiritual and physical. For spiritual cleansing, usually Meditation, prayer and Mantra chanting are required. But I'm going to concentrate on the physical cleansing, which encompasses the body, mind and emotional cleansing. For the astral body cleaning you need to go deeper and requires spiritual cleansing, because the astral body has past life memories.

PHYSICAL KRIYAS
Pranayama—(See chapter 10)
Neti (Nasal cleaning)
There are three ways to clean the nostrils and sinuses. The first is Sutra Neti (String). In this form of Neti, a thin string or catheter lubricated with antiseptic jelly is used. It is passed upward into one nostril until its end comes through the throat and out of the mouth. Next with the thumb and index finger grab the end of the string that has come out of the mouth. Now gently and slowly pull the string by its two ends to and fro a few times. Go through the same procedure on the other nostril. Practice to get used to Sutra Neti.

The second method is the water Neti. Boil some water; let it cool down and become lukewarm; then add a pinch of salt. Now draw in the water from your cupped hands or your teacup and let the water come out through your mouth. This cleans your sinuses and also improves your vision and concentration.

The third technique is to use a neti pot, prepare water as in the water neti. Then pour the water into one nostril and allow it to flow out from the other nostril, while tilting your head in the direction you want the water to flow out.

Dhouti (Washing)
This practice should not be done by just reading a book. You should learn from a practicing Dhouti before starting on our own. Dhouti Kriya is for cleaning the stomach. Take three or 4 four-inch cotton gauze that has been

soaked in water or milk and swallow it slowly. Keep the gauze in your stomach for 15 minutes and no longer.

A second technique for practicing Dhouti is vomiting. You perform this technique by drinking a full 8 oz glass of slightly salty water. Then put your index and middle fingers into your throat and induce vomit to clean the stomach. This technique is preferable when you have eaten something extremely disagreeable with your body and you need to get it out.

The Hatha Yogi, Pradipika says "There is no doubt that cough, asthma, enlargement of the spleen, leprosy, and 20 kinds of diseases born of phlegm disappear by practice of Dhouti Karma."

Uddiyana and Nauli Bandhas (Abdominal retraction)

Swami Sivananda says, "Uddiyana Bandha is a blessing to mankind, it brings health, strength and a long life to those who practice it. For abdominal exercises, nothing can compare with Uddiyana and Nauli. They stand unique, unrivalled and unprecedented amongst all systems of physical exercises in the East and the West."

Technique—First stand and keep your legs shoulder length apart and your knees slightly bent. Then place your right hand on your right thigh and your left hand on your left thigh and your body bent forward. Now empty your lungs as fast as you can, and relax the abdominal wall while keeping the lungs empty. Feel the full vacuum created. In the Nauli Bandha, the abdominal muscles roll from the left to the right and then from the right to the left. This rolling requires practice.

Trataka (Cleansing your mind)

It is the practice of gazing at an object or a candle without blinking until the eyes begin to water. It is gazing without staring at the object. This is also a type of Meditation; more precisely it could be called contemplation. Here one is focusing on a candle or a flower. Usually people gaze at a candle. When your eyes begin to water stop the Tratak. This technique will give your mind great peace.

Over 35 years of teaching Yoga I have often tried Tratak. I would ask the students to sit in a circle, light a candle and set it in the center of the circle and ask the students to gaze at the light without blinking their eyes. We did this exercise for about ten minutes. Afterward, I would tell them to place their palms over their closed eyelids and ask them if they could see the light within themselves. After this exercise, I would ask if they were relaxed. Almost everyone used to say they were.

Fasting—(See chapter 24)

Mouna (Silence)
During their weekly or fourth night fasting, many Yogis maintain complete silence. I have even heard some Yogis maintain total silence for a complete year or even longer. This difficult spiritual practice helps them attain God-realization faster.

Savasana (See chapter 9)

Brushing Teeth—(Danta Mula-Dhouti)
In India you can buy a wood stick called a "Datan," which you chew to clean your teeth. Next you split the Datan in half and use it to clean your tongue. In the West people use a brush and toothpaste, which is also good. Use your index finger to massage and strengthen your gums. You can also gargle with Listerine to kill the germs. It is good to clean your teeth twice a day, in the morning and before you go to bed. Some people brush their teeth after every meal.

Cleansing the Tongue (Jiva Sadhana)
Uliu, or a thin, narrow stainless steel strip, should be used to scrape your tongue, after brushing your teeth. This eliminates bad breath that is caused by bacteria. Using an Uliu will make you feel fresh.

Bandhas
Bandhas are a part of Pranayama and Kriyas. They prevent loss of energy or Prana. It is a process of conservation attained by advanced Pranayama. Even though Bandhas are related to Pranayama, each of them needs to be

practiced separately. There are three types of Bandhas. They are, Jalandhara, Moola or Uddiyana Bandhas.

Jalandhara Bandha—When you inhale deeply, press your chin firmly against your chest (chin lock) to prevent the Prana from escaping from the body. When you are ready to exhale, raise your head and let the air out.

Moola Bandha—In this bandha also, inhale deeply and contract the anal sphincter and abdominal muscles. This Bandha prevents the apana from escaping from the lower body and draws it up to unite with Prana (see Kundalini Fig. 9.3, page 70).

Uddiyana Bandha—After exhaling completely, pull the abdomen up and back toward the spine. This forces the Prana up the Sushumna Naadi (Fig. 10.9, page 71).

Taking a Bath
Begin your day with a hot shower or hot bath. Then start your Yoga Sadhana. The body will stretch better after the hot water bath. Use a good natural soap if you can.

Colon Cleansing
If you are young, eat some "All Bran" cereal or take some Harde an aryuvedic pill once a week. If you are 60 or over, you should take an anemia or a teaspoon of Metamucil every night before you go to bed. If you are a meat eater, it is very essential to keep your colon clean.

Cleaning the Ears (Karna Dhouti)
You should clean the ears with Q-tips and use some mineral oil once a week or once a month.

Cleansing (Kapalarandhra—Dhouti)
For this a small pot, called a nasal cup, is used sometimes. Sinusitis is often treated with drugs. A natural remedy is available and many people find it much more beneficial. Place the spout of this specially designed cup in one nostril and pour water. Let the water come out of the other nostril. This clears up clogged passages and prevents the build-up of irritants that lead to infection.

Detoxifying the Body

Detoxification means cleaning the blood. It does this mainly by removing impurities from the blood in the liver, where toxins are processed for elimination. The body also eliminates toxins through the kidneys, intestines, lungs, lymph and skin. However, when this system is compromised, impurities aren't properly filtered, and every cell in the body is adversely affected.

How should one detoxify the body? Eliminate alcohol, coffee, cigarettes, refined sugars and saturated fats, all of which act as toxins in the body and hinder your healing process. Also, minimize the use of chemical-based household cleaners and personal health care products (cleansers, shampoos, deodorants and toothpastes), and substitute them with natural alternatives. Sweating through your pores also helps in detoxifying the body. Too much use of make-up is not good, because it clogs your pores. A good vegetarian diet and fasting one day a week are also recommended.

Take a good vacation

In this fast, modern world people carry excessive tension. They should take a couple of good vacations when they do not have to constantly think and be under pressure. A good vacation is essential for relaxation. But for a Yoga practitioner it is good to stay at a Yoga camp or a Yoga Ashram, participate in activities and learn more about Yoga and Meditation. Some people like to go on a pilgrimage. That is also good.

Chapter 19

Siddhis

Sadhana or Yoga practice will get you siddhis or spiritual powers, like mind reading ability, knowing the past or the future, walking on water, living without food, etc. But these siddhis are not to be squandered; they are to be used wisely. There is a beautiful story illustrating this that I heard while on my spiritual path. In ancient India it was custom for the King or his daughter to announce a contest to determine the worthiness of her hand in marriage. This particular princess was a runner. She decided that whichever man catches her while running would be her husband. The princess's only condition of the contest was that she would get a mile's head start. She cleverly dropped a golden brick every so often. She knew that if the competitor who stopped to pick up the bricks will not be able to run fast enough to catch her, because of the weight of the golden bricks. However, one young man decided not to pick up the bricks. He knew that if he caught her, all her golden bricks would become his anyway. He caught her and married her.

This applies to Siddhis as well. God drops powers as distractions. If you get involved in the power game you will not be able to reach the Lord. Yogis stress that the powers you get along the way should not be used for personal gain. They should be used only to help the needy and for world peace.

The word "Sutra," means a thread in a fabric. Maharishi Patanjali presented the Yoga Sutra very concisely. There are many interpretations of this book. I have given Swami Vishnu's (Devananda's) translation of the Sanskrit sloka and also given Swami Venketa's interpretation for an understanding in depth. An even greater and deeper understanding can be had by reading B.K.S. Iyengar's, "Light on the Yoga Sutras of Patanjali," published by Harper Collins Publishers of India.

The third chapter of Maharishi Patanjali's Yoga Sutra is about Siddhis. In this chapter one word, "samyama," is used frequently and, it needs to be understood. In an earlier chapter, Maharishi Patanjali talks about Ashtanga Yoga, which means the eight steps leading to the highest level, Samadhi (1.Yama, 2. Niyama, 3. Asana, 4. Pranayama, 5. Dharana, 6. Dhyan, 7. Pratyahar, 8. Samadhi).

"Samyama" is a three-fold inner discipline. The three steps are Dharana and Dhyana and Samadhi. Dharana means withdrawal of the senses and/or contemplation, Dhyana means Meditation and Samadhi means oneness with all.

Chapter Three: Divine Manifestations of Power

In Chapter Three of the Raja Yoga Sutras it elucidates the last three limbs of Raja Yoga, dharana, Dhyana and Samadhi. These three highest levels of Meditation practiced together are called samyama, which is also explained in detail. Patanjali also describes many of the siddhis, or powers, that are attained through the protracted practice of Meditation.

1. Dharana is fixing the mind on one object. 2) An unbroken flow of perception between the mind and objects is Dhyana, on Meditation. 3) When consciousness of subject and object disappears and only the meaning remains, it is called Samadhi. 4) The practice of these three together is samyama. 5) Mastery of samyama brings direct knowledge. 6) Samyama's application should be in stages. 7) These three, i.e. dharana, Dhyana and Samadhi, are more internal than the preceding ones. 8) But even these are external compared to the "seedless" state. 9) Through the constant replacement of disturbing thought waves by ones of control, the mind is transformed and gains mastery of itself. 10) The mind's flow becomes undisturbed through repetition. 11) The transformation leading to the ability to enter Samadhi comes gradually through the elimination of distractions and the rise of one-pointedness. 12) One-pointedness of the mind occurs when the contents of the mind that rise and fall at two different moments are exactly the same. 13) By this what has been said in the previous sutras, changes in the form, time, and condition of the

elements and sense organs are explained. 14) There is a substratum that remains consistent through all changes, past, present and future. 15) The various transformations are caused by the different natural laws.

16) Performing samyama on the three kinds of changes (form, time and condition), brings knowledge of the past and future.

*"Therefore, knowledge of the past and of the future (and such knowledge as not already possessed) follows the practice of the three-fold inner discipline (concentration, Meditation, and illumination together) in relation to the fundamental principle of the three stages of the movement of thought—the movement of restraint, the non-arising of distractions, and the perfectly balanced state."

17) Sound, meaning and corresponding ideas are usually confused to be the same in the mind; but performing samyama on the sound makes the meaning and ideas clear and the sounds of all living beings is comprehended.

*"Language, meaning and conceptualization are always superimposed on one another, causing habit-patterns in communication. By the practice of the three-fold inner discipline on their differences there arises an understanding of the sounds uttered by all beings."

18) Perception of samskaras brings knowledge of the previous birth.

*"By the practice of the three-fold discipline on the inherent tendencies, and by the direct perception of such tendencies, knowledge of previous existence arises."

19) By performing samyama on another's mind, its mental images are known.

*"In an intimate knowledge of the ground of the Mind, there is what at first sight appears to be a supernatural knowledge of 'other' minds too, because in fact the intelligence, which is misunderstood as the mind, is indivisible.

"When the *citta* is made calm and peaceful and the *Prana* is concentrated, the *Prana* acts upon the *citta* and you get subtle vision. If you practice *Pranayama* and Meditation every day you will get this very soon. If you watch yourself when you talk to other people your *citta* will be clean and crystal-like and also extremely subtle. Because it is like a crystal it will reflect whatever object comes near it. You may develop powers of thought reading, because when someone comes near you, you may reflect his thoughts. (Therefore, because the mind is like a crystal, it is very necessary that you select your company. The thoughts and desires and motives of your friends will be reflected in your own mind.)

"You will spontaneously be able to love and to understand everybody. Understanding is looking at the other man as he looks at himself. The result is that you will always be peaceful, (at peace,) you will not be upset by anybody. If a man comes and scolds you, you know why he does it. You will look at it not as someone else looks at it, but as he himself will look at it. Only the Yogi who has reached the stage of true *dharana* will be able to understand everybody and love everybody. That is what we all are interested in, though Patanjali extends it to other objects.

"Any power that you get or use will take you away from God. Therefore, turn the whole practice towards God."

20) Mental factors which are not the subject of samyama cannot be known.

21) Samyama on one's physical body suspends another's ability to see it. The reflected light (from the body) does not come into contact with another's eyes; hence the power of invisibility.

*"By the practice of the three-fold inner discipline on the form and the substantiality of the body, one can comprehend directly the energy that makes it possible to 'grasp' it with the eyes and so forth (for the flow of light waves is the form). When this energy function is suspended, the dynamics of perception is made inoperative, the link between the perceiving eye and light is severed as it were and invisibility occurs. (Some editions have an additional Sutra here, suggesting a similar phenomenon with the sense of hearing.)"

22) Thus can also be explained the disappearance of sound and other physical phenomena.

23) Karma may be either dormant or active. By performing samyama on both, and through omens, the Yogi may know the time of death.

*"Action performed here yields results either immediately or in course of time depending on the degree of intensity. Through the practice of the three-fold inner discipline on the intensity or on the chain of action-reaction or the law of cause and effect, comes knowledge of death though not knowledge of the ultimate extinction of the ego-sense or liberation. This knowledge can be gained also through such discipline being directed towards omens and portents."

24) By performing samyama on friendliness, mercy, love, etc., their strengths are gained.

*"By the practice of the three-fold discipline on qualities like friendship one becomes an embodiment of such qualities naturally, and thus one gains great moral, psychic and spiritual strength."

25) From performing samyama on the strengths of various animals comes the power of an elephant (or any other species).

*"By the practice of the three-fold discipline on various kinds of strength (physical, mental, moral, psychic and spiritual) one grows to be as strong as, say, an elephant."

26) By performing samyama on light comes intuitive knowledge of that which is subtle, hidden or distant.

*"By correctly directing and focusing the light of perception in which the senses and their objects (the whole of nature) function, knowledge can be gained of the subtle, and the hidden, and even the remote objects or phenomena."

27) Through performing Samyama on the sun comes knowledge of the world.

*"By the practice of the three-fold discipline on the sun, a knowledge of the physical universe is gained.

When this *Samyama* is directed towards the sun, one's consciousness becomes one with the sun; and the universe and the composition of the solar system—and therefore the entire universe—is known. For instance, if you direct your Meditation at the tape recorder you will know exactly how this tape recorder is assembled, how it works. Now, here comes the mischief. Patanjali himself says, 'Please don't do this. I have described it to you in order to be truthful and scientific, but these are distractions'."

28) Performing samyama on the moon gives knowledge of astrology.

*"By the practice of the three-fold discipline on the moon, there arises a knowledge of the stellar system."

29) Performing samyama on the pole star gives knowledge of the movement of the stars.

*"By the practice of the three-fold discipline on the pole star, there comes a knowledge of movement (or the movement of the stars)."

30) Performing samyama on the navel center gives knowledge of the organization of the body.

*"By the practice of the three-fold inner discipline at the psychic center at the navel (the Manipura Chakra) the knowledge of the physiology of the body is gained."

31) Performing Samyama on the hollow of the throat causes cessation of thoughts of hunger and thirst.

*"By the practice of the three-fold discipline at the pit of the throat (or, the psychic center known as the Visuddha Chakra) freedom from hunger and thirst is gained."

32) Performing Samyama on the nerve centers, which control Prana, steadiness is achieved.

*"By the practice of the three-fold discipline on the kurmanadi, steadiness of the body and the mind is gained."

33) From performing samyama on the light at the crown of the head comes the power to perceive perfected beings.

*"By the practice of the three-fold discipline on the light that appears in the crown of your head during Meditation, one has the vision of sages who have attained perfection.

"When you are proficient in *Samyama* and direct this to the light in the crown of the head (which means after the *Kundalini* has awakened and is taken Chakra by Chakra to the *sahasrara*—the topmost center of your consciousness) then you will have a vision of the *Siddhis,* sages, enlightened ones. You can see Jesus Christ, Buddha, Krishna or whomever you want. You can also have a vision of the object of your Meditation. This can be a guide, a lamp unto your feet.

"This one Sutra in this section dealing with psychic accomplishments is sensible. But, in a way, Patanjali regards even that as a sort of distraction.

"The accomplishments listed in the other Sutras can happen spontaneously, but if you are going to struggle hard to attain perfection in concentration, Meditation and *Samadhi,* why must you waste all that talent to get knowledge of the stellar system, for example, or the ability to read other's thoughts? What for?"

34) Through intuition all knowledge is available.

*"All these can also be gained by direct intuitive perception. Or, by the practice of the threefold discipline on the inner light all knowledge is gained."

35) Samyama on the heart leads to the understanding of the nature of the mind.

*"By the practice of the three-fold discipline on the spiritual heart (or the psychic heart center, *Anahata*) there arises knowledge concerning the mind-stuff or the undivided intelligence."

36) Enjoyment results from a lack of discrimination between Purusha and Sattwa. Knowledge of Purusha comes from performing samyama on the interests of the Self rather than on the individual's interest.

*"The external object is totally distinct and different from what the experiencing personality thinks it is. When, in a state of ignorance, the personality forgets this, and as the object is imagined to be external for the enjoyment of another (which is the enjoyer), he experiences pain and pleasure. When the three-fold discipline is directed towards the substance of this self or personality (or, towards the selfishness), there arises the knowledge of the indwelling intelligence, with its' conditioning which is the ignorance."

37) From that comes intuitional hearing, thought, sight, taste, and smell.

*"Thereupon (since knowledge of ignorance is the dispelling of ignorance, and the intelligence that comprehends the mental conditioning is unconditioned) there come into being enlightened hearing, feeling, seeing, tasting and smelling—free from the perversions, limitations and distortions born of ignorance."

38)   These are obstacles to the state of Samadhi, though the mind, which is worldly, considers them to be powers.

39) When the cause of bondage is eliminated, the mind can enter another's body through knowledge of its channels.

*"When there is loosening of the bondage of the consciousness to the body, as also an understanding of the proper channel of the consciousness's entry into and its withdrawal from the body, the mind acquires the ability to enter another body."

40) With mastery of Udana comes levitation and the ability not to come into contact with water, mire, thorns, etc. (Udana = The nerve current of Udana).

*"When the anti-gravitational vital force that has an ascending flow is directly understood, there follow powers of levitation, and passage over water, mud, thorny bush, etc., without coming into contact with them."

41) Through mastery of samana comes blazing fire. Samana is another type of prana, which relates to digestion. From control of samana comes radiance.

*"When the vital force which maintains equilibrium and which fills the entire body with light, life and power, is directly perceived and understood, there is effulgence and radiance of one's personality."

42) By performing samyama on the relationship between the akasha and the ear is gained super physical hearing.

43) By performing samyama on the relationship between akasha and the body and on the buoyancy of lightweight objects is gained the ability to pass through space.

*"Beyond all these is the state of consciousness which is not the product of thought; and that is the cosmic intelligence which is independent of the body (or bodies—physical, astral and causal). By the practice of the three-fold discipline upon that, the veil that covers that light of cosmic intelligence is removed."

44) Through performing samyama on mental modifications that are beyond the ego and intellect comes the ability to remain outside the physical body. Hence all that hides illumination is removed.

45) By performing samyama on the elements in their gross, constant, subtle, pervasive and functional states, the Yogi controls them.

*"By the practice of three-fold discipline on the relation between space, as the medium of sounds, and the sense of hearing, supernatural hearing is gained (since the flow of sound waves is identical with ether or space)."

46) From the ability to control the elements come the eight Siddhis, such as making the body as small as an atom as well as perfection and invincibility of the body.

*"Thence follow psychic powers like the ability to reduce the body to the size of an atom, etc., and perfection of the body and immunity from the ravages of the elements of nature."

47) Perfection of the body is beauty, fine complexion strength and absolute firmness.

48) Mastery of the sense organs is attained by performing samyama on their power of perception, true nature, and relation to the ego, pervasiveness and function.

*"What constitutes perfection of the body? Beauty, grace, strength, and firmness."

49) From that proceeds the immediate ability to have knowledge without the use of the senses, and complete mastery over Prakriti.

*"When such understanding has been gained, the senses function with the speed of the mind, and there is direct perception without the need of intermediary instruments (even the sense organs) and the realization of oneness with the entire cosmic nature."

50) Only through realization of the difference between Sattwa and Purusha will come omnipotence and omniscience.

*"The direct realization of the independence of the indwelling intelligence from the mind, that is from the conditions to which the psychic and the physical

nature is subject, brings with it superintendence over all states of being, and omniscience.

This is the stage of 'I know.' The Yogi knows the sense, the answers to these questions of what the senses are, what their functions are, how the ego-sense arises, what the world is. There is also the feeling at that point that therefore one is neither dependent upon, nor a slave to, the outside world, and need not suffer or behave foolishly as ignorant people act. One is the master of one's mind and destiny, because the body, mind, etc., are all under one's perfect control—which implies a division within oneself—a dualism."

51) Non-attachment to even the omnipotence and omniscience of Purusha comes the destruction of the final seed of bondage, and liberation is attained.

*"When there is no craving or attraction even for such supremacy and for such omniscience, all of which suggest a division in consciousness, and when the sense of duality which is the seed for imperfection, impurity, or conditioned existence ceases, there is total freedom and a direct realization of the indivisibility and hence the independence of intelligence.

"Vairagya is dispassion or disinterestedness. The Yogi has now arrived at the point where he is neither distracted nor subject to psychological distress, because he has the feeling (or realization) that he is beyond their reach. He is, therefore, able to know all these things and superintend all these situations. He suddenly realizes, 'I am aware of this, I am alert and therefore I think I am free from all that. If that is so, if this is freedom, how did I lose it in the first place? As long as this dualism exists the possibility of my falling into this trap also exists, but as long as I am alert I am all right. If I lose that for one minute, I'm going to be lost'."

52) On being invited by a celestial being, the Yogi should feel neither pleasure nor pride, for there is the danger of revival of evil.

*"Invitations that involve the demonstration of such powers or of the characteristics of enlightenment, even when extended by those in authority, whether on earth or in heaven, are summarily rejected without being swayed by attachment or even curiosity. Otherwise, undesirable consequences may arise again, by the revival of duality, superiority, hope and despair, etc."

53) By performing Samyama on a moment and its succession comes discrimination.

*"Undistracted by these, one should proceed to transcend time. By the practice of the three-fold discipline in relation to the truth of the moment,

without the interference of thought which creates the false sequence of time, there arises understanding which is born of the faculty to perceive the false as false and hence truth as truth."

54) It (discrimination) also leads to knowledge of the difference between two similar objects, when their difference cannot be ascertained by class, characteristics or location.

*"From such understanding flows knowledge or the natural ability to distinguish between reality and appearance, even where they do not have other obvious distinguishing marks related to their species, characteristics and location and hence seem to be similar. The possibility of confusion is thus completely overcome."

55) The highest knowledge, born of discrimination, transcends all; it perceives all simultaneously in time and space and transcends all, even the World Process.

56) Kaivalya (liberation) is attained when there is equality between sattwa and Purusha.

* Taken from "the Yoga Sutras of Patanjali with commentary by H. H. Swami Venkatesananda, (a disciple of Swami Sivananda) published by The Divine Life Society, India, 1998 edition."

Chapter 20

The Mystique of Yoga

Yoga and Meditation have fascinated people for thousands of years. They bring the third dimension into our life. What I now write is knowledge that I have gained from various Yogis and from experiences with students during 40 years of teaching Yoga.

Yoga and Meditation Develop the Sixth Sense

Humans have a similarity to animals, who have a sixth sense. But we humans have lost it because our minds have become insensitive to nature. A striking example of the animals' sixth sense was that right before the Tsunami hit South Asia in 2005 all the land animals sensed danger and ran to higher ground. Even the birds flew away before the Tsunami hit. Elephants broke their chains, ran away and survived.

In Indonesia, one tribe of people ran with the animals and survived. Someone asked them why they ran away, they replied, "Our parents had told us that when animals go to higher ground you should follow." In Sri Lanka, one man had read about tsunamis and when he saw the signs of the approaching tsunami, he told everyone to run away and those who did survived. The devastating tsunami dragged entire villages into the sea. In India alone 10,000 people died. To regain our sixth sense we must practice Yoga and Meditation. Another example of an animal's sixth sense is the look on a cow's face when she's being taken to the slaughterhouse to die; she knows she's going to her death. Some cry.

An example of your sixth sense in action is before you pick up the phone you know your loved one is calling. Yet another example is a husband thinking about something and the wife starts talking about that subject. We lose this

YOGI BHARAT J. GAJJAR

sixth sense when our mind is too strong. So to be tuned in to our sixth sense we need to turn off the chattering mind. Yogis say that the mind is part of this material world, but your atman or "self" is part of God and that part knows everything you need to know.

Another example of tuning into your sixth sense would be your buying a house based not only on the price and location, but also on your gut feeling and the energy in the house. Yoga and Meditation help you develop your instincts and gut feelings because your soul knows everything you need to know. My personal feeling is that Meditation is the key, and I believe that if you have a Guru in the spirit, he will always guide you.

Yoga When Planning Pregnancy

Yogis say in order to attract a spiritual soul or good soul purposely, a couple should pray and invoke the Lord before conception. Now if somebody gets an ignorant or lower being, that child will make their life miserable. Of course, life is karma running down. Even if you're supposed to suffer it can be minimized by loving God and praying. When children are young, a family should get them involved in Yoga and Meditation.

Yoga During Pregnancy

I advised a student who came to my Yoga classes throughout her pregnancy to talk to the child and send loving vibrations. We used to chant the Mantra, "Shakti Ma." When the child came out of the womb, the doctor noticed he was smiling. This was unusual. So the doctor asked the mother if she had done anything special to cause the child to come out smiling. She told him she was going to Yoga classes. This same student told me that every time her baby cried she would chant the same Mantra and the baby immediately quieted down.

In Japan they begin teaching mathematics, etc., to fetuses (children in the womb). Now special Yoga classes are being held for pregnant women, which are worth looking into. You should also become aware that the baby's soul is old and that that it is listening. So you should communicate your feelings to the child in the womb.

Pets in Your Home

To have a pet outside your home is one thing; to have one indoors is another subject. If you love animals, you can have a pet and take care of it. However, advanced Yogis feel that it is not a good idea to have an indoor pet because it can be a human soul whose karma was to be reduced into the animal kingdom and might have lower vibrations. Also, what you feed the animal can raise or lower its consciousness.

Once you take on the responsibility for an animal, it's like having a child and that animal will require a lot of your time. And that maybe time taken away from your Sadhana, or your spiritual practice. It is difficult enough without a pet to regularly do your spiritual practice. There are instances of a very evolved soul in an animal's body and that can be a beautiful thing.

Chapter 21

Yoga and the Bhagavad Gita

The Bhagavad Gita is the essence of the Vedas and Vedanta. In the Bhagavad Gita, Yoga teaches how to attain Moksha through merging with God. The Gita doesn't talk about Hatha Yoga, because it is assumed that everybody will practice Hatha Yoga. At the time it was written, Hatha Yoga was too commonplace to be mentioned.

At a Meditation seminar, I told everyone to sit on the floor when practicing Meditation. One girl raised her hand and said that no ancient scriptures ever said that one had to sit on the floor, and asked what's wrong if she Meditated sitting in a chair? I told her that in ancient times there were no chairs and so everyone sat on the floor. So there was no need to say, "sit on the floor." It was understood. You can sit on the chair as long as you don't fall asleep. Most likely you will fall asleep, that's why you sit on the floor. If you sit on the floor, you cannot fall asleep. The first step of Yoga is Hatha Yoga, which leads to good health and peace of mind and ultimately happiness.

To understand this philosophy one has to understand samsara, which means when a person dies he takes birth again, continuously over and over again (reincarnation). The objective of a human is to come out of this Maya (illusion) and Lila (play) and this Samsara, and merge with God, therefore not come back anymore. The first step is to follow 10 commandments—given as Yama and Niyama. Swami Sivananda says, "Be good, do good." Then, of course, non-violence and do one's own Dharma. When you bring children into the world it is your Dharma (duty) to take care of them. If you do not do your Dharma it is a sin and you have to come back again and you develop bad Karma. If you help your neighbor's children, it is called Karma Yoga, selfless service (good karma), which reduces your bad Karma.

What Krishna says about Yoga in the Bhagavad Gita

Moksha
    Leads to
Bhakti Yoga (God Realization, Love God)
    Leads to
Raja Yoga (Self Realization, Meditation, know thyself)
    Leads to
Jnana Yoga (Enlightenment, know the scriptures, gaining knowledge)
    Leads to
Mantra Yoga and *Japa Yoga* (Devotional singing, remembering God)
    Leads to
Karma Yoga (Selfless service, be kind and compassionate)
    Leads to
Hatha Yoga (Good Health, discipline & happiness)

Human Journey at Death

Gita 8-24. Fire, light, daytime, the bright fortnight, the six months of the northern path of the sun (the northern solstice)—departing then (by these) men who know Brahman go to Brahman.

Swami Sivananda's commentary: "The northern path or the path of light, by which the Yogis go to Brahman. This path leads to salvation. It takes the devotee to Brahmaloka. The six months of the northern solstice is from the middle of January to the middle of July." It is regarded as the better period for death.

Seven Heavens

Do Not Return   7. Absorbed in Brahman—Om (Moksha)
                              6. Live with Prajapati* (God in Heaven)
                              5. World of Indra* (King of Gods)
Return When Merits   4. World of Varuna* (Rain Deity)
Are Finished (Take   3. World of Vayu* (Air Deity)
        Birth again)   2. World of Agni* (Fire Deity)
                              1. Path of Gods* (Deity)

"Having reached the path of the gods he comes to the world of Agni (fire), to the world of Vayu (air), to the world of Varuna (rain), to the world of Indra (king of the gods), to the world of Prajapati (the Creator), to the world of Brahman.

From the moon to the lighting; there a person that is not human who leads him to Brahman."

After Bhishma was mortally wounded, he lay on the bed of arrows till the onset of the northern solstice and then departed from here to the Abode of the Lord.

Gita 8-25. Attaining to the lunar light by smoke, nighttime, the dark fortnight also, the six months of the southern path of the sun (the southern solstice), the Yogi returns.

"Those who do sacrifices to the gods and other charitable works with expectation of reward go to the Chandraloka through this path and come back to this world when the fruits of the Karmas are exhausted."

*Deities

Three Worlds and You

Brahman is a nameless, formless eternal reality that we call the birthless and deathless eternal being, God of the Universe and all that is beyond. Brahman is Om, and it is All. Brahman decided to create the material world, which we call She or Mother (Shakti). Then the dance of Siva and Shakti started and thus Light (Knowledge) appeared, which we personify as the Guru. Darkness, which we call ignorance, also came.

In reality, the material world is the extension of Brahman or God (Paramatman or Big Soul). In the material world there is matter and the living being. In living beings we include all that takes birth, gets old and dies, e.g. humans, animals and vegetables. Their bodies are matter but their soul, (Atman) or self, is part of God. If God or Paramatman is an ocean, then my soul (Atman) is a drop of water. So they are the same. The Atman in the living being is eternal and it never dies. It is the same as God (Brahman).

Brahman, when it enters into the material world, enters into Maya. He split into three, Brahma, (not Brahman), the Creator, Vishnu the preserver and Mahesh (Siva) the transformer and they all were given forms. We can worship them. A Hindu can worship only Brahman, or Brahma, a formless reality, or a form like Vishnu the preserver, or Mahesh (Siva) the transformer. Some call Siva the destroyer of negative energy. There is no temple of Brahma, except one in Rajasthan. All other Gods are worshipped in form.

In the Universe there are three parts. One is the material world. The second is the Astral World and third is the Eternal spiritual world. The material world and astral world are Maya and Lila (play). The Astral world is divided into three parts also, Heaven, Hell and limbo (a temporary place) (Fig. 15.1). When a human dies his soul could go, according to his/her karma to Heaven, Hell, limbo or Moksha. A person can also enter into Brahma lok (live eternally with God's family) or merge into Brahman. This is called Moksha or Mookti (ultimate freedom). When one receives Mookti, the samsara or circle of birth and death ends.

Heaven and Hell are temporary. If one goes to Heaven, after his good Karma is finished, he will have to come back to earth again. Those who are dragged into Hell come back to earth again, after paying for their bad Karma. Hell is like a prison.

Lord Jesus and Lord Buddha said, "Once a person is dragged into Hell, it is difficult to come out." Lord Krishna mentioned Hell in the Bhagavad Gita seven times, but mostly he says, "I do not want to talk about it." They all tell humans to be good and do good. Those who live in limbo are just waiting to take birth again. God is loving and does not punish anyone. Our dreams are not given by God. When you see a really bad TV show or movie and you have a nightmare, it is not given by God, but is created by yourself. This earth and its' astral world are both Maya or Lila (play). They are not real. When a person dies, he goes to Heaven or Hell. Heaven is like a good dream and Hell like a bad dream.

We are responsible for our actions and thoughts. Some people who suffer in the human body or a soul can also go down into the animal kingdom, which also is a kind of Hell. Your present life is a combination of the actions of your last life, your actions from this life and what you do in the future. God gives you free will. Everyone creates his own destiny.

Every human being has three bodies. They are the physical body, which can be seen, the astral body, which cannot be seen, and the subtle body, which is the soul (Atman). When a birth takes place, the baby comes with a soul, a physical body as well as an astral body. The astral body keeps the soul's memories from all past lives. When that child grows old and dies the soul leaves with its astral body. The physical body is left on earth for cremation.

Saints do not have astral bodies; they are pure love because they have only the soul. To be in the material world, you must have a physical body, and to be in the astral world, you must have an astral body. When a person dies, his body becomes dust and the soul leaves with it's astral body. When a person does not leave the material plane, the soul with its' astral body is what we call a ghost. Ghosts suffer a great deal, because they have no physical body and yet have physical desires. For example, if a man had been an alcoholic prior to death and becomes a ghost, he will still have his desire to drink. So when a man in the material world drinks and gets drunk, his ghost enjoys drinking through someone else's body. Christians believe that a person should not create a vacuum, and they believe when a person sneezes a vacuum is created. This is why people in the west say, "God bless you," when somebody sneezes. Some fundamental Christians believe that if you Meditate, you create a vacuum as well, so they do not believe in Meditation.

The question is, "Can one attain Mookti or Moksha from the astral world?" The Hindu scriptures say, "No, Mookti is attained only from the material world." God does not intervene in our life. He does only twice in a person's life. The first time, when the soul wants to come into this material world, God gives permission. The second time, as the Bhagavad Gita says, is "at the time of death. If you ask the Lord to take you away from this Samara (circle of life and death), God will give you permission."

Some people believe that God does intervene and others believe that God will intervene if you ask Him to do so. This is why Hindus chant God's name, so that at the time of death you will remember God's name. Your last thought before you die determines your next birth. God gives you whatever you want. As long as you have desires, you will be back because of your own desires. However, if you are fed up with this material world and during the last moments before you die, you say, "Lord, please take me out of this samsara," God will end the chapter and you can merge with God or Brahman. Another way to come out of samsara is to attain knowledge of the self or atman. Or you can do karma Yoga or selfless service.

A person may ponder why a human would want to come into this material world? It is because you wanted to be God, to enjoy, and fulfill selfish desires. This is the biggest problem of human beings. Humans seek pleasure and have ego. Hindus say, "If you pursue pleasure and ego you will suffer. The remedy is to surrender to God, and eat food after blessing it with a prayer. Let God eat the food and enjoy it, and decide if you will eat the crumbs. Prasad is food, which has been blessed.

Hindus say that the goal of life should be Dharma (Duty), Artha (Material Progress), Kama (Passion), and Moksha (Freedom or merging with God). Hari Om Tat Sat.

Chapter 22

Yoga Cures Back Pain

Introduction

In the U.S.A. 75 million people have back problems. There are 7 million new victims each year. Together they cause nine million workdays to be lost annually. There are 200,000 disc removal operations per year and one-third of them require additional surgeries. Eight out of ten people on earth suffer back pain some time in their life. I hope you are one of the lucky ones spared of the problem. I do not know how many people are making visits to the chiropractor, acupuncturist and other doctors for relief from back pain. What I do know is that the least expensive and most effective method for ridding back pain is the practice of Yoga.

Appropriate Hindu Fable

There was a great King who had many servants and doctors coming and going out of the palace when his Queen was pregnant. One day he went out to the woods to hunt. On the way he came across a village girl who was in labor. She sat down and delivered her baby right there in the woods. Then she put the baby in her basket, set it on her head and went on with her business. The King wondered, "What is all this fuss over my pregnant Queen?" The king came home that night after his hunting trip and ordered everyone pampering his wife to leave. The Queen was shocked and asked what was going on. The King then told her about his watching the village girl deliver her baby in the woods.

The next day the Queen called the brilliant Prime Minister, and explained her situation. The Prime Minister told her not to worry, he would have the solution to the problem. He went to the King's prestigious and beautiful garden and ordered all the gardeners to go home. A week later all the beautiful flowers and bushes began to die. The King saw that and was outraged. He asked a servant, "Where have all the gardeners gone? My garden is dying!" The servant replied, "The Prime Minister sent them all home." The King then angrily called the Prime Minister and asked him to explain his actions. The Prime Minister said, "When I heard that you sent home everyone who was taking care of the Queen, I was very impressed. And then I thought, "Why are we spending all this money and making all this fuss over these flowers in the garden when beautiful flowers grow in the woods without any pampering." The King understood the difference between his Queen's situation and that of the girl in the woods.

In olden days, people didn't have cars and walked a great deal to get around. They had to work much harder, cutting wood, and doing a lot of other chores by hand. Today we have to do exercise or our bodies will fall apart. We were built to work harder than we do. We are consuming more fuel than we are burning. There are exercise machines, but Yoga is a very inexpensive way to get in shape.

There are three basic causes for back pain. The first is a damaged disc, the second weak back muscles, and the third high mental tension. There are three remedies for the above problems. For the damaged disc, you need to see a physician. For weak back muscles, you have to begin Hatha Yoga with proper breathing. For tension, you should start Meditation.

My experience with back pain began when I was in college. One summer vacation, I got a job in a dyeing and finishing mill where I had to open the machine, put the yarn in to set up for dyeing, and then close the dyeing machine. It was a huge and heavy machine that required a lot of strength. It was while doing this work that I hurt my back. I could no longer continue to do that job. The doctor gave me an injection and some medicine and told me to rest.

After that, because of the weakness in my back, I had one or two flare-ups every year for many years. After college, I began playing golf and tennis, but still I had the one or two flare-ups to deal with every year. In 1965, I started practicing Yoga. During my first Yoga class I was not able to sit on the floor, I had to sit near the wall. At 34 years of age I began learning and practicing Yoga regularly. After that, I have never gone back to the doctor for my back. I'm 76 years old now, and my back is strong.

In 1974, when I was working at DuPont. At that time, each office had two engineers per room, and my colleague used to make jokes about my Yoga practice. Around Christmas that year he was shaving. While bending down over the sink, he hurt his back and could not stand up or walk. He was taken to the hospital and put in traction. After a week, he was discharged. He underwent physical therapy at $100 per visit. When he came back to the office and told me he was going for physical therapy, I asked him to show me the exercises he was doing. He showed me 10 different postures, eight of which were Yoga postures.

What Causes Back Pain

A person's lifestyle, with its tension and stress, along with weak back muscles, are the causes of back pain. Even outstanding athletes, such as football and tennis players, develop back pain from being too stiff and not being flexible enough. The Philadelphia Eagles football team started Yoga-type stretching exercises and found that they helped their game and decreased the number of injuries.

A leading cause of back pain is poorly built, too soft mattresses. Another common cause is sofas that are too soft, poorly made and too large giving no back support to the person sitting in them.

Here is an old Hindu fable by Yogi Surjit called "The Primal Cause."

"For millions of years Man walked on all fours, foraging the Earth for food. Then one day he looked up. 'God lives up there,' he thought. So he stood on his hind legs, and brought his hands together in prayer. The act of prayer reduced his body support from four to two. He 'found' the Lord, but 'lost' his back." Some other causes for back pain are lack of exercise, incorrect lifting, high heels, bad posture and weak abdominal muscles.

Medical recommendations for back pain are to see your doctor, have bed rest, take an aspirin or muscle relaxant and use a heating pad or ice treatment. Dr. George Hyatt says "most back problems will correct themselves within three weeks no matter what a doctor does. So the object is to make the patient as comfortable as possible." A common theory about back therapies is that 1/3 is art, 1/3 science and 1/3 guessing.

Orthopedist Leon Root says, "Once your back is injured, it is never cured. Low back pain is your warning sign that something is wrong. The next time it hits it will be worse." My personal belief is that if a problem has not gone too far, it can be cured with small lifestyle changes. Keep in mind that orthopedists and other doctors prefer that people use the pills, drugs, surgery, corsets and braces only they can provide. They do not want people to exercise and do stretching. Due to laziness and boredom with exercise, many people prefer the easy way out, rather than change their lifestyle and work needed to heal the back. Yoga is growing in popularity because it is spiritual, occupies the mind while doing the exercises and combines stretches with breathing. Stretching without breathing is not Yoga. Doctors can relieve your pain but can never completely cure your injured back. Yoga is a preventive medicine.

Other Types of Treatments Available*

1. Surgery: A surgical operation or procedure, especially one involving the removal or replacement of a diseased organ or tissue.

2. Gravity Traction: Traction is defined as the act of drawing or pulling apart by application of a weight or force. Gravity traction is applied almost exclusively in the lumbar region.

3. Psychiatry: See a physician who specializes in psychiatry.

4. Pain Clinics: There are a number of steps in getting the pain relief that's right for you. The choice of treatment depends on the type and severity of pain, and how you respond to your pain therapy.

The following is a list of therapies that doctors may consider when treating chronic pain. (Not all treatment options are applicable to all types of pain.)

- Medication
- Physical Therapy
- Psychological Therapy
- Corrective Surgery
- Therapeutic Nerve Blocks
- Medical Devices

5. Hypnosis: An artificially induced altered state of consciousness, characterized by heightened suggestibility and receptivity to direction. Hypnotism is a sleeplike condition. Meditation is not hypnosis.

6. Biofeedback: The technique of using monitoring devices to furnish information about an autonomic bodily function, such as heart rate or blood

pressure, to gain some voluntary control over that function. It may be used clinically to treat certain conditions, such as hypertension and migraine headache.

7. Acupuncture: A procedure used in or adapted from Chinese medical practice in which specific body areas are pierced with fine needles for therapeutic purposes or to relieve pain or produce regional anesthesia.

8. Killing Nerves: Desensitizing the nerve that is transmitting the pain.

9. Chiropractic Care: Is a health care discipline that claims to prevent and treat health problems by using spinal adjustments in order to correct spinal dysfunction, or subluxations. Chiropractic asserts that the brain and nervous system control and co-ordinate all the body's functions in part through nerve branches that exit from the spinal cord between the vertebrae. Some chiropractors infer a causal relationship between nerve interference or compression at the spine and subsequent problems in more distant parts or organ systems regulated by the nerve.

Practitioners of chiropractic are called *chiropractors* or *chiropractic physicians*. In the U.S. they receive the degree *Doctor of Chiropractic, (D.C.)* and commonly refer to themselves as doctors. Chiropractors are licensed in all jurisdictions of the U.S., in addition to many other countries throughout the world. Many chiropractors have incorporated Yoga into their treatment.

10. Meditation: Is a part of the Yoga discipline (Chapter 13).

11. Cortisone Injection: An adrenocorticoid hormone, a naturally occurring hormone made by and secreted by the adrenal cortex, the outer part (the cortex) of the adrenal gland.

Cortisone was the first of the "miracle drugs" for the treatment of rheumatoid arthritis. This historic feat was achieved by Edward C Kendall and Philip S. Hench at the Mayo Clinic in Rochester, Minnesota. Their discovery stemmed from the astute clinical observation that a woman with severe rheumatoid arthritis felt much better during pregnancy, thanks to a hormone from the outer part (the cortex) of the adrenal glands. So they called it "cortisone." On Sept. 21, 1948, Hench gave a synthesized version of cortisone developed by Kendall to a patient with arthritis. Kendall and Hench shared the Nobel Prize in Physiology or Medicine in 1950 with Tadeus Reichstein from Switzerland "for their discoveries relating to the hormones of the adrenal cortex, their structure, and biological effects."

Synthetic cortisone is converted (metabolized) by the body to cortisol before it can exert its powerful anti-inflammatory (and other) effects. Its many uses include the treatment of adrenal deficiency and conditions associated with inflammation.

12. Massage: Healing touch, Eastern massage, Western massage, therapeutic manipulation, soft-tissue manual therapy, effleurage, deep friction massage, percussion massage, deep pressure, Shiatsu, acupressure, reflexology, are all types of massage that may be helpful.

Remedies for Back Pain/Prevention
1. Take a Yoga class and practice Yoga Asanas regularly.
2. Use a firm mattress, sleep on the floor or put a board under your mattress.
3. Lose excess weight.
4. Sit straight on a firm chair.
5. When lifting, squat with the knees and keep the back straight.
6. Do not wear high-heeled shoes.
7. Adjust the car seat if it is improperly tilted.
8. When standing, regularly shift your weight from one leg to the other.
9. Always wear a seat belt in your car; it gives support to your back.
10. Take breaks from sitting when you have a sitting job.
11. Play sports with caution, know your limits, and remember how old you are when playing, but be sure to get exercise.
12. Make time to take it easy and learn to relax.
13. Once you start your exercise program, keep up with it and do not slack off.

Recommended Exercises
The two best exercises are swimming and brisk walking. Traction is great for your back. If you feel the most agonizing pain, like a stab in the lower back, coming from a pinched nerve, you can put yourself into traction. You need something that you can hold on to for a few seconds, such as a bar that is high enough to let your body hang. It's as if you were about to do a chin up but decided not to. Unless you have very strong arms and hands, it is not possible to hang for more than a few seconds. Try this only when no other help is available.

The Following Yoga Postures Are the Most Beneficial For Back Pain

Yoga Mudra, Suryanamaskar, Cobra, Head to Knee Posture, Half Locust, Full Locust, (Pavanmuktasana) Supine Knee Squeeze Posture (this is part of the Wind Relieving Posture), and (Navasana) Boat Posture.

*The definitions are adapted from the online Website

Chapter 23

Yoga and Health

Yoga means physical and spiritual well-being. It is a science of good health. We like to age gracefully and we like quantity with quality, meaning living longer with a good quality of life. I worked for a large corporation for which the statistics stated that when a company employee retires they live about 2 years. The reason is that they give up on life and spend their time in a rocking chair. However some employees live a lot longer, their secrets are that they stay physically active, keep their mind active and stay involved in society instead of becoming withdrawn from it.

Yogis say that a human being has so many heartbeats to live, and when they are used up that person dies. In the modern world, the medical community says that a healthy person should have about 60 pulses per minute, 70 pulses per minute is ok, 80 pulses per minute is border line and 90 pulses per minutes is high and unhealthy. Yogis also say a high pulse is not healthy.

In the US Army when a new recruit comes, they check their pulse, and then they make them run 3 to 4 miles a day. If a young person's pulse is about 80 per minute, it will drop to 60 per minute within 3 to 4 months. When a person runs, they get out of breath and start deep breathing. Yogis say you don't have to run 4 miles to do deep breathing. If a person practices Pranayama properly their pulse will go down.

Phytochemicals

"Newsweek reports that there are some amazing trace substances in vegetables called 'phytochemicals.' Essentially, phytochemicals are the army that protects plants from disease, injuries, insects, poisons or pollutants in the air or soil, drought, excessive heat and ultraviolet rays. They form the plants' immune system.

Since most plants are food for humans, it's no wonder that scientists found that phytochemicals prevent and relieve a variety of diseases in humans as well as boost our immune systems.

Phytochemicals lower cholesterol, reduce blood pressure, stimulate regular heartbeats, detoxify the blood and rebuild the liver, heal ulcers and skin sores, and relieve allergies. For good health a person should eat fruit, along with vegetables, preferably colorful fruit such as blueberries, etc.

Vitamin E also has amazing health benefits. A British study concluded that a dime's worth of vitamin E seems to reduce heart attacks by 75 percent when taken daily by people with bad hearts. Vitamin E is one of a group of nutrients known as antioxidants. Heart disease often results from the accumulation of lumps of fat in the walls of blood vessels.

However, this fat in the blood may be harmless unless it is oxidized. Oxidation is one of the steps that put fat and cholesterol into a form that is deposited in the arteries. The differences in the amount of antioxidants in the diet might help explain why people who live in Mediterranean countries have less heart disease than Northern Europeans and Americans.

Hindu Press International Says (September 10, 2004): "Scientists confirm benefits of Turmeric against Leukemia, Alzheimer's and Other Diseases. The growing popularity of Indian food is evident from the increasing number of Indian restaurants. But it is not merely the lure of the palate that ensures the success of the cuisine; now health benefits will add to the charm of a well-cooked dish. Scientists have found that spicy food could protect the body against damage that leads to cancers, in particular leukemia. Most children in India grow up with the knowledge of the benefits of turmeric. In addition, in a childhood leukemia conference in London it was reported that the root that gives yellow color to Indian dishes is an antioxidant, which can protect against environmental chemicals that damage DNA. Scientists now increasingly believe that lower rates of leukemia in Asia may be due to the difference in diet. Turmeric is also said to slow the rate of diseases such as Alzheimer's and to possess anti-inflammatory properties that could help with Crohn's Disease. Professor Moolky Nagabhushan of Loyola University Medical Center in Chicago said while speaking at a conference that turmeric blocks some of the harmful effects of cigarette smoke, protects against chromosome damage and prevents dangerous chemicals from forming after eating processed food. It has been seen that curcumin, the compound that gives turmeric its yellow color, stops leukemia cells from multiplying. He said: 'Our studies show that turmeric—and curcumin—in the diet mitigate the effects of some of these risk factors.' Ken Campbell, of the Leukemia Research Fund, said leukemia was rare in people of Asian descent. 'This suggests that lower rates of childhood leukemia in India, China and Japan may, at least in part, be due to differences in genetically determined susceptibility'."

Yoga Therapy for Heart Diseases

A study conducted at the All India Institute of Medical Sciences (AIIMS) in New Delhi has shown that the practice of Yoga can help treat coronary heart disease.

Dr. S.C. Manchanda, who is studying the effects of Yoga on heart patients at the AIIMS, told a plenary session of 'new biosciences' at the Indian Science Congress Jan. 7 that he had obtained 'positive results.'

Forty-two patients were divided into two groups of 21 each, and one of the groups was made to lead a 'Yoga Lifestyle,' while the other was not. After some time, coronary angiography showed that the cardiac condition of those who practiced Yoga remained stable, while that of the others had worsened.

Dr. Dean Ornish wrote the famous book called, "Program for Reversing Heart Disease." He was a student of Integral Yoga, studying under Swami Satchitananda of Yogaville, VA and was a disciple of Swami Sivananda of Rishikash. Dr. Ornish says: "At least half of the men and women waiting to have bypass surgery or angioplasty today could escape their hospital rooms and never look back."

A landmark study shows that only small changes in the size of coronary artery blockages are needed to restore blood flow to the heart.

That means many patients—if willing to make tough sacrifices involving diet and exercise—can stop or reverse their own heart disease, the USA's leading killer.

A new finding that has come out today in the Journal of the American Medical Association proves for the first time that blocked arteries can be opened enough to avoid surgery when patients adhere to a low-fat diet, stop smoking, lose weight, exercise and reduce stress. But this program is not easy. It involves eating a 10% fat diet, no meat, no fish, no chicken, and no nuts. It also requires practicing Meditation and stress-reducing techniques based on Yoga, exercising a minimum of an hour three times a week and participating in group support sessions.

A man named Victor Karpenko opted for Ornish's method 10 years ago after his doctor told him he needed bypass surgery, and his chest pain disappeared in a month. Today he hikes and climbs the equivalent of 130 floors on the Stairmaster three days a week.

Insurance companies advise that, with bypass procedures costing $50,000 each, Ornish's program costing $5,000 to $6,000 per patient appeared to offer an economic alternative." This shows that the benefits of Yoga and Meditation are proven by science and accepted by the medical community of the West.

Even Fit Men Add Fat with Age

Jane E Brody wrote in the New York Times on May 7, 1997 that it is not only sedentary men who are finding that the pants they wore comfortably at 40 are hard to button at 50. Middle-age spread seems to be a near inevitable consequence of advancing age, even among men who regularly run long distances. A study of nearly 7,000 male runners 18 years old and older has shown that even those who run long distances and maintain their youthful level of exercise can expect to accumulate abdominal fat when they reach middle age.

And since flab around the waist is associated with changes in body physiology and increases the risk of heart disease, even physically active men should be concerned about their expanding girth. Weight gain occurred at the same rate regardless of the number of miles the runners ran each week. Dr. Williams's reports in the American Journal of Clinical Nutrition, "We aren't seeing a big difference in the rate of gain between those who run fewer than 10 miles a week and those who run more than 40 miles a week. For each decade, the average six-foot-tall man put on 3.3 pounds and his waist grew by about three-fourths of an inch. In other words, by 50 a physically active man can expect to weigh about 10 pounds more and to have a waist about two inches bigger than he had at 20. Physical activity should be gradually increased each year, starting at around 30. For example, an annual increase in weekly running distance of 1.4 miles should make up for the age-related decreases in metabolic rate and permit a 50- or 60-year old man to fit into the tuxedo he wore to his wedding at 30. In other words, a man who ran an average of 10 miles a week at 30 should, by the age of 40, be running 24 miles a week and, by the age of 50, 38 miles a week to maintain his youthful physique. Of course, knees and ankles and backs may be starting to weaken at the same time. Any sustained vigorous activity will do, including swimming laps, cycling and working out in a gym, as long as the workout is sustained and vigorous. Another approach is to eat less, while making more nutritious food selections." As for why these changes occur in physique, Dr. Williams suggested that age-related declines in the production of testosterone and growth hormone might account for the gradual accumulation of body fat." Dr. Williams is now looking into patterns of weight gain in women who are runners. Before menopause, he noted, women tend to gain fat around their hips and thighs rather than their waists. But after menopause, when estrogen levels drop precipitously, women tend to switch to the male pattern of weight gain, accumulating fat around the abdomen. What effect hormone replacement has on this pattern has not yet been well studied. Dr. Williams concludes, that "Either we should allow for the fact that people gain some weight as they get older, or we should tell them they must increase their activity level to prevent weight gain with age."

Since 1935 researches have known that when laboratory rats and mice are fed a very low-calorie diet—30 to 50 percent of their normal intake—they live about 30 percent longer than their well-fed siblings, as long as they get sufficient nutrition. Again, free radicals seem to be responsible: the less food consumed, the fewer free radicals are produced—possibly because on a low-calorie regimen cells' power-generating machinery operates at high efficiency, as it does during exercise.

One of the Yogic Techniques for Losing Weight

Vevekanand Kendra of Banglore India (Yoga Center) has developed a new way of dieting to lose weight. It has five points. They are as follows:

1) A person needs the desire to lose weight and has to set a goal e.g. I want to lose 10 lbs.

2) Eat half the food you would normally eat in the course of a day.

3) Drink about 8 glasses of water.

4) Increase your walking or other exercise.

5) Do 1 hour of Yoga 3 times a week.

6) Do right nostril breathing. It is done as follows. First close your left nostril then inhale through the right nostril. Hold your breath and exhale also through the right nostril. This is called right nostril breathing. Repeat this 28 times in morning, afternoon and evening. The right nostril is called Surya Naadi or Sun Naadi. By breathing this way one burns body fat.

Vevekanand Kendra has proven that doing these five things can help you successfully loose 3 to 4 pounds per month.

Diabetics and Their Problems

The 10 key symptoms of diabetes are 1. Always tired, 2. Frequent urination, 3. Sudden weight loss, 4. Wounds that won't heal, 5. Always hungry, 6. Sexual problems, 7. Blurry vision, 8. Vaginal infections, 9. Numb or tingling hands or feet, and 10. Always thirsty.

Medical statistics have shown that Indians, and African-Americans have at least 30% diabetes while all other races have at least 10%. Obesity also causes diabetes. If you find you have these symptoms please see your doctor immediately and have your blood sugar checked. Forty years ago I developed diabetes. The symptom I had was an earache that wouldn't go away. Keep your blood sugar under control and you will keep your eyesight, your kidneys and your limbs by not developing gangrene. If diabetes is not kept under control it has very dangerous consequences.

Here is an interesting story about health. The source is unknown. Once upon a time, there was a rich merchant who had 4 wives. He loved the 4th wife the most and adorned her with rich robes and treated her to delicacies. He took great care of her and gave her nothing but the best. He also loved the 3rd wife very much. He was very proud of her and always wanted to show her off to his friends. However, the merchant was always in great fear that she might run away with some other man. He loved his 2nd wife also. She was a very considerate person, always patient and in fact was the merchant's confidante. Whenever the merchant faced some problems, he always turned to his 2nd wife and she would always help him out and tide him through difficult times. Now, the merchant's 1st wife was a very loyal partner and had made great contributions in maintaining his wealth and business as well as taking care of the household. However, the merchant did not love the first wife and although she loved him deeply, he hardly took notice of her.

One day, the merchant fell ill. He knew that he was going to die soon. He thought of his luxurious life and told himself, "Now I have 4 wives with me, but when I die, I'll be alone. How lonely I'll be!" Thus, he asked the 4th wife, "I loved you most, endowed you with the finest clothing and showered great care over you. Now that I'm dying, will you follow me and keep me company?" "No way!" replied the 4th wife and she walked away without another word. The answer cut like a sharp knife right into the merchant's heart. The sad merchant then asked the 3rd wife, "I have loved you so much for all my life. Now that

I'm dying, will you follow me and keep me company?" "No!" replied the 3rd wife. "Life is so good over here! I'm going to remarry when you die!" The merchant's heart sank and turned cold. He then asked the 2nd wife, "I always turned to you for help and you've always helped me out. Now I need your help again. When I die, will you follow me and keep me company?" "I'm sorry, I can't help you out this time!" replied the 2nd wife. "At the very most, I can only send you to your pyre." The answer came like a bolt of thunder and the merchant was devastated. Then a voice called out: "I'll come with you. I'll follow you no matter where you go." The merchant looked up and there was his first wife. She was so skinny, almost like she suffered from malnutrition. Greatly grieved, the merchant said, "I should have taken much better care of you while I could have!"

Actually, we all have 4 wives in our lives… The 4th wife is our body. No matter how much time and effort we lavish in making it look good, it'll leave us when we die. The 3rd wife is our possessions, status and wealth. When we die, they all go to others. The 2nd wife is our family and friends. No matter how close they had been, always there for us when we're alive, when death comes the furthest they can take us is up to the funeral pyre. The 1st wife is in fact our Atman (self), often neglected in our pursuit of material wealth and sensual pleasure. Guess what? It is actually the only thing that follows us wherever we go. Perhaps it's a good idea to cultivate and strengthen it now rather than wait to lament until we're on our deathbed.

Chapter 24

Yogic Diet

To a Yogi, food is a vehicle in his journey toward good health, self-realization and God. To him, one is what one eats, as food partially affects mind, body and soul, (the soul is perfect, but it could be covered with impurities). The question arises; does food affect the body, mind and soul? Yogis say, "Yes."

If we examine history, all cultures have used food in one way or another in purifying life in general. Food does affect the mind. If you do not believe this, drink a glass of wine or whiskey and you will have proof. We all know that food affects our health. Americans say, "You are what you eat." In general, heart disease, high blood pressure, obesity, and some forms of cancer tend to develop less often in vegetarians than in non-vegetarians.

Dr. George Watson, in his book entitled "Nutrition and Your Mind," theorizes, "faulty diets are a leading cause of mental illness. He says, "What you eat determines your state of mind and, in a sense, the sort of person you are." Answering questions in McCall's magazine, he says that mental or emotional disorders may stem from your rate of oxidation, or the speed with which your body breaks down food to create energy. He also says hundreds of mental patients, who failed to respond to psychotherapy, electroshock and drugs, showed significant improvement when given large dosages of certain vitamins and minerals.

The Bhagavad Gita says about the Yogic diet in **Chapter 17ᵗʰ Verse #7:** "The food also, which is dear to each, is threefold, as also sacrifice, austerity and alms-giving. Hear thou the distinction of these."

Commentary by Swami Sivananda "All foods have different properties. Different foods exercise different effects on different compartments of the brain or the mind. A confection of sparrow, meat, fish, eggs, onion and garlic excites passion. Fruits, barley, etc., render the mind calm and serene. The nature of food greatly influences the being of a man. Man feels a desire for particular foods according to his Guna or temperament. "There is an intimate connection between the body and the mind."

"Everything in this world is threefold. The food is either Sattvic, Rajasic or Tamasic according to its character and effect upon the body and the mind."

Chapter 17, Verse #8: The foods which increase life, purity, strength, health, joy and cheerfulness (good appetite), which are savory and oleaginous, substantial and agreeable, are dear to the Sattvic (pure) people.

Commentary: "Pure food increases the vitality and strength of those who eat it. It augments the energy of the mind also."

"Sattvic food produces cheerfulness, serenity and mental clarity and helps the aspirants to enter into deep Meditation and maintain mental poise and nervous equilibrium. It supplies the maximum energy to the body and the mind. It is very easily assimilated and absorbed.

"Eat that food which will develop Sattva in you. Milk, butter, fresh, ripe fruits, almonds, green Dal, barley, Parwar, Torai, Karela, Plantains, etc., are Sattvic. Abandon fish, meat, liquors, eggs, etc., ruthlessly if you want to increase Sattva and attain Self-realization. The mind is formed of the subtle portion of the food. 'As is the food, so is the mind'-says a Hindi proverb. If you take Sattvic food, the mind also will be Sattvic. The seven elements (Dhatus) of the body (chyle, blood, flesh, fat, bone, marrow and semen) are formed out of food.)"

Chapter 17, Verse #9: The foods that are bitter, sour, saline, excessively hot, pungent, dry and burning, are liked by the Rajasic and are productive of pain, grief and disease.

Commentary: "Food of a passionate nature produces restlessness in the mind, evil thoughts, excitement, craving now for one thing and then for another, pain, trouble and disease. The Rajasic man always plans to prepare various kinds of preparations to satisfy his palate."

Chapter 17, Verse #10: That which is stale, tasteless, putrid, rotten, refuse and impure, is the food liked by the Tamasic.

Commentary: "Cannabis indica (Ganja), Bhang, opium, cocaine, Charas, Chandoo, all stale and putrid articles are Tamasic. The man whose taste is of a Tamasic nature will eat food in the afternoon that has been cooked on the previous day. He also likes that which is half-cooked or burnt to a cinder. He and all the members of his family sit together and eat from the same dish or plate, food that has been mixed into a mess by his children.

"The food eaten by Tamasic people is stale, dry, without juice, unripe or overcooked. They do not relish it, till it begins to rot and ferment. They take prohibited food and drinks."

Diet and Longevity

Now let us talk about people who live long and happily. If we talk about diet and long life, we must talk about (1) Abkhasians, who live in the Soviet Republic of Abkhasia, and (2) the Hunzas, who live in the Himalayan mountains—and Dr. Allinson's monkey.

Abkhasians and Hunzas are beautiful, rugged people, most of who live for more than 100 years. Some reasons attributed to their longevity and good health: They are physically active (walk and climb mountains)—the Hunzas think nothing of walking 60 miles. They eat fresh vegetables, fruits, wheat, milk, yogurt and very little meat. They will not eat leftover foods. They marry late. They do not eat white sugar; instead they use honey with their tea and coffee. They are proud people who live as a joint family and never retire. There is a high degree of integration in their lives as also a high sense of group identity. Fasting is part of their lives. They are religious.

Both groups attribute their longevity to their work, sex and diet. The mountains, fresh air and water also add years to their lives.

An English doctor who lived for seven years among the Hunzas was astonished by their endurance, good looks and health. He found no cases of ulcers, dyspepsia, appendicitis, cancer, insomnia, or even nausea. The Hunzas' only problem was smoke in the eyes. They tended to sit too close to their fires and suffered from inflammation of the eyes and granulated eyelids.

Rats fed on the Hunza diet have grown rapidly, mated young and produced healthy offspring. They lived to a serene old age and, when autopsied, showed no signs of disease.

Dr. Allinson's monkey enjoyed good health too. The doctor kept a rhesus monkey in his room when he was a young man and allowed the creature to choose his own diet. The monkey chose raw wheat grains, fresh fruit, green vegetables and occasionally potatoes. He preferred his potatoes, unsalted, and his rice without sugar. His weight was steady and perfect. **This is the exact diet that Yogis recommend!**

Famous Vegetarians
Some famous vegetarians were Henry David Thoreau, Benjamin Franklin, Voltaire, Leonardo da Vinci, John Milton, Pope John Paul II, Mahatma Gandhi and George Bernard Shaw.

FOURTEEN YOGIC RULES OF GOOD EATING
1. EAT SATTVIC FOODS.
2. EAT HEALTHY, VEGETARIAN FOOD.
3. EAT PURE, FRESH, RAW FOOD.
4. EAT WELL-BALANCED MEALS.
5. EAT ONLY PRASAD OR FOOD AFTER IT'S BLESSED.
6. FAST ONCE A WEEK OR A FORTHNIGHT.
7. DO NOT EAT AFTER SUNSET OR BEFORE SUNRISE.
8. COOK AND EAT IN PROPER UTENSILS.
9. EAT TO MAINTAIN YOUR PROPER WEIGHT.
10. EAT FOOD COOKED BY YOUR FAMILY OR BY A GOOD PERSON.
11. EAT TO NOURISH THE BODY, AND NOT TO ENJOY ONLY.
12. ORGANICALLY GROWN FOODS ARE BETTER.
13. DRINK AT LEAST 4 GLASSES OF WATER.
14. IF YOU NEED VITAMIN, TAKE THEM.

Now lets take a closer look at the 14 rules listed above.

RULES OF EATING

1. Eat Sattvic Food—There are three kinds of food. One is Sattvic, the second is *Rajasic*, and the third is Tamasic. They are explained as follows:
Sattvic foods are those in the mode of goodness.

*	milk products	*	vegetables
*	sugar	*	freshly cooked food
*	rice and other grains	*	dals, beans, and legumes
*	fruit and nuts	*	food spiced in moderation
*	food eaten in moderation	*	whole grain bread, etc.

Rajasck foods (those in the mode of passion)

*	very hot foods	*	onion, garlic
*	very salty foods	*	very spicy foods
*	very oily foods	*	very bitter foods
*	processed foods	*	food that is over-eaten
*	bleached white bread		

Tamasic foods (those in the mode of darkness)

*	meat, fish, fowl	*	putrefying foods
*	eggs	*	coffee, tea
*	rotten foods	*	harmful drugs, tobacco
*	food partially eaten by others	*	alcoholic drinks and drugs

There is an entire science on diet called Ayurveda. It covers food, special herbs, spices, and medicines for curing various diseases. It also determines the best diet based on various assessments of a person's body. For spirituality, some say, onions and garlic are not good.

David Eifrig Jr., M.D., M.B.A. wrote a wonderful article that I saw on the Internet about not eating trans-fats shown below:

Avoid Eating Trans-fats for Your Health
Disney World and even the makers of Oreo cookies have decided no more. No more to the substance that was once pitched as the perfect food filler. I am shocked at how much of Oreos' white filling was made from this stuff.

Certainly, the calories were bad, but it turns out the foodstuff in the filling was literally killing me. This stuff is so bad that municipalities have started to outlaw it. Restaurant owners in the town of Tiburon, California, just banned the substance.

This substance is deadly—and most food manufacturers don't want you to know it. What is this killer? It's called "trans-fat." Some food producers claim that trans-fatty acids are natural and thus harmless. And while it is true that the fat exists in animals -specifically ruminants, such as cows and sheep - manufacturers, especially in the U.S., use far too much.

For almost 100 years, food manufacturers have altered the structure of fat by bubbling hydrogen through it, increasing its shelf life and decreasing the need for refrigeration. The original Crisco was simply hydrogenated cottonseed oil. Other products made from this process were pitched as healthy alternatives. In the '50s and '60s, margarine was promoted as a safer alternative to the saturated fats of butter. However, studies have now shown that trans-fat has contributed significantly to the increases in heart disease.

What is so bad about trans-fat? It turns out that fat is just a huge chain of carbon atoms. Saturated fat is a chain of carbon that has two hydrogen atoms attached to each carbon atom. This kind of chain is wobbly and is usually liquid at room temperature.

Well, nature needs a stronger kind of fat. So some animals have fat with double bonds between carbon atoms, leaving room for only one hydrogen atom per carbon atom. If the hydrogen atom gets stuck on the wrong side of the chain, we get trans-fat, which is much more stable and harder to melt at room temperature. Margarine is a great example.

Eating trans-fats will increase your risk of coronary events—heart attacks. This is probably due to the fact that it raises the bad cholesterol, LDL, and decreases the good cholesterol, HDL. It also stimulates inflammatory cascades (and we all know that uncontrolled inflammation is bad for our health.) There is ongoing research that links diabetes and even cancers to trans-fats.

The fact is that we all need some fat in our diet—we would die without it. Those kinds of fats are called essential fatty acid. Trans-fatty acids are not essential. True, trans-fat appears in milk and meat, but be careful.

Many other foods contain it. Until this year, food manufacturers were not required to label the amount of trans-fat in their foods, and even now the print on the packaging remains small.

When it comes to trans-fatty acids... What do I do?

1. I try very hard to avoid them.
2. I read food labels very carefully—and if I see trans-fat listed, I put it down and walk away.
3. I avoid bakery goods since most of them still have trans-fat, especially ones commercially prepared in large quantities.
4. I try and cook with olive oil, which is a monounsaturated fat and easy for the body to break down.
5. I ask and encourage the restaurants I regularly frequent to avoid using trans-fat.

Vegetarian Diet Is Healthier
There are many reasons why one should refrain from a meat diet. Medical reports say "much of the fat of meat is in the saturated fat Continuing research into diets is being made to lower cholesterol levels of the blood and thereby reduce the risk of developing heart disease.

Eating a non-vegetarian diet is good, but eating a vegetarian diet is healthier. There are four types of vegetarian diets listed below:

1. The **Vegan** is a pure Vegetarian who excludes all animal products (dairy) and eats plant-based foods.
2. The **Ovo Vegetarian** eats **eggs and plant-based foods,** but no dairy products.
3. The **Lacto Vegetarian** includes in his diet **dairy products** and plant-based foods, but not eggs. Most Yogis fall in this category.
4. The **Lacto-ovo vegetarian** eats **dairy** products (like **milk** and **cheese**) as well as eggs and all plant-based foods (veggies, grains, fruits, etc.)

Health and Science Correspondent Maggie Fox of Reuters in Washington wrote of the Vegan diet, "People who ate a low-fat vegan diet, cutting out all meat and dairy, lowered their blood sugar more and lost more weight than people on a standard American Diabetes Association diet, researchers said. They lowered their cholesterol more and ended up with better kidney function, according to the report published in Diabetes Care, a journal published by the American Diabetes Association.

Participants said the vegan diet was easier to follow than most, because they did not measure portions or count calories. Three of the vegan dieters dropped out of the study, compared to eight on the standard diet.

'I hope this study will rekindle interest in using diet changes first, rather than prescription drugs,' said Dr. Deal Barnard, the president of the Physician's Committee for Responsible Medicine, which helped conduct the study, at a news conference.

An estimated 18 million Americans have type-2 diabetes, which results from a combination of genetics and poor eating and exercise habits. They run a high risk of heart disease, stroke, kidney failure, blindness and limb loss. Barnard's team and colleagues at George Washington University, the University of Toronto and the University of North Carolina tested 99 people with type-2 diabetes, assigning them randomly to either a low-fat, low-sugar vegan diet or the standard American Diabetes Association diet.

After 22 weeks on the diet, 43 percent of those on the vegan diet and 26 percent of those on the standard diet were either able to stop taking some of their drugs such as insulin or glucose-control medications, or lowered the doses.

The vegan dieters lost 14 pounds on average, while the diabetes association dieters lost 6.8 pounds. An important level of glucose control called a 1 c fell by 1.23 points in the vegan group and by 0.38 in the group on the standard diet."

I'd like to speak of my own lacto vegetarian diet. When I was 70 years old, I used to feel dizzy at night. So I went to my cardiologist. He did a catheterization on me at the hospital. After the operation, he showed me my heart on the computer screen. He told me my heart was like that of a young man. He said, "I know you are a vegetarian, but I cannot believe the great condition of your heart." But my dizziness didn't disappear. So he checked my heart's rhythm. It was irregular, because I've had diabetes for the last 40 years. Subsequently, he installed a pacemaker next to my heart. That solved the problem.

Dr. J. Gomey writes, "Cardiovascular—renal disorders (heart, arteries, kidneys) account for 52% of American deaths." Swamiji writes, "The inevitable result of a meat diet is arthritis in its many varieties, because of the accumulation of uric acid and other products in one's blood tissues." Recent studies suggest that other data also have shown a possible correlation between beef consumption and cancer of the colon. Among U.S. blacks and in the South, where poultry and pork have been major animal protein foods, colon cancer risks are low. Seventh Day Adventists, many of whom eat no beef, have a colon cancer death rate 20% lower than expected in Canada and Uruguay, which have a high incidence of colon cancer, also consume large quantities of beef. An estimated 99,000 new cases and 48,000 deaths from colon and rectum cancers are expected to be reported in the U.S.A. in 2006.

In 1973 two key cancer researchers postulated that substances eaten and inhaled by Americans may be causing as much as 85% of all cancer. Irving Selifkoff of the Mount Sinai School of Medicine, said in a paper, "Our food has chemicals designed to improve its taste, freshness, appearance, but which are strange to one's intestines, livers, kidneys, blood… There is literally no place to hide." Too much animal protein causes bodily stiffness and makes kidneys and skin work excessively to discard so much uric acid. The Bible says, Thou shalt not kill." it means all man and animals. On a non-vegetarian diet, spiritual progress is not possible. All Buddhist monks, all Yogis, and many Christian monks are vegetarians. Dr. Albert Schweitzer, wrote, "A man is ethical only when life, as such, is sacred to him, that of plants and animals as that of his fellow men, and when he devotes himself helpfully to all life that is in need of help." Animals eat grains and vegetables and develop muscles. Why can we not develop beautiful muscles by eating grains and vegetables? The vegetarian diet offers strength. Look at a bull or an elephant—they are strong. A vegetarian diet compared to a non-vegetarian die, is very economical. Also, it offers better health and fewer medical bills. Vegetarians live healthy, long lives. Yogis have proved that and also the Abkhasians and Hunzas, who are basically vegetarian. "If this, world is to feed all its people, a vegetarian diet is the only answer. A cow has to eat 14 lbs. of grain to produce one pound of meat. If Americans cut down 10% of their meat consumption, India can eat for one year on the amount of grain saved," says TV commentator John Chancellor. The above-mentioned are just a few of the reasons one should follow a vegetarian diet. Practice vegetarianism for moral, ethical, spiritual, aesthetic, scientific, healthful, ecological, economical and humanitarian reasons. A real Yogi or Yogini is a vegetarian.

HPI says:

HUMANE SOCIETY OF US REPORT ON THE WELFARE OF ANIMALS IN THE FOOD INDUSTRY

WASHINGTON D.C., UNITED STATES, October 28, 2006: Each year in the United States, 10 billion land animals are raised and killed for meat, eggs, and milk (this works out to a staggering 1.14 million animals killed per hour, not counting fish, which are killed in equal number.) Statistically, farm animals comprise 98 percent of all animals in the country with whom we interact directly, and that staggering percentage does not even include the estimated 10 billion aquatic animals killed for human consumption. Indeed, the numbers of animals killed by trappers and hunters; in classrooms, research laboratories, and animal shelters; and on fur farms; and those animals raised as companions or used for entertainment by circuses and zoos, collectively make up only 2 percent of the animals in some established relationship with humans.

These farm animals—sentient, complex, and capable of feeling pain and frustration, joy and excitement—are viewed by industrialized agriculture as mere meat-, egg-, and milk-producing machines, and their welfare suffers immensely as factory farm profit outweighs their well-being. Yet, despite the routine abuses they endure, no federal law protects animals from cruelty on the farm, and the majority of states exempt customary agricultural practices—no matter how abusive—from the scope of their animal cruelty statutes. The welfare of farm animals often loses out to the economic interests of factory farmers who can make larger profits by intensively confining animals and breeding them for rapid growth with little regard for the amount of suffering the animals endure.

Many in the West ask, "Is a vegetarian diet a balanced diet? Without meat, how are you going to get enough protein?" In answer, it can be said safely that a vegetarian diet is not only a balanced diet but also offers good health, supple body and longevity.

Split beans, nuts and cottage cheese are rich in protein, and far superior to meat protein in quantity as well as quality, as they are free of animal fat and disease. But if one eats an unbalanced vegetarian diet, it is as bad as eating a non-vegetarian unbalanced diet.

I would like to tell you about the following recent incident, though a part of me is hesitant. But I must to guide and help others on this noble path.

When my son was 11-1/2 years old and my daughter 10, the pediatrician who had been caring for them since birth became concerned about their health, because they were being fed a vegetarian diet (no eggs, fish or meat). My wife assured her that the children would be fine, and revealed that her 94-year-old father was a vegetarian and in excellent health. My wife did agree to give the children vitamins.

As time passed the pediatrician noticed that the children weren't getting as sick as children on non-vegetarian diet. She finally asked my wife to write down one week's menu. My wife sent her a copy of the Vegetarian cookbook she had written. The Doctor finally was convinced that the vegetarian diet was much better than the non-vegetarian diet. She told me, "I am going to study this book and then would like to ask questions to know more about your diet." When I told my wife, she said she already knew that her children's health was far better than that of many others, because over the years our children did not have any stomachaches, diarrhea or vomiting and rarely even colds. Of course, they did have minor Influenzas.

Many doctors now recognize that there is no need to eat as much meat as typically Americans do, and that animal fat and heavy diets are harmful.

1. Eat Fresh, Raw Foods
If possible, eat lightly cooked or raw foods. Yoga says eat live fresh food. Cooked foods are half dead. Eat fresh salad daily. Mr. Anand Garde and Mr.

N. W. Walker wrote the following report on raw vegetable juices in 1982. "Drinking raw vegetable juices are a great source of nutrition. There are many chemicals that are affecting the human body on a regular basis. We need to eliminate the waste in our bodies and cause regeneration of cells bringing about balance to our system."

Our lungs, skin, kidneys and bowels all have waste that must be eliminated. The vibrations of our thoughts affect our enzymes. We need to create an efficient environment for the rebuilding of our body cells. Changing from non-organic foods to organic food transforms our body system.

When food is cooked at below 130 degrees Fahrenheit, it is digestible, has fiber and vitamins, and the enzymes have not been destroyed. When food is raw and not heated, it has vitamins and enzymes still intact, but its fiber is indigestible.

Vegetables contain natural vitamins and enzymes and fibers, which have toxic elements. Raw vegetable juice contains natural vitamins and enzymes without fiber. It efficiently and quickly transfers energy from food, cleansing all waste in the disposal systems, and is a food supplement. It also has chlorophyll, which enhances mucus elimination.

Juicers will grind your vegetables to a fine consistency by either grinding them or hydraulically pressing them. When you drink this juice, you will digest fresh, clean vegetables, which are ready for immediate absorption. Consumed regularly, juice from vegetables will revitalize your body.

Juice therapy is highly recommended. Carrot juice offers beta-carotene, and improves eyes; Beet juice offers red blood cells and purifies blood. Spinach juice improves digestion; alfalfa juice ensures better hair growth; cabbage juice cures ulcers; celery juice offers organic sodium and combats the effects of heat; string bean juice is good for diabetes. Start today, be a juiceatarian and live vibrantly for a century."

2. Eat a Well-Balanced Diet
Eat in moderation and have a balanced diet (fat, proteins, and carbohydrates). Eat fruits, vegetables, grains and milk/soy milk daily. Keep in mind that soy inhibits absorption of other proteins and most soymilk is loaded with sugar. But a little soy is OK.

When eating your meal, do not go for the second and third helpings. This way you can eat what is needed and in a measured quantity. The more you eat, the more you will want to eat.

A California study covering more than 10,000 disabling injuries found injury peaks between 10 and 11 o'clock in the morning and between 3 and 4 o'clock in the afternoon—accident surges that have been attributed in part to the fall off in blood sugar levels after inadequate meals. An Indian belief is that if a person talks about going out, they must eat some food. The idea behind the belief is that you should not drive on an empty stomach.

Many nutritionists and doctors believe that it is better to eat in small quantities more frequently than to eat too much at one time. Or eat more protein, as it releases energy slowly.

Many people eat an unbalanced diet; which causes their blood sugar to go down. Again, if your blood sugar is low, eat fruit or drink juice, but do not eat heavy foods. Eating protein exclusively is not healthy. That does more damage than good in the long run. If you desire to eat between meals, a piece of fruit, or a glass of juice or milk is best.

A friend of mine told me that when he was in college, he was eating only meat and bread. At one point, his mouth began to smell so bad that even he could not stand the odor. So he decided to go to a dentist. The dentist asked him some questions and one was about his diet. The doctor figured out that the odor was from his diet and he told him to eat 2 oranges a day and some spinach. He had a vitamin C deficiency. After a week of correcting his diet, his problem disappeared. This explains why we should eat fruit and green vegetables everyday.

In other words, eat in moderation. You must decide how much to eat, depending on your need at a given time and place, as also your own physical condition.

Patanjali, in his book, "Yoga Sustra," gives an explanation. He writes, "Half (the stomach) for food and condiments, the third quarter for water, the fourth quarter should be reserved for free movement of air."

3. Eat Only Prasad or After you Say a Prayer
Eat prasad only, i.e. blessed food. Before eating, chant a Mantra or pray. Chant Om or any Mantra or a prayer. It is best to chant the following verse:

"brahmapanam brahmahavir brahmagnau brahmana hutam,
brahmaiva tena gantavyam brahmakarma Samadhina"
Gita IV, 24

It Says: "Brahman is the oblation; Brahman is the melted butter (ghee); by Brahman is the oblation poured into the fire of Brahman; Brahman verily shall be reached by him who always sees Brahman in action."

The food you eat and you who eat food are both life. The food you eat does not become part of your body until you first unite with it with all your mind, body and soul. Also thank God for giving you the food. This way when you offer the food to God, the food is blessed and becomes "Prasad." That means it is not ordinary food, but is a spiritual or Godly food. By eating such Prasad, you will enjoy the following advantages: (1) you will be able to get more nourishment while eating, and (2) you will not get attached to the food.

Many people eat a lot, but still lack energy and have vitamin deficiencies. The reason is that they do not eat Prasad. The best way to bless food is by "Kirtan" (chanting Mantras and prayers), but the simple way to do it is to say "Om" or your Guru Mantras in your mind to unite with the food and then eat it.

Eating Prasad heals one's body, mind and soul. Some Yogis do not eat any life; they eat only by products like milk and fruits.

Bhagavad Gita, Chapter 3, Verse 13 says "The righteous who eat the remnants of the sacrifice are freed from all sins; but those sinful ones who cook food (only) for their own sake verily eat sin."

Swami Sivananda explains the above in his commentary "Those who, after performing the five great sacrifices, eat the remnants of the food are freed from all the sins committed by these five agents of insect slaughter, viz., (1) the pestle and mortar, (2) the grinding stone, (3) the fireplace, (4) the place where the water-pot is kept, and (5) the broom. These are the five places where injury to life is daily committed. The sins are washed away by the performance of the five Maha-Yajnas, which are listed below:

1. Deva-Yajna: Offering sacrifices to the gods which will satisfy them,

2. Brahma-Yajna or Rishi-Yajna: Teaching and reciting the scriptures which will satisfy the Brahman and the Rishis,

3. Pitri-Yajna: Offering libations of water to one's ancestors which will satisfy them,

4. Nri-Yajna: The feeding of the hungry and the guests, and

5. Bhuta-Yajna: The feeding of the sub-human species, such as animals, birds, etc.

Fasting once a week or a fortnight

Did you know that all animals fast? All major religions recommend fasting of one kind or the other and Yoga is no exception. Proper food and fasting are part of the Yoga discipline. Fasting is important for spiritual progress. A Yogi's fasting includes milk and fruit or just water for 24 hours. A Hindu's fasting includes milk and fruit or just water for 24 hours. A Jain's fasting allows only water for 24 hours. A Catholic's Fasting means no meat or poultry for 24 hours every Friday. A Muslim's Fast allows only water for 12 hours. Hindus Jains and Buddhists believe there is a soul in animals, and to kill them and eat them is a sin.

The effects of fasting are as follow:

• Accelerates our momentum towards spiritual life.
• Brings Om consciousness (loving feeling for all).
• Heals the body and calms the mind.
• Purifies the body and relieves mental anguish.
• Awakens the inner faculties.
• Cures many desires.
• Brings longevity.
• Changes the consciousness.
• Relieves pains (arthritis, etc.)
• Improves will power
• Effectively lowers weight.
• Removes body stiffness.
• Opens the door to spiritual worlds.

Fasting gives longevity. In his famous study on rats, Dr. McCoy of Cornell University found that rats slightly underfed in calories, though not in quality of diet, matured more slowly, but usually lived twice as long as those who were given all they wanted all their life. The underfed rats were smaller and youthful, and well-fed rats were bigger. In other experiments, he fasted adult mice two days each week and their life span increased by 60%. Fasting helps even when started after maturity.

Fasting is not recommended when one is going to drive long distances or if one is sick. Yoga fasting lasts 36 hours, which is two nights and one day. It is done drinking water, and/or milk, or milk and fruit. Yogic fasting is done on any one day of the week, but many do it on Thursdays, as it is Guru's day. Some people pick the day recommended by their horoscope.

Fasting is recommended if your body can handle it. It is done on the 11th day in the Indian Lunar calendar (i.e. once very two weeks) by the vaishnavas (worshipers of Vishnu). It is done on the 13th day of the Indian Lunear calendar by Shaivites (Worshipers of Shiva). Alternatively, fasting can be done on every Thursday. The purpose of fasting is to save time normally used in preparing, cooking and eating food (and washing dishes) and dedicating it to spiritual activities. It is a way to squeeze some time out of our busy schedules and using it for Yogic practices.

Do Not Eat After Sunset or Before Sunrise

Yogis say one should not eat after sunset or before sunrise, as it is the time to rest. If one eats after sunset, the body collects fat and that is not good for your health. The main meal should be eaten at noon or in the afternoon. The best time to Meditate is also in the morning, before you eat your breakfast.

Cook and Eat in Proper Utensils

Cook in stainless steel vessels, if possible. Many Yogis cook in mud pots. They use their hands in eating. You must first feel before you eat. One should not cook in aluminum pots.

Eat to Maintain Your Proper Weight

If you want to do good Hatha Yoga, then proper weight is essential. My father-in-law lived to be 99 years old, and my own father who got diabetes at 50, lived to be 94. Both were lacto-vegetarians with excellent health. My father used to ask, "Have you ever seen a fat old person?" I said, "No." He said it's because they all die early. It is good to remain slim or middleweight. One should maintain one's weight from the time one is 21 years of age.

My father used to say "When you are under 50, eat three to five meals a day, after 50 eat three meals and after 60, eat only one meal. My father-in-law stopped eating food and ate only fruit and milk after he was 75.

One nationally televised diet called the "3-hour Diet" Plan has caught people's attention. Nadine Kaylor lost 40 pounds on this diet without cutting out carbohydrates, fat and sugar. This diet was developed by Fitness guru Jorge

Cruise. "What it does is by eating every three hours you constantly re-set your metabolism and as it slowly gets stronger, you burn fat at the rate of two pounds a week," Cruise said. In addition he said you should drink eight glasses of water a day and he recommends that you eat on time in order to lose weight.

Eat Foods Cooked by You, Your Family or by a Good Person

A Yogi will only eat food cooked by a person he knows. Have good, loving thoughts or chant Mantra (God's name) while you are cooking. Food absorbs vibrations. We like our mother's cooking because she loves us.

I used to teach children's Yoga classes to which I used to bring bananas. Before eating them at the end of the classes, the children and I chanted Mantras. Some children's mothers used to ask me, "What kind of bananas are you feeding the children in your class?" I asked why they were asking me this question. They told me that their children said they were the best bananas.

Whenever my students came to my home I would give them Bombay Chai (tea). They would always ask me to teach them how to make that tea. I would show them. They later they would tell me, "Your tea is the best." I told them, "When I make tea I chant Mantras given by my Guru at my Mantra initiation. Your tea will taste the best, if you chant your Mantra while making your tea."

Eat to Nourish Your Body and Not Merely to Enjoy

Eat to live, but do not live to eat. There is nothing wrong in eating good, tasty food, but do not get attached to it. Otherwise, you will over eat and suffer. So many people cannot control their eating. They get fat and unhealthy and consequently shorten their lives. Eat good, healthy, nutritious food to nourish the body and you will enjoy life. If you eat to enjoy, you will suffer. Overeating can drain one's energy. Keep your mind on God and/or Mantra chanting and, not on food; it will help you avoid over-eating. Scientists say it is better to eat six small meals than one or two big meals.

Organically Grown Foods Are Better

It is good to eat organically grown food; also unprocessed foods are healthier than processed foods, e.g. whole wheat vs. white bread. Many packaged foods use too many harmful chemicals. It is best to buy organically grown vegetables and fruits or produce from your local farmer's market. Unprocessed foods also are much healthier. Avoid white flour and white rice.

Whole wheat is preferable. It is better to eat breads that are and say "Whole Grain" on the package.

Drink at Least Six to Eight Glasses of Water a Day

Our body needs cleansing. A good amount of water is needed to remove the toxins from the body. I have noticed that American and European people do not drink much water. In cold weather, one might not need much water, but well-heated homes and offices certainly are not that cold. Water is needed to remove impurities from the body. A large glass of water in the morning is quite good. One should drink at least six to eight glasses of water daily and stay away from sugary drinks like soda.

If you need to take vitamins, do take them

After a certain age some people need vitamins. Take the Natural vitamins like Vitamins E, C or multi-vitamin.

Vegetarianism broken down into a few different traditions:

Yogi—No meat, fish, poultry, eggs, onions and garlic

Hindu—No meat, fish, poultry and eggs

Vegans—No meat, fish, poultry, eggs and no milk or milk products

Jain: No meat, fish, poultry, eggs and any root (i.e. potato, onion, etc.)

Advanced Yogi—Only milk and fruit

Chapter 25

Yoga Vegetarian Menus and Recipes

BY RUPAL B. GAJJAR

In the last four decades, Yoga has become a household word in the West, and America in particular. More and more people are practicing Yoga postures, breathing, Meditation, philosophy and diet. Many people are changing to the Yogic way of life and living it. As Yoga is gaining popularity, so is an interest in the Yogic vegetarian diet. There are many cookbooks available on this subject, but few focus on everyday eating. Unfortunately many are too fancy for daily meals. They are written more or less for fancy dining.

In view of this, I have attempted to compile simple menus and recipes for those who want to follow a vegetarian diet. The menus can be modified to suit your individual needs.

It goes without saying that health food is preferred in a Yoga diet. Whole wheat flour is preferred to bleached flour, honey or brown sugar to refined white sugar, pure butter is to margarine, and steel pots and pans to aluminum vessels.

Yogis hold three different views about milk. Some prefer milk and milk products. Some recommend only milk products, like butter, yogurt, cheese, cottage cheese, etc. and do not recommend milk or milk products. However, if you are allergic to milk or milk products, you should avoid them.

If you eat a heavy American diet with meat and desserts, medical doctors recommend skim milk. But if you are a vegetarian, whole milk, or 2% fat milk, yogurt, cottage cheese and butter are good and nourishing.

Yogis do not recommend eating eggs of any kind. They also do not consider fish and chicken as vegetarian. If someone wants to become a vegetarian, I recommend trying the following menus. They may be changed and combined in various ways.

The following are my suggested menus:

Monday
Garden cottage cheese
Roti (bread)
Rice
Dal Tuar (Lentils)
Green vegetable—Italian beans
Chickpeas potatoes curry

Tuesday
Cottage cheese
Salad
Bhakhri (bread)
Dal Moong (Lentils)
Green vegetable—Broccoli
Potato curry

Wednesday
Fruit cottage cheese
Rayta (Yogurt)
Roti (bread)
Khichadi (rice and dal)
Green peas
Black eye peas or kidney beans

Thursday
Salad
Rice
Bhakhri (bread)
Dal split pea or lentils
Cabbage—potatoes
Eggplant—peas

Friday
Cottage cheese
Rayta (Yogurt)
Puri (bread)
Rice Pulav (rice and vegetables,
Peas, etc.)
Kadi (Yogurt dish)
French beans
Baby lima beans
Cauliflower or cauliflower and potatos

Saturday
Garden cottage cheese
Salad
Paratha (bread)
Rice
Dal Tuar
Mixed vegetables or Okra
Dry potatoes

Sunday
Cheese
Salad
Whole wheat Bati (bread)
Lentil Dal and Rice
Spinach or turnips or carrots

Use yogurt with your dinner every day

Additional menus:

Breakfast
Orange juice or half grapefruit
Hot or cold cereal
Whole wheat toast
Cream of wheat upma
Fresh fruits

Lunch
Salad
Fruits
Whole wheat breads
Sandwich, soups or vegetarian meal like roti and vegetables

RECIPES

Plain Rice
1 cup rice
2 cups water
1 tbsp butter

Presoak rice 15 minutes after washing. Heat water and rice to boil, cover. Simmer over low heat until water is absorbed and rice is tender. Butter may be added for flavor if desired.

Brown Rice (From Yoga Camp Ashram)
2 parts water
1 part unpolished brown rice
Dash of salt to taste

Wash rice several times, add salt and water and bring to boil. After boiling, lower heat, cover and simmer approximately 30 minutes.

Kichdi (Rice with Beans)

¾ cup rice   cumin seeds

¼ cup Dal or dry soup mix* (Tuar) asafoetida powder

           butter

Wash and soak

2 cups water

1 teaspoon salt

¼ teaspoon turmeric

Melt butter in a sauce pan over a low heat, then add cumin seeds, a pinch of asafoetida powder. When the seeds are brown, mix rice and soup or Dal together. Add turmeric and water. Salt according to taste. Heat to boil, stir and cover. Let simmer over low heat until water is absorbed.

• You can use dried Minestrone soup mix for a substitute for Moong Dal.

Rice Pulav

1 cup peas   small cinnamon stick

1 cup potatoes cut in small pieces 2 cloves

1 cup cauliflower cut in small pieces butter

1 cup rice

Melt butter, add 2 cloves and one small cinnamon stick. When slightly brown, add vegetables and rice. Simmer, then add the following spices:

1 teaspoon sugar

2 teaspoons salt

1 teaspoon paprika or chili powder

1 teaspoon cumin and coriander powder

½ teaspoon turmeric

Add 2-1/2 cups of water, boil, then simmer on low heat for 10—15 minutes until rice and vegetables are tender.

Home Made Hard Bread

Bhakri
2 cups whole wheat flour
4 tablespoons oil
1 cup water

Measure flour, add oil, mix with hands. Sprinkle water and mix. Gather dough together. Make balls the size of walnuts. Press it between your palms. Roll out ¼" thick. Grill on both sides until brown. Turn as you would pancakes, and butter.

Bati
½ cup Wheatina
½ cup Cream of Wheat
1 cup whole wheat flour
½ cup brown sugar
1 tablespoon butter

Combine ingredients with lukewarm water. Make walnut-size balls. Boil water in a saucepan. Add balls to boiling water. Cook for 15 minutes. Touch batis with the spoon; When balls come to the top, they are cooked. Place bati in a casserole dish with 4 tablespoons of butter. Bake at 300° for 15 minutes.

Add brown sugar if desired. May be served with Dal. Batis are also good when broken, with sugar added.

Puri (Fried puffed bread)
Puri may be made in many ways. Use whole wheat flour or mix it with all-purpose flour. 1 cup of all-purpose flour and 1 cup whole wheat flour. It may be made plain or with spices.

Spice Puri
Add:
¾ teaspoon salt
½ teaspoon black pepper or paprika

4 tablespoons oil
12 cups lukewarm water.

Combine flour and spices and make a mound. Make a hole at the top of the mound and add oil. Mix slowly and little by little add water. Set aside. Make balls any size you want. Roll it and fry in deep oil. This is used for special occasions.

Roti (Fire Bread)
2 cups whole wheat flour
1 cup lukewarm water

This is a very healthy, everyday bread. Slowly add water to the flour, a little at a time. Use your hand to knead the dough. Set aside for ½ hour. Make pieces of dough into balls and then roll in dry flour. Roll out flat, grill, and turn like a pancake. Put Roti on a fire (gas). When it is puffed, it is ready. Eat it with butter

Paratha (Grilled Bread)

Make a roti dough. Make pieces of dough into balls, roll in dry flour, roll out flat, spread surface with a small amount of oil. Fold in half, spread again with oil then flour. Fold again into quarters, spread with oil and flour. Roll out to medium thickness and form a triangle shape. Grill. While cooking, butter both sides.

Rayta (Yogurt Dish)

1 cucumber
½ tsp salt
1 ½ cups yogurt
½ tsp paprika
¼ tsp ground black pepper
¼ tsp cumin powder
½ tsp sugar
½ ripe banana—mashed before serving

Peel and grate cucumber. Add salt. Let stand for several hours. Drain and squeeze out water. Beat yogurt and fold in cucumber. Garnish with paprika, black pepper, cumin powder, sugar, salt if needed. Yields 8 servings.

May be served with bread and rice. You can also add boiled potatoes to Rayta spiced yogurt, cooked chickpeas are delicious in yogurt Rayta also.

Dal (Tuar & Moong)
Dal means split beans or lentils. The two types of dal used are Moong dal called Mug and Tuar dal.
2 cups dal—Wash and Soak overnight
Cook in a pressure cooker or for several hours in a regular pot. Add 4 cups of water or as needed.

3 ½ tsp salt
1 tsp turmeric
1 ½ tsp chilli powder
2 tsp cumin and coriander powder
10 tsp sugar
1 ½ tsp cream of tartar

Combine all these spices and add to dal. Heat two tablespoons oil over low flame in a small saucepan. Add the following:

1 tsp mustard seeds, 1 pinch of hing (asafetida), 2 cloves, 1 whole red chili, 2 tsp lemon juice.

Combine with dal. Boil for 10 minutes.

You can add peanuts and coconut to Tuar dal but not to Mug. Dal may be frozen or refrigerated.

Yogurt Kadhi
1 cup yogurt
1 cup water
Blend these two ingredients to make buttermilk

2 tsp all-purpose flour or chickpea flour
1 tsp sugar
¾ tsp salt
¼ tsp. turmeric
½ tsp ginger

In a cup, add a small amount of buttermilk to the 2 tsp chickpea flour and beat to make a paste. Heat one tablespoon butter and add ½ tsp cumin seeds, two cloves, one whole red pepper, when lightly done, add to buttermilk (Heat to a boil).

Note: Yogurt has to be kept outside for an hour before you start making kadhi.

Vegetables

Broccoli
In a pan, heat one tablespoon oil, then add ½ tsp mustard seeds and a pinch of hing (asafoetida). Now, carefully add one box of frozen broccoli, ¼ cup water, ½ tsp salt, ½ tsp baking powder, ½ red pepper, one tsp coriander and cumin seeds. Cook until tender.

Peas & Potato Curry
1 tbsp oil
1/2 tsp mustard seed
1-1 ½ tsp chili powder
1 tsp coriander & cumin powder
½ cup water

Cook all the vegetables the same way.

Eggplant and Peas

Dice one eggplant and two boxes frozen peas or 1 cup dried peas that have been soaked overnight and cooked, or fresh peas. Take 3 tbsp of oil; heat the oil, add mustard seeds (1 tsp) and hing (asafetida) (1 pinch).

Add eggplant and peas. Add about ½ cup water and cook until vegetables are tender. Season to taste. (Add salt, red pepper, cumin and coriander powder, and a little soda).

Frozen Okra

Place enough oil in a pan to cover the bottom of it. Add ½ tsp mustard seeds. Let them burst, then add a pinch of asafoetida powder. Add ¼ tsp turmeric and okra. Add ½ tsp salt, ½ tsp paprika, ¼ tsp cumin, ¼ tsp coriander powder. Add a little oil (about 2 tablespoons) as this vegetable will be cooked in oil. Cover the pan and keep it on low heat. Check every 10 minutes. Now separate the okra. Cook for another 10 minutes.

Upma
(From the Hare Krishna Cookbook)

4 tbsp ghee
½ cup peas (frozen, if necessary)
2 medium green peppers (cut small)
1 small cauliflower or cabbage (diced)
pinch of hing (asafetida)
½ tsp turmeric
½ tsp cayenne pepper
1 cup farina (cereal)
strained juice of 1 lemon
2 tbsp butter
1 tsp sugar
2 cups water

Put the ghee in a deep pot and heat it well. Add the chopped cauliflower or cabbage until it becomes clear, and slightly soft. Add green pepper and sauté it about 5 minutes. Stir constantly. Add water, peas and spices. Bring to a fast boil, then turn the heat slightly lower and cook for several minutes until the vegetables are tender. Add farina by pouring it slowly with one hand and stirring with the other to avoid lumps. The farina may be either dry roasted beforehand or plain, according to personal preference. Add the lemon juice and butter. Stir firmly until upma is perfectly blended. Not mushy. This is very tasty and easy to prepare.

Serves 4

Dahi Bara
1 cup blackeyed peas or moong or Urhad dal
Ginger
Salt to taste

Yogurt

1 tsp sugar	½ tsp cumin powder
½ tsp salt	½ tsp black pepper
½ tsp paprika	½ or 1 tsp fresh ginger & green (hot pepper) mixture

Soak the blackeyed peas overnight and blend it the next day. Add salt, hing, ginger, hot green pepper. Heat oil for deep frying. Drop the batter with a teaspoon. After all the baras are done, put them in a bowl of water. Take them out, press them between the two palms of your hands to flatten. Arrange in a deep plate. Add yogurt on top of baras. You can garnish by whipping a little apple butter and drizzling it on top or into the yogurt adding some sweetness.

DESSERT

Carrot Halvah (from the Yogi Cookbook)
2 cups carrots, washed, skin removed, and shredded
2 quarts milk
2 cups sugar
4 tbsp ghee or melted butter

Almonds, blanched and slivered. Pistachio nuts, peeled and halved. Rose water.

Grate carrots. Scald the milk and add the grated carrots to it. And stir. Cook over very low heat, stirring—and it must not scorch at any time. 40 minutes should be allowed to reduce the milk and carrots to the proper consistency. At the end of that time, add the sugar. Continue to stir, and when sugar has all dissolved, add the ghee or melted butter. Stir until the ghee has been absorbed. The halvah will be a deep orange red. Turn out into an ungreased platter and sprinkle rosewater lightly over it. Then add almonds and raw pistachio nuts. Cut into bite-sized squares.

Wheatena and Cream of Wheat Shiro
½ Cream of Wheat
½ Wheatena
3 cups hot water
1 cup sugar (brown) or white
Raisin, almonds, coconut
Cardamon seed powder, if you like

Melt one stick of butter and add Cream of Wheat and Wheatena. Stirring constantly over low heat until brown, add water. Add sugar after water is completely blended into shiro. Decorate with cardamom powder and almonds. Shiro may be made with cream of wheat only, using one cup.

Gulabjamun
1 cup Carnation powder milk
½ cup Hungry Jack pancake flour
¼ stick of butter
½ cup whole milk

Mix the ingredients by adding a little fresh milk at a time. You may need about ¼ cup. Mix well. You can add 1 or 2 tablespoons instant strawberry powder (which children mix with milk and drink). Make into small balls.

Heat enough oil for deep frying. Fry until well browned. Put them in the syrup.

Make a thin syrup in a deep pot with 1-1/2 cup sugar and 3 cups water. Boil and simmer very slowly about 15 minutes.

Homemade Yogurt

Boil one quart milk on high flame. Remove from heat and let it set for about 2 hours (lukewarm). Make sure pot is covered. It is best to use a heavy pot that holds the heat. Add 1 tablespoon (store bought) yogurt and mix well. Let it sit covered for about 6 hours on a pilot light or a gas stove. For best results, yogurt should be kept at a temperature of 115° for the entire 6 hours. Remove and refrigerate. If you don't have a gas stove, then put yogurt in an oven that is a little warm (200°). Preheat oven for 10 minutes then shut off and put pot into oven wrapped heavily in toweling for 6 more hours.

RECEIPES FROM THE SIVANANDA YOGA CAMP ASHRAM

Date Nut Loaf
1 cup chopped dates
1 cup walnut pieces
½ lb butter
1 cup honey
¾ cup boiling water
1-1/2 tsp baking soda
2-1/2 cups whole wheat flour

Mix dates, nuts, butter, honey and boiling water and let stand for 15 minutes. Mix flour and baking soda together and add to date mixture. Bake in lined, buttered pan for 1 hour at 350°. Yield = 1 loaf

Ashram Bread (6 loaves)

Add 8 tsp activated yeast to 1 1/2 cups warm water.

In a large bowl:

2 cups sugar or 1-1/2 cups honey
10 tsp salt
3/8 lb butter (3/4 cup oil can be used)
Add 7-1/2 cups hot water or milk to mixture.

Add flour to the consistency of oatmeal. Then mix in yeast. Add more flour to the consistency of a ball (when the dough is not too sticky and you are able to knead it).

Remove from bowl and knead for 15 minutes. Grease bowl and place dough back in it. Turn around and over so it is all greased. Let rise for 1-1/2 hours then cut into six individual loaves and place in greased bread pans. Let rise for 1-1/4 hours. Bake for about 1 hour at 350°.

To test for doneness, take out of pan and tap the back; if it gives a hollow sound, it is done.

Handvo
¾ cup cream of rice
¼ cup cream of wheat
2 tbsp oil
½ cup yogurt
2 tbsp hot water
1 cup grated cabbage
¾ tbsp oil

Add salt, chilli powder, hing (asafetida), turmeric. Combine cream of wheat and rice, oil, spices and refrigerate aside overnight. Add oil and spice and set out for a few hours. Just before baking, add cabbage. Heat oil, together with mustard seed, hing, chilli and pour over top.

Bake at 400° for 15-20 minutes.

Handvo (large serving)

Measure about 2 cups cream of wheat and cream of rice. Add enough yogurt (about 2 cups) to mix well. 4 tablespoons oil, 1-1/2 tsp salt, 2 tsp chilli powder, 2 green peppers (hot) blended or chopped, ½ tsp turmeric, ½ tsp baking soda.

Keep for an hour or two just like this or overnight in refrigerator. Bake at 400°.

Handvo is always served with yogurt chatni
1 cup yogurt add the following:
½ cup planters cocktail peanuts crushed, crunchy or powdery
1 tsp ginger and green hot pepper fresh or powder
½ tsp turmeric if you want to give color
1 pinch of hing (asafetida)
Mix and serve with Handvo

HOW TO BREAK FRESH COCONUT

Heat the oven or after use, shut it off and leave the coconut in the oven for 15 minutes. Take it out and hit it with a hammer. It will break easily.

HOW TO MAKE GHEE OUT OF BUTTER

Place four or five pounds of butter in a huge pot. Heat it on a low flame for about an hour. Remove as much of the foam as possible. When the ghee is clear, it is done.

The unused portion of the butter can be used in puri and bhakhri dough. It will give a salty, buttery flavor. It will last for six to eight months.

HOW TO EAT BREAD AND RICE

Break a little part of the bread. Pick the vegetable up with it or dip it in the Dal and eat it.

Top your rice with vegetables, Dal and yogurt.

HOW TO MAKE YOGURT (II)

Use a hot plate for very low heat. Boil one quart of milk. Cool to lukewarm. Add one tablespoon yogurt; mix it first with a little milk so that it will blend easily with the remainder of the milk. Yogurt will be ready in 6-8 hours. Without a hot plate, cover and leave overnight in a warm place. Make in a glass or enamel bowl.

WHAT SEEDS TO USE WHEN COOKING WITH GHEE

When you want to cook vegetables in ghee, use cumin seeds. When you are cooking in oil, use mustard seeds. Some Yogis prefer cumin seeds to mustard seeds.

BEST TASTING YOGURT (III)

1 cup whole milk	1 tbsp yogurt
1 cup dry non-fat dry milk-Instant	2 cups water

Mix dry milk with whole milk and water in the blender. Heat to boil. Then cool to lukewarm. Add one tablespoon yogurt to a little milk and blend it good. Now add to the milk. Keep it on the hot plate or in a hot place.

Places where you can buy the following items:
You can buy all these spices and beans in any Indian grocery store in your area. Some items can be purchased in international grocery stores as well.

Spices: Some of the spices used are cumin seeds, which are also called jira, cardamom, saffron and coriander powder. Coriander seeds can be sowed to grow into a small plant. Their leaves add flavor and taste to curries. In addition, they have vitamins you need. Mustard seeds are also called 'rai'. Hing is another name for asafoetida. Chickpea flour has a great deal of protein.

Chapter 26

Yoga Messages in the Gita

A great deal is discussed about Yoga in the Bhagavad Gita. This knowledge is vital to an aspiring Yogi. These passages and commentaries are from Swami Sivananda's book on the Bhagavad Gita. His explanations are very meaningful and precise. The following verses talk about Yoga and Meditation.

Second Discourse, section 48: Perform action, O Arjuna, being steadfast in Yoga, abandoning attachment and balanced in success and failure. Evenness of mind is called Yoga.

Commentary: Dwelling in union with the Divine performs actions merely for God's sake with a balanced mind in success and failure. Equilibrium is Yoga. The attainment of the knowledge of the Self through purity of heart obtained by doing actions without expectation of fruits is success (Siddhi). Failure is the non-attainment of knowledge by doing actions with expectation of fruit.

Section 49: Far lower than the Yoga of wisdom is action, O Arjuna. Seek thou refuge in wisdom; wretched are they whose motive is the fruit.

Commentary: Action done with evenness of mind is Yoga of wisdom. The Yogi who is established in the Yoga of wisdom is not affected by success or failure. He does not seek fruits of his actions. He has poised reason. His reason is rooted in the Self. Action performed by one who expects fruits for his actions is far inferior to the Yoga of wisdom wherein the seeker does not seek fruits; because the former leads to bondage and is the cause of birth and death.

Section 50: Endowed with wisdom (evenness of mind), one casts off in this life both good and evil deeds; therefore, devote thyself to Yoga; Yoga is skill in action.

Commentary: Work performed with motive towards fruits only can bind a man. It will bring the fruits and the performer of the action will have to take birth again in this mortal world to enjoy them. If work is performed with evenness of mind (the Yoga of wisdom, i.e., united to pure Buddhi, intelligence or reason) with the mind resting in the Lord, it will not bind him; it will not bring any fruit; it is no work at all. Actions that are of a binding nature lose that nature when performed with equanimity of mind, or poised reason. The Yogi of poised reason attributes all actions to the Divine Actor within (Ishvara or God).

Section 53: When thy intellect, which is perplexed by the Veda text, which thou hast heard, shall stand immovable and steady in the Self, then thou shalt attain Self-realization.

Commentary: When your intellect, which is tossed about by the conflict of opinions regarding the Pravritti Marga (the path of action) and the Nivritti Marga (the path of renunciation), has become immovable without distraction and doubt is firmly established in the Self, then thou shalt attain Self-realization or knowledge of the Self (Atma-Jnana).

Section 66: There is no knowledge of the Self to the unsteady, and to the unsteady no Meditation is possible, and to the unmeditative there can be no peace, and to the man who has no peace, how can there be happiness?

Commentary: The man who cannot fix his mind in Meditation cannot have knowledge of the Self. The unsteady man cannot practice Meditation. He cannot have even intense devotion to Self-knowledge nor can he have intense longing for liberation or Moksha. He who does not practice Meditation cannot possess peace of mind. How can the man who has no peace of mind enjoy happiness?

Desire or Trishna (thirsting for sense-objects) is the enemy of peace. There cannot be an iota or trace of happiness for a man who is thirsting for sensual objects. The mind will be ever restless, and will be hankering for the objects. Only when this thirsting dies, does man enjoy peace. Only then can he Meditate and rest in the Self.

Fifth Discourse, Section 1: Renunciation of actions, O Krishna, Thou praisest, and again Yoga. Tell me conclusively that which is the better of the two.

Commentary: Thou teachest renunciation of actions and also their performance. This has confused me. Tell decisively now which is better. It is not possible for a man to resort to both of them at the same time. Yoga here means Karma Yoga.

Section 2: Renunciation and the Yoga of action both lead to the highest bliss; but of the two, the Yoga of action is superior to the renunciation of action.

Commentary: Sannyasa (renunciation of action) and Karma Yoga (performance of action) both lead to Moksha or liberation or the highest bliss. Though both lead to Moksha, yet of the two means of attaining to Moksha, Karma Yoga is better than mere Karma Sannyasa (renunciation of action) without the knowledge of the Self.

But renunciation of actions with the knowledge of the Self is decidedly superior to Karma Yoga.

Section 4: Children, not the wise, speak of knowledge and the Yoga of action or the performance of action as though they are distinct and different; he who is truly established in one obtains the fruits of both.

Commentary: Children: the ignorant people who have no knowledge of the Self, and who have only a theoretical knowledge of the scriptures.

Children or ignorant people only say that knowledge and the performance of action are different and produce distinct and opposite results. But the wise who have the knowledge of the Self say that they produce the same result only, viz., Moksha or liberation. He who is duly established in one, he who truly lives in one, Sankhya or Yoga, obtains the fruits of both. Therefore there is no diversity in the result or the fruit.

Section 5: That place which is reached by the Sankhyas or the Jnanis is also reached by the Yogis (Karma Yogis). He sees who sees knowledge and the performance of action (Karma Yoga) as one.

Commentary: Those who have renounced the world and are treading the path of Jnana Yoga or Vedanta are the Sankhyas. Through Sravana (hearing of the Srutis or Vedantic texts), Manana (reflection on what is heard), Nididhyasana (constant and profound Meditation) they attain to Moksha or Kaivalya directly. Karma Yogis who do selfless service, who perform their duties without expectation of the fruits and who dedicate their actions as offerings unto the Lord also reach the same state as is attained by Sankhyas indirectly through the purification of their heart and renunciation and the consequent dawn of the knowledge of the Self. That man who sees that Sankhya and Yoga are one, as leading to the same result sees rightly.

Section 6: But renunciation, O mighty-armed Arjuna, is hard to attain without Yoga; the Yoga-harmonized sage quickly goes to Brahman (formless reality or God).

Commentary: Muni is one who does Manana (Meditation or reflection). Yoga is performance of action without selfish motive, as an offering unto the Lord.

Brahman here signifies renunciation or Sannyasa, because renunciation consists in the knowledge of the Self. A Muni, the sage of Meditation, the Yoga-harmonized, i.e., purified by the performance of action, quickly attains Brahman, the true renunciation which is devotion to the knowledge of the Self. Therefore Karma Yoga is better. It is easy for a beginner. It prepares him for the higher Yoga by purifying his mind.

Section 27: Shutting out (all) external contacts and fixing the gaze between the eyebrows, equalizing the outgoing and incoming breaths moving within the nostrils,

Commentary: The verses 27 and 28 deal with the Yoga of Meditation (Dhyana). External objects or contacts are the sound and the other sense-objects. If the mind does not think of the external objects, they are shut out from the mind. The senses are the doors or avenues through which sound and the other sense-objects enter the mind.

'Muni' is one who does Manana or reflection and contemplation. If you fix the gaze between the eyebrows, the eyeballs remain fixed and steady. Rhythmical breathing is described here. You will have to make the breath rhythmical. The mind becomes steady when the breath becomes rhythmical. When the breath becomes rhythmical, there is perfect harmony in the mind and the whole system.

Section 28: With the senses, the mind and the intellect controlled, being free from desire, fear and anger, and having liberation as his supreme goal, the sage is verily liberated forever.

Commentary: If one is free from desire, fear and anger, one enjoys perfect peace of mind. When the senses, the mind and the intellect are subjugated, the sage does constant contemplation and attains forever to the absolute freedom or Moksha.

The mind becomes restless when the modifications of desire, fear and anger arise in it. When one becomes desireless, the mind moves towards the Self spontaneously; and liberation or Moksha becomes one's highest goal.

Sixth Discourse, Section 2: Do thou, O Arjuna, know Yoga to be that which they call renunciation: no one verily becomes a Yogi who has not renounced thoughts.

Commentary: *Sankalpa* is the working of the imagining faculty of the mind that makes plans for the future and guesses the results of plans so formed. No one who plans and schemes and expects fruits for his actions can become a Karma Yogi. No devotee of action who has not renounced the thought of the fruit of his actions can become a Yogi of steady mind. The thought of the fruits will make the mind unsteady.

Lord Krishna eulogizes Karma Yoga here, because it is the means or an external aid (Bahiranga Sadhana) to Dhyana Yoga. It leads to the Yoga of Meditation in due course. In order to encourage the practice of Karma Yoga it is stated here that Karma Yoga is Sannyasa.

Section 3: For a sage who wishes to attain to Yoga, action is said to be the means; for the same sage who has attained to Yoga, inaction (quiescence) is said to be the means.

Commentary: For a man who cannot practice Meditation for a long time and who is not able to keep his mind steady in Meditation, action is a means to get himself enthroned in Yoga. Action purifies his mind and makes the mind fit for the practice of steady Meditation. Action leads to steady concentration and Meditation.

For the sage who is enthroned in Yoga, Sama or renunciation of actions is said to be the means. The more perfectly he abstains from actions, the more steady his mind is, and the more peaceful he is, the more easily and thoroughly does his mind get fixed in the Self. "For a Brahmana there is no wealth like unto the knowledge of oneness and homogeneity (of the Self in all beings), straightforwardness and renunciation of all actions."

Section 4: When a man is not attached to the sense-objects or to actions, having renounced all thoughts, then he is said to have attained to Yoga.

Commentary: Yogarudha: "he who is established in Yoga" When a Yogi, by keeping the mind quite steady, by withdrawing it from the objects of the senses, has attachment neither for sensual objects such as sound, nor for the actions knowing that they are of no use to him; when he has renounced all thoughts which generate various sorts of desires for the objects of this world and of the next, then he is said to have become a Yogarudha.

Do not think of sense-objects. The desires will die by themselves. How can you free yourself from thinking of the objects? Think of God or the Self. Then you can avoid thinking of the objects. Then you can free yourself from thinking of the objects of the senses.

Renunciation of thoughts implies that all desires and all actions should be renounced, because all desires are born of thoughts. You think first and later act (strive) to possess the objects of your desire for enjoyment. "Whatever a man desires, that he wills; And whatever he wills, that he does."

Section 18: When the perfectly controlled mind rests only in the Self, free from longing for all the objects of desires, then it is said, 'He is united'.

Commentary: *Perfectly controlled mind*: The mind with one-pointedness. When all desires for the objects of pleasure seen or unseen die, the mind becomes very peaceful and rests steadily in the Supreme Self within. As the Yogi is perfectly harmonized, as he has attained to oneness with the Self and as he has become identical with Brahman, sense phenomena and bodily affections do not disturb him. He is conscious of his immortal, imperishable and invincible nature.

Yukta means 'united' (with the Self) or harmonized or balanced. Without union with the Self neither harmony nor balance nor Samadhi is possible.

Section 10: Let the Yogi try constantly to keep the mind steady, remaining in solitude, alone with the mind and the body controlled, and free from hope and greed.

Commentary: The Yogi who treads the path of renunciation can practice Meditation in a solitary cave in the mountains. He should renounce all possessions.

A householder with Yogic tendencies and spiritual inclination can practice Meditation in a solitary and quiet room in his own house or any solitary place on the banks of any holy river (during the holidays or throughout the year if he is a whole-time aspirant or if he has retired from service). The practice must be constant. Only then can one attain Self-realization surely and quickly. He who practices Meditation by fits and starts and for a few minutes daily will not be able to achieve any tangible results in Yoga. The Yogic aspirant should be free from hope, desire and greed. Only then will he have a steady mind. Hope, desire and greed make the mind ever restless and turbulent. They are the enemies of peace and Self-knowledge. The aspirant should not have many possessions either. He can only keep those articles, which are absolutely necessary for the maintenance of his body. If there are many possessions, the mind will be ever thinking of them and attempting to protect them.

If you are well established in the practice of Pratyhara, Sama and Dama (withdrawal of the senses, control of mind and the body, respectively), if you have the senses under your full control, you can find perfect solitude and peace even in the most crowded and noisy place of a big city. If the senses are turbulent, if you have not got the power to withdraw them, you will have no peace of mind even in a solitary cave of the Himalayas.

He who has reduced his wants, who has no attraction for the world, who has discrimination and a burning aspiration for liberation, and who has observed Mauna (the vow of silence) for months together will be able to live in a cave.

You should have perfect control over the body through the regular practice of Yoga Asanas before you take to serious and constant Meditation. Aparigraha means 'non-covetousness,' 'freedom from possession.'

The spiritual aspirant need not bother himself about his bodily needs. Everything is provided by God. Everything is pre-arranged by Mother Nature. She looks after the bodily needs of all very carefully in a more efficient manner than they themselves would do. She knows better what the requirements are and provides them then and there. Understand the mysterious ways of Mother Nature and become wise. Be grateful for Her unique kindness, grace and mercy.

Section 11: In a clean spot, having established a firm seat of his own, neither too high nor too low, made of a cloth, a skin and kusa-grass, one over the other,

Commentary: In this verse the Lord has prescribed the external seat for practicing Meditation. Sit on a naturally clean spot, such as the bank of a river. Or, make the place clean, wherever you want to practice Meditation.

Section 12: There, having made the mind one-pointed, with the actions of the mind and the senses controlled, and seated on the seat, let him practice Yoga for the purification of the self.

Commentary: The self means the mind. The real supreme Self is the Atma. This is primary (Mukhya). Mind also is the self. But this is used in a secondary sense. Mukhya Atma is Brahman or the highest Self. Gauna Atma is the mind.

Make the mind one-pointed by collecting all its dissipated rays through the practice of Yoga. Withdraw it from all sense objects again and again and try to fix it steadily on your center or point of Meditation. Gradually you will have concentration of the mind or one-pointed-ness. You must practice very regularly. Only then will you succeed. Regularity is of paramount importance. You should know the ways and habits of the mind through daily introspection, self-analysis or self-examination. You should know of the laws of the mind. Then it will be easy for you to check the wandering mind. When you sit for Meditation, and when you deliberately attempt to forget the worldly objects, all sorts of worldly thoughts will crop up in your mind and disturb your Meditation.

You will be quite astonished. Thoughts you had entertained several years ago, and memories of the past will bubble up and force the mind to wander in all directions. The trap door of the vast subconscious mind will be opened, the lid of the storehouse of thoughts within will be lifted up and the thoughts will gush out in a continuous stream. The more you attempt to still them, the more will they bubble up with redoubled force and strength.

Be not discouraged. Never despair. Through regular and constant Meditation you can purify the subconscious mind and its constant memories. The fire of Meditation will burn all thoughts. Be sure of this. Meditation is a potent weapon to annihilate the poisonous worldly thoughts. Be assured of this.

Section 13: Let him firmly hold his body, head and neck erect and still, gazing at the tip of his nose, without looking around.

Commentary: You cannot practice Meditation without a firm seat. If the body is unsteady, the mind also will become unsteady. There is an intimate connection between the body and the mind. If you keep the body, head and neck erect, the spinal cord also will be erect and the Kundalini will rise up steadily through the subtle 'nerve-channel' (Naadi) called the Sushumna. Sit in the Lotus Posture. This will help you in maintaining the nervous equilibrium and mental poise. You should steadily direct your gaze towards the tip of your nose. This is known as the Nasikagra Drishti. The other gaze is the Bhrumadhya Drishti or gazing between the two eyebrows where the psychic center known as the Ajna Chakra is situated. If you practice this with open eyes it may produce a headache. Foreign particles or dust may fall into the eyes. There may be distraction of the mind also. Do not strain the eyes. When you practice concentration at the tip of the nose you will experience various aromas. When you concentrate your gaze at the Ajna Chakra you will experience perception of supra-phenomenal lights. This is an experience to give you encouragement, push you up in the spiritual path and convince you of the existence of transcendental or supra-physical things.

Section 14: Serene-minded, fearless, firm in the vow of a Brahmachari, having controlled the mind, thinking of Me and balanced in mind, let him sit, having Me as his supreme goal.

Commentary: The spiritual aspirant should possess serenity of mind. The Divine Light can descend only in a serene mind. Serenity is attained by the eradication of Vasanas or desires and cravings. He should be fearless. This is the most important qualification. A timid man or a coward is very far from Self-realization.

Section 16: Verily Yoga is not possible for him who eats too much, nor for him who does not eat at all, nor for him who sleeps too much nor for him who is awake, O Arjuna.

Commentary: You must observe moderation in eating and sleeping. If you eat too much, you will feel drowsy, and sleep will overpower you. You will get indigestion, and diseases of the bowels and the liver. If you eat too little you will get weak and will not be able to sit for a long time in Meditation.

Section 17: Yoga becomes the destroyer of pain for him who is moderate in eating and recreation, who is moderate in exertion in actions, who is moderate in sleep and wakefulness.

Commentary: Too much of austerity is not necessary for Self-realization. Austerity should not mean self-torture. Then it becomes diabolical. Always adopt the happy medium or the middle course. Take measured food. Sleep and wake up at the prescribed time.

Section 20: When the mind, restrained by the practice of Yoga, attains to quietude and when seeing the Self by the self, he is satisfied in his own self,

Commentary: When the mind is completely withdrawn from the objects of the senses, supreme peace reigns within the heart. When the mind becomes quite steady by constant and protracted practice of concentration, the Yogi beholds the Supreme Self by the mind which is rendered pure and one-pointed and attains to supreme satisfaction in the Self within.

Section 21: When he (the Yogi) feels that infinite bliss which can be grasped by the (pure) intellect and which transcends the senses, and established wherein he never moves from the reality,

Commentary: The infinite bliss of the Self (which is beyond the reach of the senses) can be grasped (realized) by the pure intellect independently of the senses. During deep Meditation the senses cease to function as they are involved into their cause, the mind. The intellect is rendered pure by the practice of Yama (self-restraint) and Niyama (observances and disciplinary practices) and constant Meditation.

Section 22: Which, having obtained, he thinks there is no other gain superior to it; wherein established, he is not moved even by heavy sorrow,

Commentary: *Which*: the gain or the realization of the Self or the immortal soul.

Wherein: in the all-blissful Self, which is free from delusion and sorrow. The Self is all-full and self-contained. All the desires are fulfilled when one attains Self-realization. That is the reason why the Lord says: "There is no other acquisition superior to Self-realization." If one gets himself established in the Supreme Self within, he cannot be shaken even by heavy sorrow and pain, because he is mindless and he is identifying himself with the sorrowless and painless Brahman. One can experience pain and sorrow when he identifies himself with the body and the mind. If there is no mind, there cannot be any pain. When one is under chloroform he feels no pain even when his hand is amputated, because the mind is withdrawn from the body.

Section 23: Let that be known by the name of Yoga, the severance from union with pain. This Yoga should be practiced with determination and with a non-despondent mind.

Commentary: In verses 20, 21 and 22, the Lord describes the benefits of Yoga, viz., perfect satisfaction by resting in the Self, infinite and unending bliss, freedom from sorrow and pain, etc. He further adds that this Yoga should be practiced with a firm conviction and iron determination and without non-depression of heart. A spiritual aspirant with a wavering mind will not be able to attain success in Yoga. He will leave the practice when he meets with some obstacles on the path. The practitioner must also be bold, cheerful and self-reliant.

Section 24: Abandoning without reserve all desires born of thought and imagination and completely restraining the whole group of senses by the mind from all sides.

Commentary: *Without reserve:* The mind is so diplomatic that it keeps certain desires for its secret gratification. Therefore you should completely abandon all desires without reservation.

Section 25: Little by little let him attain to quietude by the intellect held firmly; having made the mind establish itself in the Self, let him not think of anything.

Commentary: The practitioner of Yoga should attain tranquility gradually or by degrees, by means of the intellect controlled by steadiness. The peace of the Eternal will fill the heart gradually with thrill and bliss through the constant and protracted practice of steady concentration. He should make the mind constantly abide in the Self within through ceaseless practice. If anyone constantly thinks of the immortal Self within, the mind will cease to think of the objects of sense-pleasure. The mental energy should be directed along the spiritual channel by Atma-chintana or constant contemplation on the Self.

Section 26: From whatever cause the restless and unsteady mind wanders away, from that let him restrain it and bring it under control of the Self-alone.

Commentary: Just as you drag the bull again and again to your house when it runs out, so also you will have to drag the mind to your point or center again and again when it runs towards the external objects.

Section 27: Supreme Bliss verily comes to this Yogi whose mind is quite peaceful, whose passion is quieted, who has become Brahman and who is free from sin.

Commentary: In this verse and in the next also the Lord describes the benefits of Yoga.

Supreme (eternal, unalloyed and uninterrupted) bliss comes to the Yogi whose mind is perfectly serene, who has calmed his passionate nature, who has destroyed all sorts of attachments, who has attained knowledge of the Self and thus become a Jivanmukta or one who is liberated while living, who feels that all is Brahman only, and who is taintless, i.e., who is not affected by Dharma or ADharma (good or evil).

Section 28: The Yogi, always engaging the mind thus (in the practice of Yoga), freed from sins, easily enjoys the Infinite Bliss of contact with Brahman (the Eternal).

Commentary: By Yogic practices, such as the withdrawal of the senses, concentration and Meditation, he loses contact with the objects of the senses and comes into contact with Brahman or the immortal Self within and thus enjoys the Infinite Bliss of Brahman.

Sensual pleasures are transitory or fleeting, but the bliss of Brahman is uninterrupted undecaying and everlasting. That is the reason why one should attempt to realize the Self within.

The Yogi removes the obstacles that stand in the way of obtaining union with the Lord and thus always keeps the mind steady in the Self.

Section 29: With the mind harmonized by Yoga he sees the Self-abiding in all beings and all beings in the Self; he sees the same everywhere.

Commentary: The Yogi beholds through the eye of intuition (Jnana-Chakshus or Divya-Chakshus) oneness or unity of the Self everywhere. This is a sublime and magnanimous vision indeed. He feels, "All indeed is Brahman.' He beholds that all beings are one with Brahman and that the Self and Brahman are identical.

Section 32: He who, through the likeness of Self, O Arjuna, sees equality everywhere, be it pleasure or pain, he is regarded as the highest Yogi.

Commentary: He sees that whatever is pleasure or pain to himself is also pleasure and pain to all other beings. He does not harm anyone. He is quite harmless. He wishes good to all. He is compassionate to all creatures. He has a very soft and large heart. He sees thus equality everywhere as he is endowed with the right knowledge of the Self, as he beholds only Self everywhere, and he is established in the unity of the Self. Therefore he is considered as the highest among all Yogis.

Section 35: Undoubtedly, O mighty-armed Arjuna, the mind is restless and difficult to control, but by practice and by dispassion it may be restrained.

Commentary: The constant or repeated effort to keep the wondering mind steady by constant Meditation on the center, ideal, goal or object of Meditation or practice. The same idea or thought of the Self or God is constantly repeated. This constant repetition destroys vacillation of the mind and desires, and makes it steady and one-pointed.

Dispassion or indifference to sense-objects in this world or in the other, here or hereafter, seen or unseen, heard or unheard, is achieved through constantly looking into the evil in them. You will have to train the mind by constant reflection on the immortal, all blissful Self. You must make the mind realize the transitory nature of worldly enjoyments. You must suggest to the mind to look for its enjoyment not in the perishable and changing external objects but in the immortal, changeless Self within. Gradually the mind will be withdrawn from the external objects.

Section 36: I think Yoga is hard to be attained by one of uncontrolled self, but the self-controlled and striving one can attain to it by the (proper) means.

Commentary: *Uncontrolled self:* he who has not controlled the senses and the mind by the constant practice of dispassion and Meditation. *Self-controlled*: he who has controlled the mind by the constant practice of dispassion and Meditation. He can attain Self-realization by the right means and constant endeavor.

Section 42: Or he is born in a family of even the wise Yogis; verily a birth like this is very difficult to obtain in this world.

Commentary: A birth in a family of wise Yogis is more difficult to obtain than the one born in a house of the pure and wealthy.

Section 46: The Yogi is thought to be superior to the ascetics and even superior to men of knowledge (obtained through the study of scriptures); he is also superior to men of action; therefore be thou a Yogi, O Arjuna.

Commentary: To all these the Yogi is superior, for he has direct knowledge of the Self through intuition or direct cognition through Nirvikalpa Samadhi.

Eighth Discourse, Section 27: Knowing these paths, O Arjuna, no Yogi is deluded; therefore at all times be steadfast in Yoga.

Commentary: Knowing the nature of the two paths (bright and dark paths) and the consequences they lead to, a Yogi never loses his discrimination. The Yogi who knows that the path of God or the path of light leads to Moksha (gradual liberation), and the path of darkness to Samsara or the world or region of birth and death, is no longer deluded. Knowledge of these two paths serves as a compass or a beacon light to guide the Yogi's steps at every moment. He strives to stick to the path of light.

Twelfth Discourse, Section 9: If thou art unable to fix thy mind steadily on Me, then by the Yoga of constant practice do thou seek to reach Me, O Arjuna.

Commentary: The practice of repeatedly withdrawing the mind from all sorts of sensual objects and fixing it again and again on one particular object or the Self. If your mind wanders much, try to fix it on the Lord through the continuous practice of remembrance.

Section 10: If thou art unable to practice even this (Abhyasa Yoga) constant steadying of the mind, be thou intent on doing actions for My sake; even by doing actions for My sake, thou shalt attain perfection.

Commentary: Even if you do mere actions for the sake of the Lord, without practicing Yoga you will attain perfection. First you will attain purity of mind, then Yoga concentration and Meditation, then knowledge and ultimately perfection or liberation. Even when you serve humanity with the feeling that you are serving the Lord is also considered doing actions for the sake of the lord. Such service should go hand in hand with worship of God and Meditation.

Section 11: If thou art unable to do even this, then, resorting to union with Me, renounce the fruits of all actions with the self-controlled.

Commentary: This is the easiest path.

Section 12: Better indeed is knowledge than practice; knowledge of Meditation is better than renunciation of the fruits of action: peace immediately follows renunciation.

Commentary: Desire is an enemy of peace. Desire causes restlessness of the mind, and is the source of all human miseries, sorrows and troubles. Stop the play of desire through discrimination, dispassion and enquiry into the nature of the Self; then you will enjoy supreme peace.

Renunciation of the fruits of action is prescribed for the purification of the aspirant's heart. It annihilates desire, the enemy of wisdom. The sage, too, renounces the fruits of actions. It has become natural to him to do so.

Thirteenth Discourse, Section 24: Some by Meditation behold the Self in the self by the self, others by the Yoga of knowledge, and still others by the Yoga of action.

Commentary: There are several paths to reach the knowledge of the Self according to the nature or temperament and capacity of the individual.

Section 25: Others also, not knowing thus, worship, having heard of it from others; they, too, cross beyond death, regarding what they have heard as the supreme refuge.

Commentary: The three paths, Yoga of Meditation, Yoga of Knowledge and the Yoga of action have all been described. Now the Yoga of worship is described.

Some who are ignorant of the methods described in the previous verse listen to the teachings of the spiritual preceptors regarding this great Truth or the Self with intense and unshakable faith, solely depending upon the authority of others' instructions and through constant remembrance and contemplation of them attain immortality. They are devoted to their preceptor. Some study the books written by realized seers, stick with great faith to the teachings contained therein and live according to them. They also overcome death. Whichever path one follows, one eventually attains the knowledge of the Self and final liberation from birth and death,—salvation. There are several paths to suit aspirants of different temperaments and equipments.

Chapter 27

Brahmachara

Brahmachara means continence or celibacy. In America, people are reluctant to talk about celibacy because it is taboo culturally, but in Yoga it is part of tradition. Beginner Yoga students do not probably need to know but it is good to know about it for your spiritual practice. Sexual energy is very important for spiritual sadhana or spiritual practices.

Maharishi Patanjali, in his Yoga Sutra book, says the first step of Asthanga Yoga is *Yama,* which consists of five things: 1) Non-injury, 2) Truthfulness, 3) Non-stealing, 4) Continence, and 5) Non-possession. In this chapter we shall explore continence.

In India Yogi's, Swami's, Sadhu's or Hindu monks observe strict celibacy. Please note that some Yogi's do marry. In the Christian tradition, Lord Jesus and his disciples were celibate and the Catholic Church has Fathers who are unmarried and celibate.

To preach religious messages sexual energy is very vital. In Jesus's time so few did so much, but now so many can do so little because the preachers are not strictly conserving sexual energy. I'd like to tell you of an incident. Two Swamis from India came to give a lecture at the Sivananda Yoga Center in Wilmington, Delaware. After Satsang or the meeting, I invited them for dinner at my home. While my wife, Rupal, was busy cooking I asked the Swamiji's why there was so much high energy at the Center when they started chanting and everyone blissed out. I asked from where does this energy come? They said it was because of their strict celibacy.

273

Mahatma Gandhi wrote in his book that, after having children, his wife and he observed celibacy. All of you know that when he gave talks he had everyone in the palm of his hands and that everyone was hanging on his every word. Maybe we should ask from where does this energy comes?

I've been teaching Yoga over the last 38 years. After one of my classes, a couple told me, "We love each other, but everything is going wrong. What is the reason?" I advised them to restrain sexual activity. I told them not to touch each other for a whole month, and then to come back and tell me if things had improved. This solved their problem. They came back and told me everything was now going well.

Spiritual energy is very essential for preaching religious and spiritual messages. I'd like to give you two examples. First, a Yogi friend from India told me that Baba Muktananda was coming to New York for the first time. He suggested that I go for his Darshan (spiritual blessing). So I went. A small gathering was waiting for him to come in the hallway. After a few minutes this old man appeared. The men and women were separated by a walkway. When Baba Muktananda walked by three or four girls near me began to cry. I asked, "Do you know Swamiji?" They replied, "No, we've never met him." By the way, Baba Muktananda did not know one word of English. Sitting in the room with him, I felt a tremendous energy, very similar to what I felt sat in the presence of my Yoga Guru, Swami Vishnu Devananda Maharaj. It was a very powerful energy they both have because of their celibacy and years of Meditation.

When a young couple asked, how often should a married Yogi have sexual activity? A Yogi he replied, "once a month, but no more than twice."

What Lord Krishna says in the Bhagavad-Gita about Brahmachara is very important. Out of the 18 chapters and 701 verses, the following three talk about Brahmachara. These are from Swami Sivananda's book:

"1. Serene-minded, fearless, firm in the vow of a Brahmachari, having controlled the mind, thinking of me and balanced in mind, let him sit, having me as his supreme goal. VI-14

Commentary: A Brahmachari (celibate) should serve his Guru or the spiritual preceptor whole-heartedly and should live on alms. This also constitutes the Brahmachari-Vrata which means taking the oath of celibacy. The aspirant should control the modifications of the mind. He should be balanced in pleasure and pain, heat and cold, honor and dishonor. He should ever think of the Lord and take him as the Supreme Goal.

Brahmacharya also means continence. Semen or the vital fluid tones the nerves and the brain, and energizes the whole system. That Brahmachari who has preserved this vital force by the vow of celibacy and sublimated it into Ojas Shakti or radiant spiritual power can practice steady Meditation for a long period. Only he can ascend the ladder of Yoga. Without Brahmacharya or celibacy not an iota of spiritual progress is possible. Continence is the very foundation on which the superstructure of Meditation and Samadhi can be built up. Many waste this vital energy—a great spiritual treasure indeed—when they become blind and lose their power of reason under sexual excitement. Pitiful is their lot! They cannot make substantial progress in Yoga.

That which is declared imperishable by those who know the Vedas, that which the self-controlled (ascetics or Sanyasins) and passion-free enter, that desiring which celibacy is practiced-that goal I will declare to thee in brief. VIII-12

Commentary: The Supreme Being which is symbolized by the sacred monosyllable Om or the Pranava is the highest step or the supreme goal of man.

The same ideas are expressed in the Kathopanishad. Yama (the God of Death) said to Nachiketas, "The goal which all the Vedas speak of, which all penances proclaim and wishing for which they lead the life of celibacy, that goal (world) I will briefly tell thee. It is Om." Satyakama the son of Sibi questioned Pippalada, "O Bhagavan, if some one among men Meditates here until death on the syllable Om, what world does he obtain by that?" Pippalada replied, "O Satyakama, the syllable Om is indeed the higher and the lower Brahman. He who Meditates on the higher Purusha with this syllable Om of three Matras (units) is led up by the Sama-verses to the Brahmaloka or the world of Brahma". (Prasnopanishad)

Pranava or Om is considered either as an expression of the Supreme Self or Its' symbol like an idol (Pratika). It serves persons of dull and middling intellects as a means for realizing the Supreme Self.

Chant Om three times at the commencement of your Meditation; you will find concentration of mind easier.

Worship of the gods, the twice-born, the teachers and the wise, purity, straightforwardness, celibacy and non-injury are called the austerities of the body. XVII-14.

Commentary: Brahmacharya means control, but not suppression of the sex-desire or sex-force. If the mind is filled with sublime thoughts by Meditation, Japa (repetition of a Mantra), prayer, study of holy scriptures, inquiry of 'Who am I?', and contemplation of the sexless, pure Self, the sex-desire will be devitalized by the withdrawal of the mind. The mind also will be thinned out. Suppressed sex-desire will attack you again and again and will produce wet dreams, irritability and restlessness of the mind. The mind should be rendered pure by Meditation, Japa singing the Lord's names, and prayer. The mind should be controlled first. Then it will be easy for you to control the senses. That is the reason why the practice of Sama or the control of the mind comes first and then comes Dama or the restraint of the senses (in the order of the six fold virtues-see page 31). The senses cannot operate without the help of the mind. So the effective remedy for lust and the best aid to celibacy is to control the mind first and then the senses."

Swami Sivananda says in his book named Sadhana: "Brahmacharya is the keynote of success in every walk of life. It is absolutely necessary for spiritual advancement. There is no panacea more potent than Brahmacharya to eradicate the dire malady, lust, of ignorant persons and to make the aspirants well established in Brahman. Brahmacharya is a vow of celibacy in thought, word and deed, by which one attains Self-realization or reaches Brahman. Veerya (semen) is the essence of thought, intelligence, life and consciousness. The energy that is wasted during one sexual intercourse is tantamount to the physical energy that is spent in physical labor for ten days, or mental energy that is utilized in mental work for three days. A Yogi always directs his attention to the accumulation of the divine energy in him by unbroken chastity and perfect celibacy. Those who have not observed the vow of celibacy become slaves of anger, jealousy, laziness, fear, etc. He, who has completely eradicated lust, is Brahman himself. There cannot be two opinions in the matter of Brahmacharya. No Viveki thinks of having many children. The life of a householder is not inconsistent with the maintenance of celibacy. As soon as the householder has one child, to continue the line the wife becomes his mother. Brahmacharya includes not only control of sex Indriyas, but also all other Indriyas. The practice of keeping the mind fully occupied is the best of all practices for keeping up of physical and mental Brahmacharya. The Japa of any name of the Lord, Sattwic food, Satsang, study of religious books, Pranayama, prayer, Kirtan, Vichara, Viveka, etc., will go a long way in the eradication of sexual desire and impulses. A proper understanding of Brahmacharya is possible when one lives in seclusion for some time. Always wear a Kowpeen or Langotee or suspender bandage. This will help Brahmacharya and make you healthy, wealthy and wise. Remember the pains of the world, the unreality of objects and the bondage that comes from attachment to wife and children. Constantly remember, "Through the grace of God, I am becoming purer and purer, every day. Pleasures come but not to stay. Mortal flesh is only clay. Everything will pass away. Brahmacharya is the only way."

India Monitor, June 1, 1997 says: "SEX, MALES—AND EARLY DEATHS?"
Lust drives males to an early grave and, if worms are anything to go by, men, wanting to enjoy a long life, should stay at home and resist their sexual urges, a British researcher reported.

Dr. David Gems said studies of a tiny worm, caenorhabdiris elegans, showed the males exhausted themselves pursuing the females. When they gave up the chase, males lived up to twice as long as females. In the majority of species, including man, males do not live as long as females. Longevity is governed by constitutional factors, covering the basic physiology of species, and sexual behavior.

Sexual behavior includes the effects of reproduction, and conflict between males including searching for mates, and holding and protecting mates and territory. The worm is normally hermaphrodite in the wild, but there are a few males. For his research, Gems classified the hermaphrodites as female, an article in the New Scientist said. 'Essentially the males are like supercharged females.'

'They move a great deal more than the females searching for mates, and their life is shortened because of this,' Gems told Reuters. When healthy males were 'crippled' by genetic mutation, they lived a great deal longer. 'It basically reversed the pattern of gender-specific longevity. Males lived up to twice as long as females,' Gems said. When males were put together with females they lived for just over 10 days.

But when individuals were isolated they lived for 20 days longer than the female average of 16 days. Isolating female worms had no effect on their life span. The genetically mutated males lived for 30 days but mutation had no effect on the life span of females. 'If you look at nature, males do not live as long. Is this because they age faster? Or is the higher mortality associated with sex? I would suggest it is because of sex,' Gems said.

'This (worm) is a basic organism but it gives ideas of what we can look at in higher organisms.' The New Scientist quoted geneticist Armand Leroi of London's Imperial College as saying Gems's work was the first time the difference in longevities between males and females in one species had been dissected in great detail. Gems said there was already evidence that males in other species live longer when sex is taken out of the equation. Male marsupial mice die in just a few sex-crazed weeks, copulating five to 11 hours a day. But if they are castrated they can live for years, he said. Human eunuchs also live considerably longer than whole males. Gems said men might be built to live longer than women if it were not for sex.

'This research lays open the fact that gender differences, as far as constitutional factors are concerned, are unknown,' Gems said. 'Man might be an instance where male constitutional factors are stronger than females.''

In "Brain Gain and Chastity," Dr. R. W. Bernard, A.B., M.A., PhD., and His Holiness Danvir Goswami write.

"Conservation of semen means conservation of sex hormones and increased vigor, while loss of semen means loss of hormones and diminished vitality; also chronic deficiency of such hormones leads to the symptoms of senility.

1. There is a remarkable similarity of chemical composition between the semen, the brain and the central nervous system, being especially rich in lecithin, cholesterol [hormones affecting sex organs] and phosphorus compounds, which would indicate that seminal emissions withdraw from the body substances necessary for the nutrition of nerve and brain tissue.
2. Loss of vital seminal fluid causes under-nutrition of the nervous system and brain.
3. [Sexual] Continence is beneficial to the brain.
4. Physiological evidence points to the fact that the seminal fluid contains substances of great physiological value (such as Poehl's Spermine, lecithin, cholesterol, vitamin E, sex hormones, etc.
5. Leading physiologists, urologists, genito-urinary specialists, neurologists, psychiatrists, sexologists, gynecologists and endocrinologists [from the early 20th Century] endorse the physiological value of continence.

Wild animals in a state of nature practice copulation only in certain mating seasons for the purpose of reproduction. Civilized man practices this act all times, and in most cases without intention to conceive. Such considerations lead to the conclusion that the sex life of civilized men is unnatural and that the excessive manifestation of the sex urge among them is due to certain aphrodisiacal stimuli rather than to natural instinct.

The harmful effects of the seminal discharge involve a sudden withdrawal from the body of calcium, lecithin and other substances necessary for the normal functioning of the nervous system. The sudden withdrawal of calcium caused by the seminal discharge biochemically produces the tetany-like symptoms of the orgasm, which are so similar to those of the epileptic attack. During the sexual orgasm of coitus symptoms occur which border on psychopathology [behavioral disorder]; and there can be little doubt that excessive frequency of such symptoms may indelibly impress themselves on the brain and nervous system.

Brain and Semen

Spermatozoa, when not discharged, are reabsorbed into the blood stream and carried to the brain. Both in their chemical composition and their elongated form, they have a remarkable similarity to brain-cells, which, like them, lack the capacity of reproduction, in contrast to most other cells of the body, which have this capacity.

Loss of seminal fluid results in lowered nutrition of nerve and brain tissue, and, when the loss is excessive, it leads to nervous and mental disorders. The concentration of lecithins and cholesterols, both of which are constituents of the semen, the brain and nerves, often vary, depending on intake and outgo. Activity of the sex glands causes withdrawal of both. This means a lessened supply available to the nervous system."

During Child Conception

There are many types of souls. Hindus believe that every person is at a different level of consciousness, so when you have children, you could have a spiritual loving child who is peaceful and intelligent or you could have an angry, miserable, cunning child which would make your life miserable and unhappy. This second type of child will bring unhappiness to the family. Sometimes such a soul will bring death and destruction. So Yoga philosophy says before husband and wife plan to have a child, prior to conception the couple should sit and pray to the lord and request the Lord to send a soul which is spiritual, loving and intelligent.

Chapter 28

Yoga, Hinduism and Depression Summarized

Three important subjects are covered in this chapter 14 essential principals. One can benefit a great deal by studying these.

14 ESSENTIAL PRINCIPLES OF YOGA

These are the key principles of Yoga, which I have learned from my Guru, H.H. Swami Vishnu-Devananda Maharaj, from other Yogis and by studying and practicing Yoga. I have been teaching Yoga and Meditation since 1967.

1. Yoga or yog means union or uniting soul with super soul or God. It is a way to your goal or God, but it is not the end. Yogis have freedom of belief. So belief in God is not essential.

2. Yoga has been practiced for thousands of years in India. But around 200 B.C. Maharishi Patanjali compiled the knowledge of Yoga into a book, called "Yoga Sutra of Patanjali." To a Yogi it is the Gita or Bible of Yoga.

3. People of any faith can practice Yoga. It is not a religion, but a way of life. A Yogi is a man or woman who practices Yoga. A woman who practices Yoga may be called a Yogini

4. The main goals of Yoga are: God realization, self-realization and life realization; a healthy, flexible, energetic, peaceful, happy long life and liberation.

5. The Asthang (eight) steps of Yoga are: a. Yama (self-discipline), b. Niyama (cleanliness, study, and other observances), c. Asana (postures), d. Pranayama (Yogic breathing), e. Pratyahara (withdrawal of senses), f.

Dharana (mind control), g. Dhyan (Meditation), h. Samadhi (the highest state of consciousness or complete oneness with all—Om).

6. The seven types of Yoga are: a. Bhakti (devotion), b. Mantra (remembering God or japa), c. Raja (Meditation), d. Jnana (knowledge), e. Karma (selfless action and service), f. Hatha (body conditioning), g. Kundalini (energy centers).

7. Dhyan or Meditation: There are three levels of Meditation a. Contemplation, b. Meditation, and c. Samadhi. There is only one way to know Meditation; that is to learn and practice Meditation from a qualified teacher. Its goals are to develop mental health, awakening, purifying, entering higher consciousness and knowing your true self.

8. Pranayama (Yogic breathing)—is Prana Shakti. Prana = Living force, and Shakti = Divine Mother. There are two basic categories, which are cleansing breath and healing breath. Within these two categories there are two major types of breathing. For cleansing breath they are: a. Kapalabhati, b. Bhastrika (bellows). For healing breath, they are: a. Ujjayi and b. Visama Virti. Cleansing means to cleanse the physical body, mind and spirit as well as the astral body.

9. Asana: There are 480,000 postures. There are 108 major postures and out of them, four are the most important. They are: a. Yoga Mudra, b. Surya Namaskar (sun prayer), c. Headstand or Shoulder Stand, d. Cobra with Head to Knee Posture.

10. Balance the practice of Hatha Yoga (Ha = sun, Tha = moon) by including: Asana, Pranayama, Nindra Yoga (Savansana or relaxation), Bandhas, Mudra, mind control, Kundalini, fasting, Tantra, Diet, Tratak, Kriyas, prayers, Abhiyas, Guru Seva, etc.

11. Maintain your proper weight, eat sattwic or healthy, good food in moderation; Follow vegetarian diet (no meat, fowl, fish or eggs) preferred by Yogis.

12. Kriyas mean cleansing the physical body, mind, spirit and astral body. There are many types of Kryas. They are: a. Pranayama (Yogic breathing), b. Neti, which is nose cleaning with Jala (water) or Sutra (string), c. Dhouti, which is stomach cleaning through Voman (vomit) or Vastra (eating cloth and taking it out, d. Uddiyana (Abdominal squeezing), e. Nauli—an exercise of abdominal recti, the muscles starting from the lower abdomen), f. Basti (cleaning of the lower intestine), g. Trataka (a gazing technique to improve

eyesight, memory and concentration), h. Fasting, i. Mouna—not speaking, j. Selected Asana, k. Uulyu—tongue scraper.

13. Important Yoga books are: The Complete Illustrated Book of Yoga and; The Hatha Yoga Pradipika, by Swami Vishnu-Devananda; Light on Yoga by Yogi B.K.S. Ivengar; The Sivananda Companion to Yoga by The Sivananda Yoga Center; and many books by H.H. Swami Sivananda Saraswati of Rishikesh.

14. Practice Yoga Sadhana. Learn Yoga from a guru or a qualified Yogi or a teacher. Practice regularly, and at one point teach and spread the word of Yoga.

YOGA IS THE HOPE OF THE WORLD

14 Essential Principles of Hindu Dharma (Hinduism)

These 14 principles have been written and revised over the last 35 years. Please teach them to your children and display it on the walls of your Hindu Temple. Visitors will also benefit from reading it.

1. Goal of Hinduism is Moksha (Mookti or freedom), which means to become one with God. To achieve Moksha, you should love God, know thyself, do your Dharma, Sadhana (spiritual practices), Yoga, Meditation, Yagna, Puja, Japa, Ahimsa, selfless service, go on pilgrimages, visit the Ganges, visit temples, be good and do good. The goal of Hinduism is also known as Dharma, Artha, Karma and Moksha.

2. Brahman is the formless Supreme reality or God, which enters the material world in three forms: Brahma (the Creator; his daughter is Sarasvati), Vishnu (Preserver, his consort is Lakskmi) and Siva (Transformer, consorts are Durga or Kali, sons Ganesh and Subramanya). God is all and all is God. (Soham or Tat Tam Asi—that thou art).*

3. God is nirguna (impersonal formless reality known as Brahman) or Om, or is Sadguna (God in a personal form who listens to prayers and also comes to earth as an Avatar (God in a human incarnation). God has many forms and names: Lord Vishnu incarnates as Ram, Krishna, et al. Surrender and love them. (Sathyam, Sivam, Sundaram)*

4. Hindus have freedom of thought and belief, but accept the conformity of Dharma (i.e. duty, conformity of proper action, care for family). With freedom of belief, even atheism can be included in Hinduism.

5. Karma is the concept that a reaction follows every action. Good results come from good actions. Karma leads to Reincarnation, which is the circle of birth and death. Everyone should advance in each life, with the goal of achieving moksha.

6. Yoga means union with God. Types of Yoga are Jnana (knowledge), Bhakti (devotional service), Raja (Meditation, Kundalini), Mantra, Karma (selfless service), Kriya (cleansing), and Japa (reciting the names of God), and Hatha (Aham Brahm Asmi—I am Brahma or spirit*).

7. Paramatman (Supreme Soul or God), Jivatman (individual souls) and the souls within all living entities are real. Everything else is Maya (illusion). Purush (Spirit) is the Father-aspect of God. Pakriti (matter or energy) is the Mother-aspect of God. There are three worlds: material, astral and spiritual. (Satchitananda—means Existence, Knowledge and bliss absolute)*

8. Truth is one, but religions are many. Some of the main divisions of Hindus are Vaishnavas, Shaivas, and Shaktas. Jainism, Buddhism, Sikhism, as well as Charvaka and Sankhya philosophy are included as a part of Hinduism.

9. Hindu Scriptures are the Vedas, Upanishads, Bhagavad Gita (which are Sruti or words of God), as well as Ramayana, Mahabharata, Puranas and many other books and commentaries written by the sages (which are Smritis, what is remembered).

10. There is no "Devil." Each person is responsible for his own actions. Wrongdoers are not evil, but are in darkness and ignorance. There are seven temporary heavens and hells. Moksha is only attainable while living in the material world.

11. It is your Dharma (duty) to challenge or fight Adharma (injustice or wrongdoing). Yet non-violence towards the weak is also Dharma. Vegetarianism is practiced to show non-violence towards animals.

12. The Scriptures say there are four castes—Brahman, Kshatriya, Vaishya, and Sudra. A person's caste was originally determined by a person's nature, but later became set by birth. Adherence to the caste system is weakening. Slavery has never been a significant part of Hindu culture or history. There are four Ashrams: Brahmacharya, Grahastya, Vanaprashta, and Sanyasa.

13. God is worshiped as mother, father, guru, friend, or in other forms. The guru is the spiritual teacher who takes you from darkness to light. A Guru's grace is essential for receiving spiritual knowledge. The Sat Guru may be

worshipped as God. Murthi (idol) worship is used to focus one's devotion on God and is considered as God in person. When a person says "I am a Hindu," he or she is a Hindu. Hindus do not have a conversion ceremony, but recently some groups do.

14. Bharat, or Hindustan, is divya bhumi matru bhumi, where people of all religions are welcome. India has never invaded any country. Hinduism is a way of living. All of humanity is one family; Respect all religions. Arnold Toynbee said, "The world will realize that the only way to salvation for mankind is the Hindu way."

* These are Mahavakyas

14 ESSENTIAL PRINCIPALS OF DEPRESSION AND HOW TO OVERCOME IT

Out of the US population of about 280 million, 12 million experience depression. I'm not a medical doctor. However, I am a Yogi and spiritual man, and these are my views and some ideas on how to overcome depression. I have never experienced deep depression, though we all experience some amount of highs and lows. I feel Yoga, which is for health, happiness and liberation, is the best help for people suffering from depression.

1. Definition—It is a darkness that takes over one's life, at that time when hope appears to have left, and life feels doomed and lost. One doesn't want to do anything, not even to get out of bed. Some feel there is no point in living.

2. There are 4 kinds of depression: Type A: sociological, physiological; Type B: post-traumatic event, and fate or illusive.

3. Type A requires heavy medication, help from a psychologist or a psychiatrist and sometimes hospitalization. Type B has brighter hope and I'm sure one can do without medical help and use the help of alternative medicine.

4. For healing, one should first forgive and forget people who have harmed one and also accept the play of karma. Take one day at a time and try to come out of this negative loop.

5. It is best to fight one's bad karma. Positive thinking helps. Believe that God, your family and friends love you, that you are needed in this world. Do not give up now, you have come a long way. This life is precious, a gift from

God, do not waste it. Get up and march on to meet your goals. Things are going to get better. Get involved in serving.

6. Suicide is the greatest sin. Do not entertain that thought. Take this opportunity to burn your bad karma or to carry your cross. Your family needs you. Do your Dharma (duty). Keep yourself busy.

7. Some problems have occurred in life as you are living in it. Come out of that negative phase and establish yourself in truth. That will bring peace. Some people say that depression is the rich man's disease.

8. Your standards are too high, seek reality, detach yourself and do the best you know how. Make your standards more realistic. The best thing is to play some games, take a good vacation or go on a pilgrimage or visit an ashram.

9. Read Spiritual books or listen to some good sermons, to some uplifting music or bhajans (religious songs). You can chant Mantras or sing them. Or sing some music that touches your heart.

10. Every human has a need to share his or her deep thoughts. So have a close friend. In the West, people have many acquaintances but very few close friends. That's why people go and pay a psychologist or psychiatrist to listen to their troubles.

11. Do Yoga regularly, Jnana, Bhakti, Raja, Karma, Mantra, Japa, and Hatha Yoga. Do Yogic breathing and learn Kundalini Yoga.

12. Love all and seek a Guru or be a disciple of a Guru in the Spirit like Lord Jesus, Lord Krishna or Swami Sivananda. Go into spirituality, but not into the psychic realm.

13. If you have to take your child to the psychologist or psychiatrist, it should be your last resort. The best thing is to love them and work with them lovingly.

14. Surrender to God, he is the only refuge. Read the Bhagavad Gita or the Bible, or the Holy Book of your faith. Pray.

Chapter 29

Freed-Om

(To Get Freed-Om,
One Has to Give Up Freedom)

All of us seek freedom, inner freedom. Yoga and Meditation offer this inner peace and freedom, besides many other things.

We are all caught in maya, in this material energy. It is an elusive force. When maya imprisons us, we forget our true selves. To get out of that bondage some people take heavy substances and liquor as palliatives. But they only become slaves to the drugs that give them a temporary illusion of freedom.

The best way to achieve inner freedom is to surrender to a Guru or God and practice Yoga and Meditation. This is not easy, it requires practice and a disciplined life. That is how a Yogi lives.

Let's see what Swami Sivananda says in his book "Bliss Divine," about Freedom.

"Losing life is not perfect freedom. Eating anywhere from anybody's hands, sleeping anywhere you like, saying anything you like; these are not freedom. You have become a slave of your body, senses, mind, creature-comforts, food and fashion.

Liberty of speech is not freedom. Liberty of thought is not freedom. To move about aimlessly is not freedom. To do just what one likes is not freedom.

To be in a nude state is not freedom. To be a king or monarch is not freedom. To have Svarajya (your own kingdom) is not freedom. To have plenty is not freedom. To have a comfortable life is not freedom. To possess immense wealth is not freedom. To conquer nations is not freedom. To shirk responsibility is not freedom. To renounce the world is not freedom.

Material independence will not give you total happiness, it cannot give you perfection. Bread and jam cannot give you real happiness. These little things of the world cannot give you eternal joy.

Real Freedom

Real Svarajya is not merely political or economic, though political and economic freedom is essential for the welfare of the people. Real Svarajya is lordship over oneself. It is Atma-Svarajya. It is immortality. It is perfection. It is attainable only by slow and steady stages.

This is freedom or emancipation. Let the mind become still. Herein lies freedom and bliss eternal.

Real freedom is freedom from birth and death. Real freedom is freedom from the trammels of flesh and mind. Real freedom is freedom from the bonds of Karma. Real freedom is freedom from attachment to body, etc. Real freedom is freedom from egoism and desires. Real freedom is freedom from thoughts, likes and dislikes. Real freedom is freedom from lust, anger, greed, etc. Real freedom is identification with the Supreme Self. Real freedom is Self-realization. Real freedom is merging in the Absolute.

Freedom is in detachment. Freedom is in desirelessness. Freedom is in mindlessness. Eradication and extinguishing of desires lead to the sublime state of supreme bliss and perfect freedom."

One way to get inner freedom is to close your eyes and start journeying within yourself. This is your commitment to seek an inner journey to self-realization. First you have to believe in your Self. You have to believe that you are a spirit soul or atman, which is part and parcel of the supreme atman or Paramatman. This will bring you here and now. Your past life is dead and the future does not belong to you. Just say "Lord I am thine and you are mine." This is the process of surrendering to the Divine Self. Once you do this you will enter the ocean of freedom. To get freedom you have to surrender your freedom.

It is very difficult to surrender to God, because God is the most difficult being to reach. For human beings the best way to reach the Supreme Lord is through a divine human being who has gone there and so they can take you there. This person is a Guru. In Sanskrit Gu means darkness, ru means light. That means that any person who can take you from darkness to light is a Guru. A Guru can be a man or a woman. He or she is an enlightened being. A Guru is one who has gone on the road that he wants you to travel. Suppose you are in a town you have never been to before. You know the address you need to reach, but do not know how to get there. What do you do? You ask a person, "Do you know how to get there?" Usually that person says, "Yes," and gives you the directions. He is your Guru, because he has been to that address and is guiding you to that address.

A Guru is not only a divine teacher, but is as good as God. In reality, he/she is God. When you have this faith in his teaching, it is very easy to walk the path he wants you to. When you surrender to a Guru, you lose your freedom, but real freedom can be achieved when he puts you into discipline and on the road to your goal. A Guru digs the ground, plants the seeds, covers the earth and then waters the earth. The seed takes root and the plant sprouts up.

A real Guru never says "I'm a Guru." Instead, he says, "I am a disciple of my Guru." He is the real Guru. The student is the one who says, "He is my Guru." When I met my Guru, Swami Vishnu-Devananda Maharaj he went past all his students and straight to the picture of Swami Sivananda, and bowed down to him. He told us that "He is the Sat-Guru and I am his disciple." When I saw how humble Swami Vishnu was I decided that he was my Guru. A Guru liberates his students, with his calling card, perhaps he gives you a lollipop. He loves you, gives you confidence, then he shows you discipline and gives you transcendental knowledge, and will liberate you so that you can be a Guru. The lollipop could be an introduction to Hatha Yoga. In the process you fall in love. Then he puts you through the discipline and pulls you into higher spirituality and subsequently liberates you.

Master Sivananda, "Bliss Divine," says the following of the Satguru.

The Sadguru

To be a Guru, one must have a command from God. Mere study of books cannot make one a Guru. One who has studied the Vedas, and who has direct knowledge of the Atman through Anubhava, alone can be enrolled as a Guru. A Jivanmukta or liberated sage is the real Guru or spiritual preceptor. He is the Sadgruru. He is identical with Brahman or the Supreme Self. He is a Knower of Brahman. A Sadguru is endowed with countless Siddhis. He possesses all divine Aiswarya, all the wealth of the Lord.

Possession of Siddhis, however, is not the test to declare the greatness of a sage or to prove that he has attained Self-realization. Sadgurus generally do not exhibit any miracle or Siddhi. Sometimes, however, they may to convince the aspirants of the existence of superphysical things, give them encouragement, and instill faith in their hearts.

The Sadguru is Brahman Himself. He is an ocean of bliss, knowledge, and mercy. He is the captain of your soul. He is the fountain of joy. He removes all your troubles, sorrows and obstacles. He shows you the right divine path. He tears your veil of ignorance. He makes you immortal and divine. He transmutes your lower, diabolical nature. He gives you the rope of knowledge, and takes you up when you are drowning in this ocean of Samsara. Do not consider him to be only a man. If you take him as a man, you are a beast. Worship your Guru and bow to him with reverence.

Guru is God. A word from him is a word from God. He need not teach anything. Even his presence or company is elevating, inspiring, and stirring. His very company is self-illumination. Living in his company is spiritual education. Read the Granthsaheb. You will come to know the greatness of the Guru.

Man can learn only from man, and hence God teaches through a human body. In your Guru, you have your human ideal of perfection. He is the pattern into which you wish to mold yourself. Your mind will readily be convinced that such a great soul is fit to be worshipped and revered. Guru is the Moksha-dvara that means Guru is the giver of the Moksha or final freedom.

Every time I see Lord Krishna's picture, I see on his forehead a "Tilak", which is like a "U." I used to wonder what it really meant. Finally, I figured out what it is the following incident. One of my friends had a drinking problem. He got drunk every night. Eventually he lost his job. His wife asked me what should she do. Then I remembered a colleague and friend who worked with alcoholics showing me a diagram in the shape of a "U" that was used in Alcohol Addiction and Recovery developed by the Wilmington Council on Alcoholism. It showed that through her behavior the wife was feeding his addiction and that he does not accept that he has a drinking problem, that because of his drinking problem he lost his job and that his family is suffering. I explained this to the alcoholics' wife. The harsh and strong message was that she had to tell her husband that he could not drink in their house, and that if he wanted to drink, he must leave the house.

Everything the chart showed happened to my alcoholic friend. He left the house, kept drinking, and nobody fed him. One day he fell down in the street and the police picked him up and put him in prison. He called from the prison and his wife went to see him. She told him sternly that if he agreed not to drink, he could come home. He promised to do that. He never drank again, and the family was saved. A person doesn't accept he is an alcoholic until he goes all the way down to the bottom of the "U." From there, if he is determined to save himself, he moves slowly but surely upwards. Then I understood that U is for freedom.

This applies in the material world too. If man starts indulging in wrong ways and destroying his life, there comes a stage when he cannot take it and goes all the way down to the bottom of the "U." At that time a Guru or teacher shows him a spiritual way of living. This person who has suffered is real qualified to learn about spirituality or Yoga. Please see the chart in Table 15.1 (page 151).

Yogic Wisdom About Gurus

• When you seek a Guru, the Guru appears
• There are many good Gurus, but a good student is one in a million
• A Guru never says, "I'm your Guru." A good Guru always say's "I'm a disciple of my Guru." Only a student says, "He or she is my Guru."

• High spiritual knowledge cannot be obtained without a Guru.

• Gu—means darkness, Ru—means light. Any person who takes you from darkness to light is a Guru.

• If one has faith in his Guru, he can move mountains.

• When you surrender to a Guru, you are aided by your Guru and his or her lineage.

• There are two kinds of Gurus, a living Guru and a Guru in spirit.

• Guru is God, and God is Guru.

• Over time, humans bring Gurus when they are needed, and when times change, they change Gurus. For example, the Chinese went to India and brought Lord Buddha, and when the time came they dropped Lord Buddha and brought Mao Se Tung.

• Guru takes you to Mother (Shakti), and Mother takes you to Father (God).

Meditation Is To Regain Our Freedom, Love, and Be Enlightened
Humans are at different levels.

1) A child is one with God, in freedom and Love, in spirit and self, in Om and all is one.

2) Society conditions the child's mind for his survival in the material world. The child eats the apple or enters into Maya. I'd like to say that Maya is like a prism that turns the white light, which passes through you, into many colors on the other side that you see. The many colors is the maya. But the white light is the ultimate reality.

3) The soul or self gives control to the mind.

4) The mind controls the human and is fragmented. Now humans have lost their freedom, love and self. They are lost and unhappy.

5) They then find a Guru; a spiritual teacher.

6) They gain power from the Divine Mother.

7) They gain discipline through Yoga.

8) Knowledge of the self (Atma Jnan) brings awareness.

9) Freedom, love, Om, enlightenment (siddha) and God Realization is attained.

They are similar and shows you the way to Om consciousness. Om consciousness is God consciousness. Om means God is everywhere, in everybody and in everything.

You Are Satchitananda

In the book "Kathapanishad" God says, "O Nachiketa (all humans), Your nature, is pure awareness and you are Sat-Chit-Ananda."

This word Satchitananda means you are SAT-CHIT-ANANDA. That means God you are existence, knowledge and bliss absolute. The word (Sat) existence means Lord you are eternal, you never took birth and you will never die. You are changeless. The material world is constantly changing, but you are changeless. Chit means knowledge. That means that you know all. Ananda means bliss absolute. You are joy. You are completely joyful and happy. My soul is part of you, the Super-soul. Because of that, my soul is also Satchitananda.

That means my soul has never taken birth and will never die. My soul needs to know all, it needs to know, because it is part of you. And, my soul is bliss absolute but, as it is in this material body, it has forgotten who he or she is because I am in maya. It is an elusive force. Because of that, I have been confused and I have forgotten who I am. To realize that I am Satchitananda, that is existence, knowledge and bliss absolute, I have to do sadhanas. That means be good, do good, read scriptures, do Yoga, prayers and Meditation. Once I do these, I will come out from this deceptive maya and come to the realization that I am Satchitananda that means existence, knowledge and bliss absolute. Once I realize I am Satchitananda, I am enlightened. That is my goal- to become enlightened. Once a person is enlightened he becomes Buddha or Siddah. Once you realize Brahman, you, the little soul, and the big soul become one, that means Om. God is the big soul and you are part of that reality. If God is the ocean, you are a drop of water. At one point you do not see any difference. We are one in the spirit; the big and the small spirit that is Om. Go beyond body and mind and stay in the center of your being. Do not forget that you are Satchitananda that means existence, knowledge and bliss absolute.
Hari Om Tat Sat

Adisankaracarya, great sage of India, says:
"The self to be known, the limitless self other than which nothing exists, who is pure, all-knowing, the seer of everything—to that self which is to be known, salutations."

You Are Complete, You Are Purna

Hindus chant prayers in Sanskrit and the last prayer which they recite is the following.

Om Purnamadah Purnamidam
Purnat Purnamudachyate
Purnasya Purnamadaya
Purnameva Vashishyate
Om Shantih Shantih Shantih

Translations:

That is perfect, this is perfect, (it is whole). This perfect world arises from perfection. If we remove the perfect world, that which remains is indeed Perfect (God). Om Peace, Peace, Peace be unto us all.

You, the world and God are perfect, so whatever God has made is perfect. If you want to be happy, you should understand that God has made you complete "Purna." That all your needs are within you. You are not in the periphery, but you are in the center. You are not lost. You are anchored. You are not in "unreality." You are in reality. You are not in darkness. You are in light. If you do not feel this purna, then you should surrender to Guru or God, Meditate regularly and seek to know who you are. You have to begin by taking charge of your life, accept your karma, fight the bad karma, do your Dharma and keep a balance between the material world and the spiritual world. Be healthy and remain strong by maintaining a good diet and doing Yoga regularly.

LIFE IS A NUMBER GAME

Human beings want to be happy so it is good to know what to expect in the future and how it helps to be flexible and change with time. It is very interesting how numbers affect our life.

Four Hindu Ashrams

Hindus have divided a humans life into four parts they are as follows:

Brahmacharya (Age 1—25)—means a young person should remain celibate and keep away from lust and study hard. Have a simple life. They should live with their parents lovingly (learn Yoga).

Grihastha (Age 25—50)—means after 25 years of age get married, earn a good living, have children, serve society and live happily (practice Yoga).

Vanpratha (Age 50—75)—means to live a simple life with your spouse and be a teacher and serve society (teach Yoga).

Sannyasa (Age 75—up)—meaning become a monk or just love God (bless Yoga)

Above is the formula to be happy and how to live a good life.

I came across this Rule of 9, which tells us how gradually a person becomes God conscious and it does this by showing how much God gets and how much you get in this material world.

RULE OF 9 (Source Unknown)

	GOD GETS	YOU GET
$1 \times 9 = 9$—$0 + 9 = 9$	0	9
Brahmacharya		
$2 \times 9 = 18$—$1 + 8 = 9$	1	8
$3 \times 9 = 27$—$2 + 7 = 9$	2	7
Grahatha		
$4 \times 9 = 36$—$3 + 6 = 9$	3	6
$5 \times 9 = 45$—$4 + 5 = 9$	4	5
$6 \times 9 = 54$—$5 + 4 = 9$	5	4
Vanpratha		
$7 \times 9 = 63$—$6 + 3 = 9$	6	3
$8 \times 9 = 72$—$7 + 2 = 9$	7	2
Sanyasa		
$9 \times 9 = 81$—$8 + 1 = 9$	8	1
$10 \times 9 = 90$—$9 + 0 = 9$	9	0

"God Gets," means serve God Society, Temple, etc. "You Get," means you and your family get.

Seven Year Itch

An American proverb says your marriage takes a shift in its seventh year; it either improves or gets worse. From my experience I feel a shift occurs every seventh year throughout a person's life. So a shift would occur at 7, 14, 21, 28, 38 and so on.

If your marriage lasts 35 years, you are doing well, and I would say that both partners are blessed. On my wedding day, my wife asked me "How much do you love me?" I was surprised, but didn't want to lie. So I showed her with my hands, "My love is this much but I have lots of lust, but I will make sure my love will grow every day we live together." She was satisfied with my answer.

After 25 years of marriage, my wife passed away. On our 25th wedding anniversary our marriage had reached its highest level. I feel when two people get married they are quite apart. Then they live together lovingly and their love grows with the years.

Your Life And Seven Years

$7 \times 1 = 7$ at 7, the child is no longer a baby

$7 \times 2 = 14$ at 14, the child becomes a teenager

$7 \times 3 = 21$ at 21, the teenager becomes an adult

$7 \times 4 = 28$ at 28, the adult develops a sense of who he or she is and some become a parent.

$7 \times 5 = 35$ at 35, the parent or competent adult begins to feel his age through his/her body's aches and pains

$7 \times 6 = 42$ at 42, come the reading glasses

$7 \times 7 = 49$ at 49, they offer you the management position, you have earned distinction

$7 \times 8 = 56$ at 56, you can be the president of the company, your children are grown up

$7 \times 9 = 63$ at 63, you can retire, you become a grandparent

$7 \times 10 = 70$ at 70, a person has become old

$7 \times 11 = 77$ at 77, one is older

7 x 12 = 84   at 84, one is very old, has become like a baby again
7 x 13 = 91   at 91, every moment of life is a blessing.
7 x 14 = 98   at 98, if you make it, you've almost lived an entire century.

Yoga and Om

In Yoga, Om or the Mantra Om is very important. Om is God and God is Om. Om means the whole Universe is one and you are part of that. The symbol Om is shown in Fig. 15.2 (page 151). Om has four parts. In the front it says "3", behind 3 there is a half moon going down. It symbolizes the earth. On the top is another half moon going up, symbolizing the Moon, then on top of the Moon there is a single star, which signifies that there are billions of stars beyond the Moon. This whole thing signifies the universe. However, Om is the unity of all yet it is divided into three. In Christianity, it is the trinity. Yoga says it's the three aspects of divinity. The following are the different aspects of Yoga in three:

Three Main Types of Yoga

| 1. Jnana Yoga | 2. Bhakti Yoga | 3. Raja Yoga |

Three Supreme Yogas

| 1. Surya Namaskar | 2. Headstand | 3. Mudra Yoga |

Types of Yoga

| 1. Hatha Yoga | 2. Mantra Yoga | 3. Karma Yoga |

Goals of Yoga

| 1. Health | 2. Happiness | 3. Liberation |

Yoga Offers

1. Good Health	2. Long Life	3. Lots of Energy
1. Flexibility	2. Harmony	3. Healing
1. Power	2. Cleansing	3. Balancing
1. Truth	2. Love	3. Enlightenment
1. Peace Within	2. Peace with Others	3. Peace with Nature

To Many, Yoga is

| 1. Asana | 2. Pranayama | 3. Meditation |

To Others, Yoga is

1. Mudra Yoga 2. Laya Yoga 3. Tratak Yoga

Three Main Pranayamas

1. Ujajjayi 2. Bhastrika 3. kapalabhati

Three Bodies

1. Gross Body 2. Astral Body 3. Subtle Body

Three Worlds

1. Material World 2. Astral World 3. Spiritual World

Three States Of Mind

1. Maya 2. Lila 3. Dreams

Types of Human Beings

1. Yogis 2. Bhogis 3. Rogis

Three Aspects of the Human

1. Body 2. Mind 3. Soul

Three Gurus

1. Maharishi Patanjali 2. Swami Sivananda 3. Your Guru

Trinity of Christianity

1. The Father 2. The Holy Ghost 3. The Son

Yoga Three

1. Spirit 2. Energy 3. Light
1. Father 2. Mother 3. Guru

I'm sure there are many other threes, but these are a good place to start.

108 Is a Divine Number

In the Oct./Nov 2005 issue of Hinduism Today, the following was written, "In numerology, 108 breaks down to 1+0+8 = 9. Nine is a mystically charged number, and the sum of the digits resulting from any number multiplied by 9 always returns to 9.

Vedic astrology divides the heavens into 27 moon signs, called *Nakshatras*, each with 4 *Padas*, making 108 *Padas* in all, giving 108 basic kinds of human nature. The *pada* occupied by the moon at the time of birth indicates the nature of one's career, pleasures, family and path to liberation.

In astronomy, Vedic seers calculated that the distance between the Earth and the Moon is 108 times the diameter of the Moon, the distance between the Earth and the Sun is 108 times the diameter of the Sun, and the diameter of the Sun is 108 times the diameter of the Earth. These numbers are remarkably close to the results of calculations based on modern scientific measurements using the average distances between the Earth and the Moon, and the Earth and the Sun.

Ayurveda tells us that there are 108 *Marmas*, points in the body, where consciousness and flesh intersect to give life to the living being. Similarly, the lines of the mystical, mesmerizing Sri Chakra Yantra intersect in 54 points, each with a masculine and a feminine quality, totaling 108.

In explaining the number of beads on a *Japa Mala*, some say that 108 are the number of steps a soul takes to reach the Divine within himself. With this sacred number appearing in so many intersections between the Divine and the human, it is no wonder that Hindus, Buddhists, Jains, Sikhs and Taoists find that offerings of 108 help us remain in harmony with God's perfect universe."

Chapter 30

Yogi, Bhogi and Rogi

There are three types of human beings; they are Yogis (good spiritual human beings), bhogis (pleasure conscious human beings) and rogies (ignorant human beings who do wrong things). If you want to be happy with high goals then you should strive to be a Yogi. First I'd like to look into our individual problems that cause negativity.

Hindus say the following are the obstacles in achieving liberation or moksha: 1. Kama—Lust (sex) you are a victim of the unreal and temporary world. 2. Krodha—Anger (Adversity). You are angry because your desires were not fulfilled. 3. Lobha—Greed (No contentment). You are not satisfied with what God has given you. Moha—Attachment (Not free). You have too much love for the material world. 5. Maya—Illusion (caught in the play). You have been caught in Maya; you have forgotten "Who you are."

In 1947, Mahatma Gandhi wrote down his list of seven causes that lead to all the violence in society today. He called them the "Seven Blunders Of The World," and he gave the list to his grandson, Arun Gandhi, when he was on his way back to South Africa. The list looked like this: 1) Wealth without work, 2) Pleasure without conscience, 3) knowledge without character, 4) Commerce without morality, 5) Science without humanity, 6) Worship without sacrifice, 7) Politics without principles. Mahatma Gandhi preached non-violence, self-sufficiency and self-reliance. He believed that truth is the answer to all human problems.

I once wrote down all the human problems that I could think of, and this is the list that I came up with 1) Feeling empty (no fulfillment), 2) Not feeling centered, 3) Looking for something to uplift a person's mood, 4) Feeling caught or stuck, 5) Looking for spiritual light and can't find it, 6) Loneliness, 7) Too much tension, 8) Fear, 9) Depression, 10) Can't let go of something, someone or a situation, 11) Confusion, 12) Stress, 13) Lack of energy, 14) Stuck in the paradigm and do not have a creative solution, 15) Boredom, 16) Waiting for others to change their life situation—don't take charge of their life, 17) Negativity and Blame, 18) Encountering disease (poor diet), 19) Losing strength, and flexibility (no posture), 20) Bodily organs loose power (kidney), 21) Body gains weight, metabolism slows down, 22) Body lacks energy, 23) Drugs (escape), 24) Laziness (no goals), 25) Not enough money, 26) No commitment, 27) No loving relationship, 28) Selfishness, 29) Violence. Yoga cannot solve all these problems, but it can help.

In my teaching I talk about three things that create problems in the lives of human beings, 1) False ego, leads to destruction of life, 2) Seeking only pleasure, leads to pain, 3) Ignorance, not wanting to study or know anything, leads one to darkness. The three solutions are, 1) be humble, and surrender internally to Guru and God, 2) do your Dharma (duty) and do your Sadhana (spiritual practices) and 3) continuous learning and improving yourself through knowledge.

All the problems shown above are the traps that Bhogies and Rogies fall into. Yogis are not trapped by these problems because Yogis are free.

How One Can Become a Yogi

In the Bhagavad Gita, Lord Krishna says, "Tasmaat Yogi Bhava Arjuna" Gita IV-46, which means, "Be Thou a Yogi O Arjuna."

If you want to be a Yogi, declare yourself to be a "Yogi." Get on the Yoga path and start walking where you stand. (You do not have to drop anything, just be a Yogi and start marching towards the goals of Yoga; the undesirable things will drop out on their own). When you declare yourself a Yogi, Yoga will follow you.

Say in your Meditation or anytime you wish "Dear Shakti Ma; Dear Lord I am yours but separated and in Darkness, I am possessed by Maya. Please help me and guide me to be a Yogi—Hari Om Tat Sat." or say whatever your heart tells you to say—Please ask Master Sivananda and/or your Guru's Grace. Then subsequently, whenever you are ready, get an initiation from your Guru.

All About Yogis

There are three kinds of Yogis. The full-time Yogi who practices and preaches and earns a living teaching Yoga. The part-time Yogi has another job but is greatly involved in Yoga and Yoga practice. The third type is a Yoga practicer who has a full time job and does Yoga practice for good health, happiness and liberation. The first kind, the full time Yogi, believes in and follows the Yoga Sutra of Maharishi Patanjali. To them, Yoga Sutra is the Bhagavad Gita or the Bible. To them it is the word of God. One of these Yogis is H. H. Sri Sri Swami Buaji Maharaj who is known as Swami Yogi Bua. He is the founder of the Indo-American Yoga-Vedanta Society, in New York. He teaches Yoga classes daily, is active in missions to South America and has never advertised himself in any publication or ever levied any fee for any Yoga class, he eats only what is offered to him, fasting if nothing comes. He was chosen for the Hindu Renaissance award in 1988. He was about 109 years old when he wrote the following article in Hinduism Today in the year 1999. As of 2007, he is still alive and active teaching Yoga.

It is very important for us to know his way of living and thinking, and for this reason, I'm including his article here.

"Like all entities in the universe, the human body is in constant change. Even the tiniest microscopic subatomic particles throughout the whole cosmos, of which the body is composed are on the move. Without change there is no life. Life itself is constant change, governed by time and space. To cover the space or span of life requires time. The shorter the time to cover the space (faster wear and tear) the shorter the life span. If you walk fast, you will reach the destination in a shorter time.

Daily stress, causing imbalance in the normal flow, accelerates the mutation and deterioration in the body cells, resulting in a short life span. Slowing down the rate or speed of mutation in the body cells prolongs the life span. Numerous factors including environmental conditions, atmosphere and the immediate surroundings significantly influence our physical and mental health. According to Ayurveda (the Science of Life), excessive use, inadequate use and improper use of food (intakes), physical activities, mental activities or behavior are the causes of all diseases. These are merely interruptions and malfunctions in the smooth flow of life, and sometimes in their advanced states some of them become so-called terminal diseases. Keeping or bringing all the above-mentioned three factors in balance will maintain sound physical and mental health for a longer, healthier life span. I have subsisted on a primarily liquid diet of vegetable and fruit juices throughout my life. I only take solid food on rare occasions.

Owing to the constant change or mutation, the body, throughout its life, goes through various phases leading to the final change or phase, so-called death. But death is not the end. It is just a transition to the next state, phase or form called rebirth. So the endless cycle of birth and rebirth continues as the law of the universe. It keeps changing its forms like every atom or particle in the universe. Disease is just another created change in the body.

Meditation, prayer, unconditional love, compassion, charity, serene music and quiet atmosphere have calming and relaxing effects on the human mind and body. Their tranquilizing affects slowdown the wear and tear of the body cells, thus contributing to prolonging the life span. Meditation is the single most powerful practice to improve quantity and the quality of human life.

Change requires time, but during the Meditation time stops. It doesn't exist. Time and space go together; therefore space also ceases to exist. So, in Meditation, time and space don't exist. Thus it creates a state of suspension. In this state, body and mind are totally relaxed and dissolve their entity. Thoughts stop. This is an altered state in which the respiration and heartbeat slow down. Thus body and mind are at total rest.

There is less feeling and a sense of weightlessness, throbbing and numbness of the fingertips and the experience of total detachment from body, mind and the surroundings. Only the awareness, the pure state of Being remains. During this state, mutation comes to an almost complete halt, giving way to the restoration and rejuvenation of the body cells, triggering the retardation of the aging process. Meditation also influences the endocrine system in the body. It regulates and harmonizes the hormonal flow, thus retarding and reversing the aging process by interrupting the mutation of the body cells. This helps extend the life span over 100 years.

Productive actions, creative thoughts, intelligence and wisdom contribute to the quality of a long life span. Wisdom is the result of intelligence and practical experience in life. Therefore, the longer the life span, the greater the wisdom, which is beneficial, if shared with others, for serving humanity. Among all other forms of life, human life has a unique purpose, and that is to serve others. Service to humanity is the ultimate purpose of life. However, if one decides to accomplish this purpose in a shorter period, then one doesn't have to have a life span of 100 years and can leave the body at will.

I wish to share with those advancing in years, a poem I have had since 1986: 'O! Adorable Lord of Mercy, Love and Compassion. Thou knowest better than I that I am growing older and older, and will someday be really very, very old. O Lord, keep me from being talkative, and particularly from the fatal habit of thinking I must say something on every occasion. O, Lord release me from the craving to straighten out everybody's affairs. Keep my mind free from the recital of endless details; give me wings to get to the point. I ask for Grace enough to listen to the tales of other's pains. Help me to endure them with patience; but seal my lips on my own aches and pains. O Lord, they are increasing by leaps and bounds and my love of rehearsing them is becoming sweeter and sweeter as the years go by. O! Immaculate One, teach me the glorious lesson that occasionally, nay often, it is possible that I may be mistaken or have blundered. Keep me sweet, friendly and loveable. I do not want to be a saint—some of them, nay most of them, are so hard to live with. A sour old person is one of the crowning works of the Devil. Make me thoughtful, O Lord, but not moody, helpful but not bossy. With my vast store of wisdom, it is a pity, not to use them at all. But Thou knowest, indeed, O Lord, that I want a few friends at the end."

Swami Vishnu Devananda, a great Yogi, summarized Yoga in five points. They are: follows:
   1) Proper Exercise (Yoga Asana),
   2) Proper Breathing (Pranayama)
   3) Proper Diet (Balanced vegetarian diet)
   4) Proper Relaxation (Tension free life)
   5) Positive Thinking and Meditation (Raja Yoga)

Tools of a Dynamic Person

It is very important to have the right kind of tools to work efficiently, properly and effectively. I learned and developed these tools during the 35 years I worked in the corporate world and during the 10 years I taught at the university.

A dynamic person can carry out many projects successfully at one time. An American proverb says, "If you want to get something done, give it to someone who is busy." Time management skills are highly important, as also being on time and being dependable. Target your goals and be attentive to the smallest details of the project on hand. A person has to take responsibility by taking charge, and take risks when necessary in order to achieve success. Organize your work, keep your files in order so that needed information will be readily and easily available. Work on your listening skills. Investigate your options and take the necessary actions to accomplish your goals. Follow your plan diligently and seek continuous improvement. Keep a pad of paper in your pocket to write down ideas and make lists of things that need to be done so that you don't forget important items. Of course, it is very important to keep a weekly and monthly calendar. Keep a separate information book, with a 3-ring binder that has sections, for example (A-Z), in which you can keep important information such as addresses, travel information, personal business and hobbies, etc., to retrieve needed information quickly. Before starting your day, make a list of things to be done and cross them off after doing them. Also next to your telephone keep a notebook in which you can write down the date, who called, and the caller's phone number. If your business or work requires new ideas, keep an idea book. Be a custodian of your main profession by keeping certain job related articles in a file. My friend used to say, "When I work hard, I get lucky."

Advice for the Yoga Practicer

As opposed to a full-time Yogi, a Yoga practicer cannot spend too much time practicing Yoga. They should do as much as they can in their limited time. Here is some advice, for dynamic Yogic living. Take charge of your own life; do not depend on others to make things happen. Be a Guru graced Yogi, by being a good disciple of your teacher and having faith in their teaching. Swami Sivananda says, "Serve, love, give, purify, Meditate and realize, Mother, Guru, and God." Have a vision in life. Do your Dharma (duty and a goal), and Sadhana (spiritual practices). First is God, second is your health, third is family, and fourth is your profession. Follow scriptures and live positively. When going through life, seek continuous improvement, seek growth and take risks. Work hard and accept what God gives you. Stand up to Adharma, be compassionate and be upright. Remember that this life is grace from God—work as if every day were your last. Seek freedom from the circle of life and death, work hard, do Yoga and walk towards liberation. Your faith and perseverance will move mountains.

These are 14 points to remember if you want to be happier:
1. Stay within your limits, 2. Seek safety and security, 3. Do not relax with drugs, 4. Do Yoga and maintain your weight, 5. Forgive and forget, 6. Be dependable and upright, 7. Be loving and compassionate, 8. Bring simplicity and beauty in life, 9. Serve and love family and friends, 10. Look before you leap, 11. Stay on top of things, 12. Plan for tomorrow, 13. Keep company of the wise, 14. Work without expectation. Know This Life Is A Gift From God.

A dynamic person has the best attitude in their work place. These are the qualities of the best workers:

Dependability: Arrive when agreed to, conscientious, dependable, communicates

Quantity and Quality: Efficient, high volume, enthusiasm, precision, follow-up

Creative: In solving problems and new ideas

Cooperation: Friendly and agreeable, willing to change

Adaptability: Adjusts to new challenges, willing to change

Housekeeping and Safety: Clean, orderly, injury free attitude

Teamwork and Leadership: Works with others, team participation, positive

Know-how: Possesses skills and knowledge

Goal / Focus: Knows the needs and is responsive

Initiative/Independence: Self motivation, self management and responsibility

Judgment/Risk taking: Understanding and effective decision making

Communications: Oral, written and effective listening

Chapter 31

The Words of Anandi Narayani Ma

Article Written by Ajay B. Gajjar

The soul has the everlasting flow of love. The soul can express love without a kiss or a hug. The Soul has the everlasting music of happiness. The soul is the bridge between the two people and the world. Soul ties are real ties. When one feels the spiritual tie with another person, real freedom begins. When mind and heart are guided by the soul—all relations are complete. Soul is not man, not a woman nor a child. The soul is not bound into the limits of childhood, manhood or old age. The love flows evenly to all.
—Anandi Narayani

Anandi Narayani (Fig. 14.3)

Anandi Narayani was the spiritual name selected by my mother, Rupal B. Gajjar, at her initiation by her guru Swami Vishnudevananda. I believe *Anandi* means the feminine form of a person who is blissful and *Narayani* means belongs to Narayan. Narayan (Vishnu) is the name and form of the Divine Spirit that she chose to worship. She did a lot of sadhana throughout her life and helped many people, especially through Yoga. She was very loving and spiritual. I believe she was self-realized while living and reached Naraayan when her spirit left her body in 1984. This chapter is a glimpse of some of the wisdom provided by my mother. Italics represent quotes from my mother's writings.

—Ajay B. Gajjar.

Guru

Spiritual life starts with a guru. As my father, Bharat J. Gajjar, would say, "When the student is ready, the guru appears." In my mother's case, her spiritual journey began when my father could not teach one of his Yoga classes, and he asked my mother to teach the class for him. At first she refused. But since she had to do it, she went to the class. Although she didn't think she knew how to teach a Yoga class, at a deeper level she was already ready for it because she had attended many Yoga classes including some at the Sivananda Yoga Camp in Val Morin, Canada. She also participated in short daily satsangs at home before dinner. When she came back from teaching the class, she said she loved it. After my mother became more involved with Yoga, she eventually asked for initiation from her guru, Swami Vishnudevananda. Here is an article she wrote about the meaning of initiation.

Bhakti-Yoga

Anandi Narayani's favorite Mantra was *om namo naarayanaaya*. She would do japa mala regularly and would repeat this Mantra mentally before falling asleep at night. She would also sing bhajans and chant Mantras during the day. She particularly enjoyed Sunday Satsangs at the Sivananda Yoga Center located in Wilmington, Delaware at the time.

Jnana-Yoga

Throughout her life, she would read books, write essays, letters, or poems, often revising them and copying them into "final" form in a notebook. Here are her notes for the philosophy portion of a Yoga class. She may have collected this information from a variety of sources:

Jnana-Yoga

When we face death, a question comes "Is the world real?" If we all have to leave this world why should we cling so much to our worldly activities? The average man has ambitions, has newer and newer forms of desires and keeps busy satisfying them. The unthinking pleasure-seeker deludes himself into a belief that he is perfectly secure in his day-to-day existence in the sense world.

Jnana Yoga says, "Reject what is false; and with a keen sense of discrimination seek what is true." The Jnani refuses to identify himself with anything that is unreal. He analyzes everything belonging to the sense world with "neti, neti"—"not this, not this." With sheer effort of the will, keeps himself unattached to anything that is of a transitory nature. He knows his physical body will perish sooner or later. He always kindles in himself the consciousness of his separateness from the body. He maintains himself on the Self or Reality.

One day his "cloud of unknowing" suddenly clears away and in a flash he actually realizes that he is the Self. His body must obey his highest thoughts as spontaneously as a supple twig bends at the touch of the wind. The Gita says, "harder is the task for those who aspire after the unmanifested. Those who have not risen above the body consciousness will have to suffer if they try to realize the unmanifested Brahman."

It is not easy to eliminate the body idea. A keen sense of discrimination between the Real and the Unreal is required. Control of the mind, control of the senses is not a simple game. One's own will power and receptiveness of the instruction of the teacher (Guru) and longing for liberation is needed. If someone has mastered the discipline in his past lives he has some hope to succeed in the path of Jnana Yoga.

Great illumination is possible if sincerely and constantly searched and reached, the strength from the Source of infinite power that lies hidden within every being. A Guru who has directly realized the Self, the true nature of his being, can help a student reach the same. One must not be lazy on this path; must not justify wrongful acts by saying the world is maya or illusion.

The Gita says "The self which is deathless does not kill, nor can it be killed." Intellectual conviction that the path of Jnana Yoga is best suited to his temperament is not enough. He has to fight out his battles alone against human weakness and tricks of the mind.

Yoga of Knowledge does not prohibit devotion to God or Guru. In the beginning when a student has to go through darkness of ignorance, the blessing of a Guru gives light and strength. Even Karma Yoga adds to the success of a Jnana Yogi. Self-purification, control of the mind and a high degree of concentration are also needed by a Jnana Yogi. Concentration is best acquired by practicing Raja Yoga. "We are the Eternal Spirit and not the body or the mind." That is the road of the Jnana Yogi.

Karma-Yoga

My mother would write letters to her friends and Yoga students. Most times, she would write a rough draft first and then write the final draft. Sometimes she would copy the letter down in her notebook before sending it. She also taught Yoga to children and senior citizens in Wilmington, Delaware. Here is Anandi Narayani's poem about service:

Man should serve his wife. Wife should serve her husband.
Parents should serve their Children. Children should serve their Parents.
This is the only act of Dharma.
Guru should serve his students. Students should serve the Guru.

Hatha-Yoga

Anandi Narayani conducted Yoga classes at the YMCA, for her neighbors, children at the Sivananda Yoga Center, senior citizens, and many others. Her classes included hatha Yoga combined with Pranayama, Meditation, Mantra chanting, and philosophy. Here is Anandi Narayani's guidance on how to reduce stiffness while practicing hatha Yoga:

1.   After sleeping 7-8 hours, one is stiffer. In other words, you are stiffer in the morning than in the evening. Take a shower and do warm up stretching.
2.   When you are tensed and under pressure, you are stiffer than when you are relaxed. Do a little Meditation and Yogic breathing, prayers, and relaxation.
3.   If you overeat, that day or the next day, you will be stiffer. A moral disciplined life will bring peace and love. Practice yama and niyama. Once you realize, use moderation in eating and sleeping.

4. *When the physical body and astral body are not going in the same direction, one is stiffer. First harmonize yourself, then mentally let the astral body go in that position, then stretch.*

5. *Postures become easier when you ask the Guru in the spirit to assist you. Be aware of your Guru in your heart, and the Guru outside who teaches you in the body, and his Guru in spirit whom you can invoke. God and Guru are one in Yoga.*

6. *Body will be stiff when the mind is not there and not in harmony with the body. Bring Om Consciousness and be in tune with your body. Be "here and now" as Ram Dass says.*

7. *When the posture is done without harmony with breath or prana. Always do postures with Yogic breathing.*

8. *When the body is stiff, you are not listening or in tune with your body. Postures will be easier to do if you do them at the same time and place, same carpet, and sit regularly with reverence.*

Remember postures are a prayer to God with your body.

Sadhana

Anandi Narayani had read in a book by Swami Sivananda that it is good to keep a spiritual diary, so she kept one. She made entries for doing hatha Yoga, writing a Mantra, number of japa malas done during the day, and interesting thoughts or spiritual concepts. Here are Anandi Narayani's notes from *Commentary on the Bhagavad Gita* by Sri Chinmoy from her spiritual diary.

Yoga Is the Secret Language of Man

Arjuna is the ascending human Soul. Krishna is the descending divine Soul. Finally they meet. The human Soul says to the divine Soul "I need you." The divine Soul says to the human Soul "I need you, too. I need you for my self-manifestation. You need me for your self-realization." Arjun says "O Krishna, you are mine, absolutely mine." Krishna says "O Arjuna, no mine, no thine, we are the same oneness complete within, without."

Yoga is the secret language of man and God. Yoga means Union, the union of the finite with the Infinite, the Union of the form with the Formless. Yoga is to be practiced for the sake of truth. The Gita demands man's acceptance of life, and reveals the way to achieve the victory of the higher self over the lower by the spiritual art of transformation—physical, vital, mental, psychic and spiritual.

Our body's Dharma is service, our mind's Dharma is illumination, our heart's Dharma is oneness and our soul's Dharma is liberation.

The body is perishable, the Soul, the real in man or the real man, is deathless, immortal. Life lives the life of perfection when it lives in spirituality. The body has death, but not the Soul.

Action binds us only when we bind action with our likes and dislikes. Sacrifice is the secret of Self-dedicated service. A man of wisdom knows what he has and what he is is the Soul. Hence to him the Soul's needs are paramount.

Purusha is the silent face; Prakriti is the activating smile.
Soul Joins the Light of God After Leaving the Body
Here is Rupal's letter to her friend who had just experienced the death of a loved one:

Dearest ____: **2-23-82**
I have been thinking about you. Without saying in so many words—heart does his thing. As long as our heart is alive and does his thing, we are OK.

Our mind keeps his link with God, there is no pain in the mind. Pain is only in ignorance. Mind needs light. Light is whatever we feel, whatever we can be thankful for.

When the Soul leaves the body—soul joins the light of God. Pure egoless, mindless light. The beauty of life is that, we can feel the same even in the body. _____ has become light. Do whatever we must do and still keep our cool. Walk our road of life with a smile on our face. Loving and happy. Make the best of the Journey to Freedom.
—Rupal

A Quotation From Swami Sivananda
Here is Rupal's letter to her friend:

Dear _____: *3-1-82*
Our teacher Swami Sivananda asks only one sentence from us "Serve,
love, be truthful, Meditate and realize God, Guru, Yoga & Dharma."
Serve means our body—take good care, keep fit, strong, healthy and
serve others. Love is Bhakti, devotion to children, God & other souls. It
is good to do these things when we are young so we can do it when we are
old.

Truth and Trust are the language of Soul. Soul knows no other
language. Meditation helps us to reach that language and our mind is
quiet and desireless. I don't expect anything from anyone. I am never
disappointed. God is your Soul, Guru is your mind if God lives in your
mind and guides the body.

Swami Vishnu Devananda says today is one day closer to death or God.
So we should not waste time. If we do something hopefully it is worth dying
for. Every soul waits in heaven or at God's home to come down to earth with
their dreams to fulfill. God asks what do you need—whatever we ask He gives.
Still when we are here many times we hate someone, for not loving us. We find
a lot of excuses for not doing what we really came here to do.

My father passed away in August, _____ passed away in August. I am
sure souls like these did so much while they were here and then left the
body because body was of no help. Death is as wonderful as birth. We are
all here to do the best we can to help and guide other Souls. Pray in action,
so we can really help someone. Those little children need help. The soul
which leaves the body goes back in God. That soul is just like God. They
all love you, always. Children will be loved through God, that soul and
other souls. They will never be neglected. Our share of hurt, pain is given
to us to teach some message. We must learn the message and our life will
be of some purpose and good cause.

Love always makes other person free. Love is not perfect unless we are free in ourselves. Most people live here like they are living in a hotel. Always thinking about themselves. They cannot be free. When we stop thinking about ourselves—life starts as real love, real freedom. Only one or two people in our entire lives, are enough to help us to make our lives something special. Like my teachers to me. I need nothing more. I hope you feel better and I hope ___ feels better. We are like pieces of a puzzle thrown away in the emptiness, we like children put it together—"Life."

Spiritual Union; God is Beyond Religion
Here is Rupal's letter to a Yoga student:

Dear ____,
They say children pick their parents. Why do they pick? How do they pick? We don't know. There is such a wide choice of parents. After selecting, sometimes they are confused. Life seems it is not making as much progress as they hoped. Parents are their Guru. It should work. But something happens in between the time of life. Everything must work.

The same selecting happens in spiritual life. Though God is the same, and we are the same, what are we selecting? What are we selecting through initiation? The light, the inspiration, the Guide, the Guru, God. Because we must unite. We must find ways to enrich our life.

Still the whole process depends on ourselves. God is beyond religion. He is not Christian, he is not Jewish, he is not Hindu, nor is he Muslim. He is in Om. We can only see Him through the eyes of Om. The eye of Shiva. Because God's message to every soul is to be transformed from his love, through his love.

Our job is to inspire you. Our job is to give you the eternal knowledge of God and Guru. Your job is to understand what we are saying. There must not be a feeling of guilt in receiving "knowledge" and living knowledge.

Krishna and Radha are one of the forms of God consciousness. They are a mirror of spiritual union. In that mirror we try to see our little image (our soul) just like them gentle, loving, respectful and full of devotion from the She and He side of life. If you are a pure soul your vision is clear and clean. Your mind is calm with love and devotion for the eternal. There is no dirt on your mirror. There is no conflict of any kind in the heart about God and Guru.

We trust you. We are offering all we have. May this picture inspire you, keep and enlighten you. Your good karmas will always protect you. So keep creating them. Do the best of your ability in life to serve your true self. See through the problems of life, be strong, be firm, and be successful. These things are very easy to attain.

Serve the Lord and Guru through simple ways, because they don't ask too much. There is no frustration on the spiritual path. Remember that.
Love,
Rupal

The Soul Has the Everlasting Flow of Love
Here is an except from Rupal's essay entitled "Happiness Always."

Mind and heart keep discussing without the leadership of the Soul forever…
Mind says, "There is no God."
Heart says, "I believe there is God."
Mind says, "There is no love in this world any more."
Heart says, "There is lots and lots of love. Take it as much as you want."
Mind says, "There is nothing but darkness here."
Heart says, "You must be joking, there is so much light around each person in this world. You sure have no idea."
Mind says, "I have lost faith in people, religion and nations."
Heart says, "Faith you must have in people."
Mind says, "There is no truth. Truth changes with people."
Heart says, "The beauty of truth is: it just is. It does not change. His truth and my truth remain the same. There are many people who are dedicating themselves for serving people and to build a happy world."

In reality we are the masterpiece of the Universe. We must recognize the Soul of the human being. The soul is the teacher, guide and unselfish giver—the loving God in human beings.

The soul has the everlasting flow of love. The soul can express love without a kiss or a hug. The soul has the everlasting music of happiness. The soul is the bridge between the two people and the world. Soul ties are real ties. When one feels the spiritual tie with another person, real freedom begins. When mind and heart are guided by the soul—all relations are complete. Soul is not a man, not a woman nor a child. The soul is not bound into the limits of childhood, manhood or old age. The love flows evenly to all.

Whenever, wherever you say, "I do" say it with body, mind, heart, and soul. Be in harmony in and out of your self. Start to feel yourself as a soul, act as a soul, and live as a soul. Go beyond the petty mind and short-lived emotions. Live in the Godly spirit of the soul, be happy and be united. The job of the body is to serve the soul. The mind delivers and instructs the message of the soul to the body. The heart is the measuring cup of all the human qualities blessed by the soul dedicated to life. Be one and be a whole human being. (Don't be just heart, or mind or body.) Hari-Om.

Here is Anandi Narayani's letter to her husband Bharat on Valentine's Day

Feb. 11, 1976
To the Valentine—whom I met on Valentine's Day 1959. To those special moments of life when I felt one. To those moments which we lived to the fullest.

My dearest Bharat:
It is just the beginning when we start living as souls. Start loving as souls. Last year I suppose was the sad year or the pain of delivering the truth. Truth is that we never looked at each other as souls. We were more like a man and a woman. We reached to our limitations. Now the time of unlimited light starts. So far our eyes did the seeing, now may our souls

do the seeing. So far our lips did the kissing. Now let the soul feel the kiss of another soul.

Now is the time for my favorite thought—perhaps now the beautiful thought can live between us—One of us comes down, one of us reaches up—and we meet. One of us says to another I need you. The other says, I need you too.

One of us says—The great one you are mine. The other one says—no mine and thine. We are one. No one can recognize us from each other. Our own selves blend in ourselves.

Let two souls be one. And we feel the real blissful positive vibrations around us. Bring the shine of your soul out let it flow into mine. Let the instrument of mind be in perfect harmony. Our minds are capable of doing that. Reach out to my soul. Let us become the source of strength, divine love, and hope for tomorrow. Let our souls make the conversation. Open up.
    Yours in Union,
    Anandi Narayani,
    Anandi the mother of Ajay and Meeta

Blissful Mother
This poem is about the Sivananda Yoga Center, but it could just as easily apply to the Divine Mother.

The Blissful Mother (The Sivananda Yoga Center)

The mother taught love being love.
The mother taught service by serving.
The mother cleaned up our mixed up minds.
The mother fed our souls around the clock.

Often the child grows up,
Learns to run faster and faster.
And never finds time for the mother.
Gives a hurried hug on Mother's Day.

317

She wipes the unhappiness
From our lives magically.
She lives in a Yogic existence.
She has the knowledge of Vedanta.

She has the music of the eternal soul.
She has the depth of Meditation.
She has the love of the deepest devotion.
Learn to love the mother deeply.

She has many loving children.
She is the proud mother of Swami Vishnu-Devananda.
She has made many lives.
Let her spiritual love flow towards you.

Give her a little special love.
Each day of your life.
Stay in Union, Go deep in Yoga.
Serve the divine mother. (Sivananda Yoga Center)

—Anandi Narayani, on Mother's Day, May 8, 1977.

Here is Rupal B. Gajjar's letter to the editor of the News-Journal entitled "Mother has many names" dated January 4, 1983.

Mother Has Many Names

Mary deserves the love and respect of every Christian. In India we have several names for God as father and several names for mother as God and also for their children as God. So we can look up to them and make our family godly.

I understand Mother Mary because in our culture God's wife is seen as mother. It is again and again expressed, "Mother, you are my Father's Shakti (strength). Mother, you are Saraswati (knowledge of the universe). Mother, you are Sita (the perfect wife and perfect mother). Mother, you are Radha (the perfect beloved to my Father)."

Man needs to understand the mother, as God understands Mary. Women need to know God, the beloved son. Bring the balance of spiritual energy in life.

Hell and sin disappear when we are in love with Mother and Son (God). Yoga means union. Once you unite with the Lord, you learn to unite with his Mother Mary. We have a name for Mother—Laxshmi, which means mother who bestows all forms of prosperity, truthfulness, non-violence, humility, spiritual understanding, contentment, serenity of mind, endurance, compassion and wisdom of the cosmic self. I understand Mother Mary. Mother is one, but she has many names. The spirit of Mary alone can bring and raise the spirit of the Lord.

Rupal B. Gajjar
Wilmington

Here is Rupal B. Gajjar's letter to the editor of the News-Journal entitled "God Never Disappoints" dated January 30, 1983.

God Never Disappoints

I read the Jan. 5 letter from Ann Costello and the Jan. 29 letter in response to it from Joann Hollinger. Does it really matter who goes to heaven? That is for God to decide. Mrs. Costello loves Jesus and she loves his mother. It seems to me that gives her just a little more grace. How can she go wrong with so much love for mother? She will make it to God's heart. Whoever seeks God finds him. God never disappoints anyone. In the past, religious solders went out with their swords to decide who was a devotee and who was not. God never wanted that…Every religion has four kinds of followers: One is lazy and ignorant; he cannot live God. The second is selfish; he does business with God, always thinking of what God will give for his prayers. The third is good but he is not thinking about God either; he worries about who will go to heaven, a waste of time. The last desires nothing; he keeps his heart and mind on God and does God's will.

Love mankind, serve mankind and love God, not matter what different names the world calls him.

Rupal B. Gajjar
Wilmington

Beloved is Watching You…

I practice Yoga. Yoga means union with God. By practice of a religion, man is trying to invoke God in his or her life. Success in knowing God depends on an individual's efforts. [To reach God,] man needs to come out of his or her prison of ego and selfishness. I love prayers and songs of devotion to God. I think every human being is a prayer to God. God brings endless energy and strength into human life. But the other day I was restless and needed comfort so I played a tape of memorable songs by a famous singer of India, whose songs are heard by every Indian at least once a day. As the tape moved on from one (sad) song to the next, suddenly I found myself getting into a strange sadness. I stopped the tape.

I thought if we make a survey of all the sad songs sung in the world or make a survey of all the sweethearts who suffered heartache or a list of disappointments of every parent in their children or a list of disappointments of children in their parents or a list of troubles of every teacher who has to work with wall-faced children or a list of student's frustration when a teacher cannot teach and only gives grades from a readymade checklist and feels his job is done. When you see so much disappointment around you, you see TRUTH in the saying of monks, "Beware mankind, this world is not real. God is. All relationships are false. They bring nothing but heartbreaks."

As I see it: Love is a One Way Street. Love is nothing but service to another human being with full devotion. When I look back and think about my parents, how much love they had for us, how much service and sacrifice they performed. Even if I tried, there is no way I could return it. Every parent does the same sacrifice—in its own way. Their love is like burning logs which give the flame of warmth in our life. Miracles like these occur all the time. Have you witnessed the times when you found yourself in a jam and someone came forward and helped you out without asking for a reward or even a thank you? We receive life, not to be disappointed but to serve another human being. When you are serving another human being there is no disappointment.

Life is a celebration, a special dance of a human being and God. One has to be in love with Him. God dances with every human being. It is an opportunity to return all the debts we accumulate from others. Life is never a burden, a pain or one big sad event. We should just get busy. Treat every day of our life as the last day of our life. Then we can do all we have to do for the beloved. Receive love, knowledge, light, energy, truth and strength, all you need and as much as you need from God and give it away freely. Remember we came empty handed and we shall return empty handed. He (and She) gives us the stage of the world to see how we play our human role and try to reach Divinity.

This article is dedicated to Yoga master Swami Sivananda and my respected Guru Swami Vishnudevananda. Rupal B. Gajjar, M.A.

Pain Is Real, Freedom from Pain Is Just as Real

There is an answer to every pain and problem.
It is always very close. When you refuse suffering,
you will find it. Find the answer. You have the answer.
No one can give it to you, even if they are very
close to you and want to give it to you, they can't.
Pain is real, freedom from pain is just as real.

—Rupal (an excerpt from a letter to a friend, August 7, 1983)

Power of Love

By giving yourself in service, you reach out to the Soul.
By serving at home, you serve the Universe.
By serving the Universe, you reach God.

Meditate and find peace.
Send love to Swami Sivananda, love will grow.
Send love to Swami Vishnu-Devananda, love will expand.
Send love to your Guru, love will Shine.
Send love those "you cannot stand," love will become dynamic.
Thoughts are mighty powerful, Positive always wins over negative.
Those you feel are a lost cause—will walk straight.
They will reach home to the Soul. Hari-Om

By Anandi Narayani Devi, January 26, 1976

Here is my mother's letter to my sister, Meeta.

Dear Meeta: *May 2, 1980*
   Learn to realize you are Sat, Chit, Anand (you are bliss). You should always keep your mind centered to truth. Where truth exists, happiness exists. You are that bliss.

   I was mad at Mrs. _____ for her meanness but perhaps to grow we need to pass by that meanness. To go beyond suffering we have to know how it feels. Perhaps we deserve it for sharing her land. It was a part of that deal. We passed by her life. We should be happy that we are not in her shoes. We are happy. God has given much more than she can grab now. It is better to be free from under her thumb.

   Problems are really our true friends. They show you a road to success, and help us go beyond pain.

   You have to understand each other (Ajay and you) and each other's personalities, and find a path of harmony, strength, and success in life. Always look at the best side of each other.

   Always respect truth and honesty in other people. Don't hurt them. Don't hurt yourself. Turn negative things around because there are only two sides of everything, negative or positive. Positive is there because negative is hiding. When negative is on your side remember positive is hiding. So, never get sad and upset or punish yourself. Self is Satchidananda. Problems make us strong. Easy life makes us soft and weak. Be a warrior like Arjun who merges in Krishna and does his duty and finds liberation.

Love you,
-Mommy- (Rupal)

Satsang with Baba Muktananda

Baba is a one of the spiritual saints. Every time you meet a saint, something happens to you. You take a few more steps on the eternal path of bliss. You feel richer spiritually than you have ever been. You can only know a saint if you are enlightened with Guru's grace.

Baba's school of philosophy is called Siddha and his Center is called Siddha Dham of America. They reach the top of the mountain by Guru's energy. Many ways you can reach there. Guru's energy uplifts you only when you deserve it and don't demand it.

[paragraphs in between removed]

My soul told Baba, "I don't want anything from you." Baba's divine Soul answered, "I don't want anything from you." His bliss reached out to me. My Soul and his Soul became one. I felt tears in my eyes and I felt very happy. I know without any words he knew my thoughts and he answered.

He told us a nice story about religious groups. How much conflict religions carry with them. Some rich people in town got together and collected a huge fund. They wanted to use it for a good cause for the human race. They decided to build a beautiful temple of Shiva, the Lord of Bliss. After they built it, only a few Shiva bhaktas [devotees] used the place. It was pretty disappointing to see 15 people using such a big place. They decided to demolish Shiva's temple and make it Krishna's temple. The same thing happened with only a few Krishna people using the place.

They decided to make a church. Only a few Christians used the place. Finally they tried to make a mosque and still no success. So finally a wise man came up with a great idea. They built a big hotel/restaurant. Everyone used the place. They welcomed each other and lots of thank you's were heard.

So he gave a message, "God dwells within you as you. See God in each other. Thou art that, that thou art." This is why Yoga is not a religion. Your Soul is the Source of enlightenment.

Happiness in Marriage Through Yoga
by Rupal B. Gajjar (Anandi Narayani)

I came to the United States at Christmas time in 1961. One day I was standing outside of my apartment and a charming girl stopped and started talking. She was very kind and warm. She was my first friend in Wilmington. One day she and her husband invited my family for dinner. I thought these two people went together so well. Two days later, she told me her marriage was not working out and she was going to be separated. It was a great shock to me. After that I heard from several friends that their marriages were not working out.

Some men feel their wives have failed them. Some women feel their men have failed them. They leave each other to find a new partner. There is no promise that a new marriage will prove successful.

Women in the liberation movement cry about the suffering men have caused them. They like to be free from man and free from suffering. How can people be free from one another? Freedom lies within. I have admired my father, brother, husband and son. I feel totally free. These men have enriched my life. I would not have been a complete woman without them. My husband's and my spiritual teacher, Shri Swami Vishnu Devananda, who has given us the knowledge of Yoga is a man.

If you are lucky you can see beyond the body to the soul. Souls have no sex. Why are we wasting our time and energy on this bodily concept?

Marriage is the union of two souls. Two souls walk toward God to unite with the Super-Soul. Love is to serve. When you love, you never have time to think about returns. You never feel lost or cheated if you are one. Like your body, all parts work together.

Many times a young girl grows up with a dream about her Prince Charming and she never grows out of this fairy tale. Outside the fairy tale, a girl or boy has many problems to solve. Nobody becomes the king or queen. Marriage is all hard work, understanding and serving for the greater cause beyond enjoyment of the senses. Fairy tales always start with suffering and end with everlasting happiness. But the average American girl starts with all the comforts and ends with suffering. She thinks marriage is a game of one-up. Nobody wins that game.

The fact is, one should not demand anything from one's husband or wife. Never ask your husband to prove his love by doing certain things like taking out the garbage or buying you a mink coat. He will give you what he can afford. But if you hurt each other, you will soon learn to hate.

Marriage is two lovely souls walking happily on the road of life, blending in love, truth and bliss. The children are pure souls, equal to parents and they receive proper education about soul, body and mind that is Yoga. The children know all freedom has boundary of right action. Without right actions, freedom loses its strength. You are free to do right or wrong.

Marriage is a wonderful, real and joyful relationship when you walk toward God. The marriage fails only when husband and wife walk toward each other. They want and demand happiness from each other. Nobody can present happiness; it is created within.

Road to a Happy Family

"Patanjali says to secure peace with family and society use four different keys to human locks: be friendly with a happy individual; be compassionate with an unhappy individual; be delighted with a virtuous person; and be indifferent to a wicked one.

Let us examine families: in the first kind, all family members feel anger and use the language of violence. In the second everyone always thinks about himself and uses the language of screams. In the third kind, all family members love and serve the whole family. Each member enjoys peace, harmony, happiness, and good health. Everyone uses the language of respect and the whole family watches over every individual.

We have these three choices. Whatever we want, we get.

Rupal B. Gajjar

Dearest _____ (a friend):   *August 5, 1983*
Life is a stage. People are the actors. Karma is the director of the play. God wants you to direct your own parts. That choice is yours. Over all, acting is a temporary situation like life is. For a short time, life is given to us to straighten out our act and reach perfection.

You and I were put together so I can comfort you, inspire you and help you to understand the situation and go above it. You still keep slipping in past memories. It is like watching an album of sad memories. Reinforcing the pain. Everything has two sides. If you are on the sad side, then walk to the happy side. Reinforce all the good things you have. Find the answer you alone can find. You alone have to try a little harder. Refuse to suffer. Make an even stronger effort and close the door to anxieties. You have been traveling into your mind all this time. Start traveling into your soul. Every time the mind invites you to travel to the past, take your mind into prayers and memorize them. When they will become your strong part, your life will come to an order. There is lots of power hidden in those prayers. Don't refuse them. Create everlasting love, peace, hope, harmony and good health which you wish to have.

Find that perfection in your life, which is there. Don't ignore it anymore. When there is an opening, move. It is very close. Very close indeed.
Love,
Rupal

Fearlessness

There are many things we can be afraid of while living our lives. But many fears disappear when we realize we are Spirit Souls and a part of God. My mother was fearless. When she was running Meeta's Discount Bazaar, an Indian/American grocery and gift store in Wilmington, she was once threatened by a man with a hammer. My mother did not react with fear in the situation. The man left the store without doing anything else.

Blessing to the Buyer of Their Home

Dear _____,

The Ganesh at your door means God is Lord Ganesh who helps and protects us. To bring success into our life. It also represents union with the animal kingdom and nature. Man uniting with the animal kingdom. Elephant trunk means elephants are sharp and man should be sharp like an elephant. When you are sharp you succeed. Success is created by hard work. All wisdom is around man, man has to tune in with wisdom. To love is the greatest wisdom. When we love we feel secure inside. To feel secure inside is the most important thing in the world.

I have a lock shaped like Ganesh in my kitchen. Ganesh is like a lock and you are the key. You alone can open the lock. With this I wish to welcome the God in you. I wish you and your family all the happiness and success in life in your new home. Moving in a new home is life-rebirth like spring flowers. After the winter, the first spring flowers bloom from the dirt. They faced cold, wind and rain, but they kept on dreaming only about the warm, shiny sun. The dream pulls them through. The tension of moving and settling down is like the death of comfort. But once you face that death, life begins. Life only gets better and better.

[a paragraph removed]

When I blessed my new home, I blessed your old home, and your new home. You have to bless your home every day to feel and fill it with the same bliss. You have to adore your home, so your home learns to adore you. You have to feel proud. Make a list of little things and finish them cheerfully.

Life is full of problems—little or big. Problems are like shoes. We wear them and they fit our feet just right. We cannot wear anybody else's shoes. My feet have their problems too. Life is like love. We should learn to smile and learn to serve whomever we love, whatever we love.
    Your Friend,
    Rupal

Thoughts After Visiting Her Father in India

As one grows up and starts calling oneself an adult, one starts worrying about tomorrow. It is funny, very funny indeed. No adult understands how to live now. I think he knows. In Yoga the body may age, but the Soul stays happy young. Even if people think you seem crazy. But you are a happy crazy. Why not? I want to be happy crazy, till the end of my journey. You may witness it.

  Now I consider my Soul the greatest poet,
  my life the greatest poem.
  I am a complete song.
  God is the music of that song.
  I am reaching out, to that wealth which the Soul,
  has handed over to life. Hari-Om.

—Rupal B. Gajjar, January 21, 1976

When the time is right, we meet.
When the time comes, we part.
So, there is not much difference—
Between meeting and parting.
They are just little events—
Of the universal play.

—Anandi Narayani

Chapter 32

Yoga and Related Subjects

YOGA WITH FAMILY

Lord Krishna says, "Blessed are those who are born in the family of a Yogi." It is good to learn and practice Yoga alone, however it is better to learn Yoga with your spouse and practice together at home. If you have children, you should teach them Yoga. My experience might give you some ideas about how to learn and teach Yoga to your family.

After I started Yoga I decided to intensify my pursuit of the Yogic path. But as I was working I did not have much free time. So during my vacation I spent one week with my family at the Sivananda Yoga Vedanta Center at 8th Avenue, Val Morin, Quebec JOT 2RO, Canada, Telephone (819) 322-3226. We drove up to Val Morin, and during that week we participated in all the programs, including Yoga twice a day, morning Meditation with Swami Vishnu Devananda Maharaj, and evening Satsang. Our first visit was in the summer of 1968, and we continued going every summer because we liked it so much. My children played with other children and learned Yoga with them.

In the late '60s, I drove to New York City for DuPont, my employer, and one evening, as I was walking to a restaurant for dinner, I saw a young American in orange clothing, like a monk's, and a girl dressed in an Indian sari chanting the Hari Krishna Mantra. I crossed the street to talk to them and give them a donation. They invited me to their Satsang that night. It was on 26th Street and 2nd Ave. So, after dinner, I went to their Krishna Temple and was told that Swamiji (A. C. Bhakti Vendanta Swami Prabupada) had gone to London to see George Harrison of the Beatles. Swami Prabupada had brought a trunkful of his Srimat (Srimad) Bhagavatam books, and I bought for $10 each two of the original copies that he had brought from India. I stayed for the chanting and invited Swamiji to our Wilmington Sivananda Yoga Center. However, he became very popular and busy, and so was never able to visit.

In his lecture, he (Prabupada) said that every family should have an altar at home, and before dinner should offer food to the Lord before eating, making it Prasad. My Mother had an altar in our home in India. So I thought it an excellent idea to have one in our home. Then every weekday evening my wife, two kids and I held an evening family Satsang. On our altar we had a picture of Radha Krishna, and eventually a picture of our Guru, Swami Vishnu Devananda, the symbol Om, some incense and a candle. Every evening we used to sing a Bhajan, then chant the Jaya Ganesha Mantra of the Sivananda Ashram, and read one verse of the Bhagavad Gita. Then we did one new Hatha Yoga posture every night and we did Arti (light ceremony). The singing of the Mantras was getting more and more powerful as we sang every night. At one point I taught my son, Ajay, to play the harmonium and I played the Indian drums (Tabla), and my daughter Meeta played the manjera while we all sang. If I had something to say to the children I would not at that time. But sometime at the end of the Satsang I would say, "Let's all say one good thing and discuss one problem which needs to be worked on." I would give my message that way. Then the children got a chance to tell their parents of one problem as well. I thought this was a nice communications technique.

Here's an interesting story. My daughter Meeta had a friend from Wales, UK, who would sit in with us during our family Satsang when she was visiting or eating with us. We learned that once when she was at home with her family, she vomited her supper and at that time "Hare Krishna" came out of her! That was the turning point for this family and the children began Sunday school in a church.

My children were able to learn Yoga and the Bhagavad Gita in depth through our home Satsang and Yoga postures that we did nightly together. See the photo of our altar with my wife Rupal in Fig. 15.3 (page 151). My son Ajay has two children and has continued the nightly family Satsang with his family.

My wife and I never punished our children we only had a talk with them. But one thing we did, was go out to dinner every Friday or Saturday night. The four of us took turns selecting where to eat; so everyone got a turn, even the children. When we went out to dinner, my wife and I would not criticize our children; instead we would build their self-esteem by telling them how great they were. They never disappointed us. Positive living is very powerful living.

Great People Remember Names
I received the following article on the Internet by an author unknown to me. It read, "During my second month in college, our professor gave us a pop quiz. I was a conscientious student and had breezed through the questions until I read the last one: "What is the first name of the woman who cleans the school?"

"Surely this was some kind of joke. I had seen the cleaning woman several times. She was tall, dark-haired and in her 50s, but how could I know her name? I handed in my paper, leaving the last question unanswered. Just before the class ended, one student asked if the last question would count toward our quiz grade. "Absolutely," said the professor. "In your careers, you will meet many people. All are significant. They deserve your attention and care, even if all you do is smile and say "hello."

"I've never forgotten that lesson. I also learned her name was Dorothy."

This message stunned me, because I could remember the names of only the people I worked with. To others around me, I would say 'Hi,' but did not know their names. After reading this message, I became more aware of how important it is to remember everyone's names. I try very hard to remember someone's name and when I address him or her by their first name, they feel I am their friend and I care.

When I was working for DuPont DeNeumors and Co., the General Director (highest level in management) would come during Christmas and shake hands with all the employees and address each one by their first name. His name is Dr. Russ Peterson. Later he became the Governor of Delaware. When I saw him 30 years later at a party, he came over to me and addressed me by my first name. I was stunned that he remembered my name.

An Indian had met Mahatma Gandhi once. When he met him again after many years, Mahatma Gandhi called him by his first name.

Once I saw a TV show in which the host asked 100 people in the audience to stand up and say their full names. The guest of the show was able to identify all the 100 audience members by their names. This is an extraordinary example, but you should remember the names of the people you come into contact with.

My brother used to travel around the world and keep a diary in which he would jot down names. When he visited a city again, he would visit friends, he would recall names of all the children's and other family details. He would give at least one meaningful compliment a day. I try my best to put this into practice.

I knew a man who tried to circumvent his difficulty in knowing someone's name by calling everyone by the same name. For example, he would say "Hi, Joe" to every man he passed by. He annoyed everyone by doing this and not taking the effort to learn anyone's name.

It is good to teach your children to remember people's name.

Even God likes to be called by His first name. We as human beings also like to be called by our first names, don't we?

When remembering someone's name, it is a sign that you really love that person.

Creativity is as important in life as your personal growth. I was very fortunate to have had a job with DuPont in the research laboratory. Out of the budget for my assigned projects I was allowed to spend 5% to 10% on my own ideas. I was recognized one year in the Patent division as one of the three top engineers with the most patents. I had 20 of them. Then someone asked me what was my secret for achieving so many patents. I replied, "That within the 10 ideas I come up with to present to the Management, I also add one curve ball, an idea that is not very logical but has potential. Often it turned out to be the winner and the new direction and eventually became a new Patent." I have my own paradigm and always want to stay within my own paradigm or field of knowledge. I go just outside my paradigm and experience it. If I like it I go a little farther the next time. Within a short time I always find my paradigm has shifted. I focus on the Supreme Being when I'm formulating my ideas. I keep all the problems in my mind. Then, during Meditation, sometimes answers and new directions are revealed to me. All my patents are a grace from God. These creative methods helped me in teaching. It made my Yoga classes more effective.

Pain and Yoga

Safety is very essential in practicing Yoga. Yoga says, "No pain, no gain." When you do Asanas, you have to come within the margin of pain to make any progress and to increase flexibility, but you have to make sure you do not cross the limit where you may injure yourself. God has given pain so that we can live happily with a long life. I heard a story about a man who had no pain. It was his greatest handicap. He had to be very careful when living in this material world. So pain is actually a signal from God to be careful. Pain can be your friend or your enemy, so you have to figure out which one it's going to be. Pain is a red light, so don't ignore it, but at the same time if you do not come into the margin of pain—you cannot make progress. When your body has pain, it means something is wrong and you need to correct it. My father used to say, "Don't pamper your pain." There are three types of pain mental, emotional and physical. All pain is experienced through the mind. Different people have a different tolerance levels for pain. There are so many sources of pain: psychological, fear, chemical imbalance, disease, temporary or permanent bodily injury, self-inflicted, and so on. I believe some mental pains or unhappiness is a sign from God that we are on the wrong path, have the wrong attitude or wrong philosophy of life. Swami Sivananda used to say, "Keep a diary and take notice if you are on the wrong path. Make necessary corrections." To solve our worldly pains we should seek answers from wise men, medical doctors, scriptures or do Meditation regularly. Prevention is the best medicine, and for that practice Yoga, breathe deeply, eat a balanced vegetarian diet and maintain your weight. Karmic pain is a different issue and I like the American proverb regarding this, "Whatever goes around comes around."

HPI reported the following in April 2006:
India's Vice President Launches Yoga University

HARIDWAR, INDIA, April 6, 2006: Vice President Bhairon Singh Shekhawat today launched the first Yoga University of the country, Patanjali Yoga Peeth, a dream project of Swami Ramdev at Bahadarabad near Haridwar. In his inaugural address, Mr. Shekhawat said, Swami Ramdev has assured the right to lead a healthy and disease-free life to all. Uttaranchal Chief Minister N. D. Tiwari, who presided over the function, declared that the University had been empowered to open colleges in all parts of the country. Railway Minister Lalu Prasad announced that a railway station would be built at the project site about 15 km from Haridwar. Swami Ramdev, who is the life-long chancellor of the university, said his mission was to provide peace, health and Sanskars (moral values) to the people through Yoga, Ayurveda and spirituality.

Yoga and Energy
One of the major points of Yoga is to work with energy. Energy offers ojes that gives off spiritual light and high, loving vibrations. This is needed in practicing Yoga and doing spiritual Sadhana. Yogic energy is very important to a Yogi or a Yoga practitioner. There are three aspects of energy in Yoga. The first is how to gain energy, the second is how to block energy or to preserve energy and, the third is how to use energy to obtain God, self, and life realization.

One may ask where does energy fit into Yogic philosophy? From my perspective, life is divided into three aspects, God the spirit (Father), God as energy (Mother or Prana Shakti) and light (Guru). The opposite of light is darkness, which is ignorance. So energy is Prana Shakti and it is the key of Yoga Sadhana. In Christianity this would represent the trinity Father, Son and Holy Spirit (ghost which is energy)(Drawing 32.1, page 339).

Prana Shakti is the breath, which is the energy Yogis work with. It is also the healing force. It heals the body, mind and soul. Many Yogis worship this powerful energy as Mother Shakti or the divine mother of the universe. One of the foremost Mantras is "Shakti Ma."

How to Gain Energy

Pranayama is the key to capturing Prana or the living force. The second thing Yogis do is to eat sattvic food or good vegetarian food with the understanding that cooked food is half dead. This compassionate food has lots of energy and is best when eaten after offering it to God. Yet another way to gain energy is to surrender to Mother (shakti) or Prana Shakti (living force). The process of surrendering is loving and letting the ego go. Mantra Yoga where God's name is repeated many times with love (Japa Yoga) also increases energy. Most Yogis practice Meditation, which is Raja Yoga. There are people who believe that Karma Yoga also (selfless service) increases energy through giving. Yogis who are at a higher level of consciousness receive energy through Kundalini Yoga (Mystical Yoga). Of course Hatha Yoga is very vital as a tool to increasing energy when the Asanas are done with Pranayama. Hatha Yoga can be further enhanced when Mudra Yoga is added to the Pranayama. Preservation of sexual energy will also enhance one's spiritual energy through abstinence. When one is very lazy one cannot gain energy. Random acts of kindness will increase your energy.

How Not to Lose Energy and Preserve Energy

To preserve energy, Yogis practice bandhas during Pranayama. Andre van Lysebeth describes Bandhas as follows: "Bandhas, like so many words of the Yogic vocabulary, cannot be translated exactly into western language. It means to tie, to control, to block, to hold, to join and to contract, all at the same time. In Yoga practice, and particularly in Pranayama, Bandhas refers to various muscular contractions intended to influence the circulation of blood, the nervous system and the endocrine glands. Most Bandhas are concerned with the control of one particular orifice of the body." Overeating causes loss of energy. So make a point to not over eat. Yogis believe one should not eat after sunset or before sunrise. Eating meat and drinking alcohol will also take its toll on your energy supply. Extremes of any kind will deplete your energy, including sexual energy. Anger, hatred and negativity will drain your energy quickly. Overdose of exercise also can deplete energy. Lack of proper sleep is a big cause of energy loss. Fear will exhaust one's supply of energy. Undisciplined living will cause loss of energy too.

There are some negative people that will suck your energy out. I call them Prana suckers; some others call them vampires. These negative people will drain your energy so be conscious of that. Do not hug and shake hands with these types of people. Women are very sensitive of this. That is why in the East we do Namaste (I bow to the God within you) rather than shake hands as people do in the West. Women in the West, have the privilege in the West to decide whether or not to shake hands when introduced to a new person, whereas men are obliged to do so.

Yogis believe that your energy goes out of your body from your thumbs and your big toes. In the east it is common for a disciple to touch his Guru's feet. Most of the time, they touch their Guru's toes and receive their Guru's energy. Some healers in Christianity will touch a person's forehead with their thumb when performing healing in Church.

I used to show my students the power of energy released through the thumb by asking my class in the winter if anyone was cold. I would go over to the cold person, inhale deeply, then, put my right thumb on his forehead and exhale. The person would immediately feel warm.

One of my students thought she would try the technique on an ill person in a hospital. She told me that the patient sucked all her energy out and she was completely drained.

How to Use Your Energy in Yogic Sadhana
It is important to understand that without energy it is very difficult to practice Yoga Sadhana.

My daughter Meeta had a student in her Yoga class for years as well, who enjoyed relaxation but never experienced the deeper level of reaching her subconscious. This is a deeper form of Meditation experienced where one feels loving energy and peace. Then one day the student found out that she had the beginning stages of osteoporosis. She changed her diet completely, becoming vegetarian and this raised her consciousness. Then one day she went to a seminar where she wasn't prepared to go into relaxation and she found herself deep into her subconscious where she had never been before. She told Meeta that it was an amazing place and that she never wanted to come back. Meeta was really surprised because all those years she thought this student had been experiencing this higher level, but she had not. It's true that once you reach there, it is such an amazing place you don't want to come back, but you have to. Some people are able to reach higher levels of consciousness and relaxation without becoming vegetarian.

Many young people go to work and experience high tension, insecurity and a negative working environment, which leads them to be completely drained of energy by the time they come home. Young people between the ages of 20—40 need a nap when they come home. They need to learn to block their energy and learn to relax. Yoga, Pranayama and Meditation can help them achieve these goals.

A lot of people would like to do a lot of things, but in reality they cannot. A person may have the talent of writing poetry but no energy to write it. To do things you would like to do requires energy, dedication, and passion to reach your goal. My experience tells me that if there is a brilliant man whom you would like to be the president of your club, but he is lazy, he would not be a good candidate. A hard working, energetic, but less intelligent person would be a better candidate for your president.

In India, as they believe in Reincarnation, they accept that all human beings are at different levels of consciousness. To gain energy and blessings they seek an enlightened being, a saint or a sat guru. They believe that if they come near the sat guru, and have darshan (in the presence) they receive blessings and high energy. They try to touch his feet or big toe to receive transcendental energy.

I believe that if you have a small temple, Chant Mantras, and do Meditation in your home, your house will have very high Satwick energy. Guests often tell me that when they come to my home and sleep over that they have the best sleep and that many times they have difficulty sleeping in other peoples homes. I also believe that if a family curses and has negativity it gets into their walls and you do not have loving vibrations. This causes suffering from this negativity in the home.

An old lady died in the house we bought from the bank, which became the Sivananda Yoga Center. There was a rumor that a ghost lived there. I experienced the presents of this ghost. The ghost eventually left because of the small temple, Mantra Chanting and Meditation that went on at the center.

Our custom in the Hindu Temples as well as at our Sivananda Yoga center required people to remove their shoes before entering the center. This Asian custom of shoe removal before entering the home is because there are positive and negative energies in the dirt that your shoes walk on outside, that can enter your home. In many Asian cultures people sit on the floor. In America, I have continued this practice of shoe removal for the same reasons. I even had a student ask me during a Yoga class, why I had everyone sit on the floor? I told her because Yoga requires one to take their shoes off and sit on the floor. Jesus and his disciplines in the Middle East also sat on the floor, but when Christianity went to Europe, the floor was so cold they had to sit on chairs.

Yogi's love animals and they are fond of cats and dogs. They like to feed animals and keep them happy. If they have pets, they like to keep them outside the house and not within their living area. One time I asked a Yogi why they have this practice of not allowing animals in their living space, and I was told that they have a different vibration and consciousness, which could interfere with Yogic practices and Meditation.

Illustration 32.1

Prana Shakti grows when one
<u>Harmonizes the mind, body and soul</u>

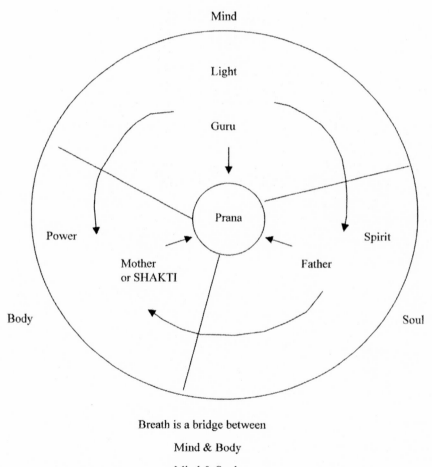

Breath is a bridge between

Mind & Body

Mind & Soul

Body & Soul

"<u>PRANAYAMA</u>" BRINGS ABUNDANCE OF PRANASHAKTI

Yogi is the one who is in harmony within him and without

Chapter 33

How to Teach Yoga

In the West, Yoga is getting more and more popular. It seems Yoga has arrived in the mainstream in America. In my hometown two hospitals used to call Yoga "Stretching Class." Now both are calling it Yoga Class. At our University of Delaware, Yoga is now a credited course. I believe, in a few years Yoga will be practiced around the world, by most people, for health, happiness and inner freedom.

This article is intended to help teachers in the West to conduct more successful and effective Yoga classes. There are 480,000 Yoga postures. However, it is better to teach thoroughly and systematically 30 to 40 important postures, which should be learned properly. Most people do not know more than 100 to 200 postures. Impress on your students that Yoga is not a religion, but a way of living that leads to health, happiness and freedom.

Objective of Teaching

Some of the many objectives for teaching are listed below. After reading these, ask yourself this simple question, "What is my objective for teaching Yoga?"

The Goals for Teaching Hatha Yoga:
1. To answer an inner calling to teach;
2. To make people healthy, peaceful, happy and free;
3. To earn some extra money or make a living;
4. To serve your Guru and spread his message or tradition;

5. To have your students attend Yoga class, practice at home regularly and recommend it to others;

6. To teach because it makes students and you happy and you meet new people.

Whatever your reason for teaching, know that it is one of the highest forms of Sadhana or spiritual practice. We all should learn, practice and teach Yoga. Teaching Yoga is one way to learn Yoga. Only teach what you know. Always remain a student. Continuously and constantly keep learning and improving your knowledge of Yoga even while passing it on to your students.

Recommended Yoga Class Routine

Speak up Time
On the first day, welcome everyone and introduce yourself. Ask each student to give his or her name and tell briefly why they are taking up Yoga.

Chant Om
Always start a class with Sukhasan or with an Easy Posture and in Vishnu Mudra (Fig. 10.6) and chant Om three times and Shanti three times.

Recite Prayer
After that, say the following prayer and/or any other prayer of your choice.

Sanskrit
Om Asato Ma Sat Gamaya
Tamaso Ma Jyotir Gamaya
Mrityor-Ma Amritam Gamaya
Om Shanti, Shanti, Shanti.

English
Om Lead us Thou, O God
From Unreal to Real
From Darkness to Light
From Death to Immortality
Om Shanti, Shanti, Shanti
Om Peace, Peace, Peace be unto us all.

This is the Universal Prayer

Surrender to Your Inner Self
Next do the swan posture. It has the Bhav or feeling of surrendering to God within you or to the God you believe in. Sitting on your knees also helps the flexibility of the knees. (Fig. 3.3, page 64)

Soorya Namaskar
On the first day of class, start with the sun prayer which is called Soorya Namaskar in Sanskrit. It is the king of Asanas (Fig. 9.1).

Every Yoga class should include at least some selected postures, at least one or two Pranayamas or Yogic breathing techniques, a brief explanation of Yoga and Savasana or relaxation (Fig. 5.4)

Rules for Practicing Asana
Before starting the Yoga class, please read or briefly mention the following rules.

REMEMBER DURING ASANAS
• Relax your body before starting Asanas
• At least 2 hours after eating must elapse before beginning Asanas
• Before starting Asanas, sit in a Sukhasan or easy (comfortable) Asana with Jnan Mudra and Chant Om
• Say a prayer or the Yoga prayer (Om Asato Ma)
• It is good to do Pranayama or Yogic breathing before starting Asanas
• I like to start Asanas with the Swan Asana and the Sun Prayer
• If you do not have much time to do Yoga, at least do the Sun Prayer (Soorya Namaskar) three times a day
• Do some Asanas at least three times and hold the other Asanas as long as you can. Hold the Asana for a minimum of three deep breaths, e.g. Go into the Cobra, inhale, deep, hold and exhale deep and do this three times and then come out of the Cobra
• During Asanas with breathing, chant "Om" silently or your Guru Mantra, or focus on the part of the body you are working on.

- Do Asanas slowly, evenly and without jerky motions
- Do Asanas Meditatively and practice mindfulness
- Work with pain and stay within your limits
- Do not compete with anyone
- Keep safety in mind and avoid sharp pain
- Take rest frequently
- Always stretch three times. Once you stretch, hold the stretched position. The second time, go a little more and the third time, come into the margin of pain. Always inhale, hold, and stretch during exhalation.
- If possible, do Asanas religiously, daily and at the same time and place, or on the same carpet or mat.
- Develop your routine, some Asanas you might do once a day, some others once a week and some others once a month
- As a general rule, during most of the Asanas when the stomach folds or contracts, you should exhale and when your stomach unfolds or expands you inhale
- Always do opposite Asanas e.g. if you do forward bend, then do the backward bend
- Never breathe through your mouth
- Remember Asanas are prayers to God with your body. Keep that feeling
- When you do Asanas, you are working with Prana Shakti, a living force which heals your mind, body, soul and your astral body.

If your class is at least 1 ½ hours long, repeat the speak-up time before starting the second class. The teacher should let each student give his or her name and then should say something inspiring to them and/or ask them if they have any questions. This speak up time will help you in teaching. If you are giving one-hour Hatha Yoga classes, speak up time will not be possible after the first class. Speak-up time doesn't have to be long, just request that the class keep it short.

Types of Yoga Classes
There are two basic types of Yoga classes. The first type is just Hatha Yoga or postures, Yogic breathing and Savasana or relaxation. It is usually of an hour class or 1 ¼ hour class. The second type is a complete Yoga class, which includes Hatha Yoga and the philosophy of Yoga, Meditation, Mantra, etc. These classes run 1 ½ hour to 2 hours long.

There are two basic types of students. One who practices at home and the other likes to practice only with a group. Of these two basic types, one likes only the physical aspect and the other likes the spiritual as well as the physical.

Some teach only beginners, while others teach beginner and advanced classes. In longer or advanced Yoga classes, one could introduce Jnan Yoga, Raja Yoga, Mantra Yoga, Bhakti Yoga, Karma Yoga, Advanced Hatha, Vegetarianism, Diet, Yogic Fasting, etc.

There are many Yoga traditions. Teach what you have learned and keep practicing. Also, keep improving your teaching so that you become more effective.

What to Teach

Teach the most important Asanas, and not the Asanas you like or are best at. You may want to show your students how good you are; there's nothing wrong with that to establish your credibility. In India it is often said, "Chamatcar Bina Namaskar Nahi", which means no one will bow to you without your showing them a miracle. When your students see your ability, they will be inspired. So a little show-off is allowed. However, make sure it is not overdone. Always teach whatever you yourself practice. If you teach what you do not practice, your students will know, and the impact of your teaching will be poor.

A man asked Mahatma Gandhi to tell his son not to eat too much sugar. He told him them to come back in a week. The man came back a week later with his son and Mahatma Gandhi told the son not to eat too much sugar. Later the man asked why he had not told his son right away and why he had made him come back after a week. Mahatma Gandhi said, "How could I tell your son not to eat too much sugar when I myself was eating too much."

In my Yoga classes I used to teach a little Kriya Yoga and requested my students to fast on Thursday, two nights (beginning Wednesday night) and one day with milk and/or fruit and/or water, and I used to fast myself. The next week I would ask my class how many fasted and 90% of them would. Now I have diabetes and I cannot fast. I still ask them to fast and when I ask them how many fasted, only 10% say they did. If you are not a vegetarian and tell your students to be vegetarian, they are not going to listen to you.

Guru

There are two basic types of Yoga teachers. One has their Guru and/or lineage or tradition. I have my Guru H.H. Swami Vishnu-Devananda and the Sivananda tradition. The second type has no Guru or tradition. Some might just have a great teacher. It is good to have a Guru and/or tradition. However, teachers without a Guru or a great teacher can also be successful.

It is said that only a good student can become a good Guru. When a student is ready, the Guru or the teacher appears. An Indian proverb says, "There is no true knowledge without a Guru."

Teaching Style

In the beginning, one can copy one's Guru or teacher in teaching technique, but at one point everyone has to develop his or her own style of teaching. Like the Vedas say, everyone is a unique individual. Also, one should remain a student forever so they can continuously learn and improve their style and teaching. Great Gurus are the ones who always remain students. Be humble and always learn and improve.

The best way to learn Yoga is to learn, practice, teach, and improve, and then learn some more. This is the best cycle and a way to perfection. Your students will also be your teacher. As you teach more, you will learn more.

Before the Class Begins

It is not a good idea to come, "just on time." The best thing is to come early for your class. If there is anything to straighten out, you can do it, then sit down and Meditate in the room to purify the vibrations. Of course if you are teaching at your own Ashram or center, you do not need to Meditate in advance, because high vibrations should already be there.

Always start your class on time so that everyone gets the message to come on time. I usually request them to come 10 to 15 minutes before the class and ask them to lie down and relax before starting the class. This helps the class in doing better Yoga.

Financial

There are two basic types of Yoga classes: 1) Classes are given continually and students pay when they attend the class. 2) The second type where 6 or 10 classes are given once a week. Students join the classes and pay up front for 6 to 10 classes. This way they commit for the whole course. I prefer the second type of class with 6 to 10 weekly classes making up the course. Also it is good to announce the first class is free. If they do not like the class they don't have to join, and if they like it they pay for the full course.

It is good to sell books and other things at your Yoga class. It brings revenue and spreads your message. Every student who takes the teacher's training course asks this question, "Can I make a living from teaching Yoga?" The next question is "Can I make a fair living, good living or excellent living?" Of course, some people learn Yoga just as a hobby or for their self-fulfillment. Some people like to teach Yoga part time. For both of these types of people's questions, I don't advise them to try to make a living at it.

For those who really want to make a living by teaching Yoga, I can say yes you can make a good living, but it is not easy. One has to make the effort or one has to have the right formula.

Without giving names, I'd like to tell you about the Yoga teachers who have made an excellent living teaching Yoga. The following are the methods:

Buy or rent a home on a main street and start a center. Live upstairs and use the living room for teaching Yoga classes. Keep one room as a store selling books, healthy vitamins and Ayurvedic medicines, etc.

Buy a house at the seashore, rent rooms as well as teach Yoga.

Buy a home and run a Yoga center. You or your spouse can have a part-time job and both of you can teach Yoga. Also allow others to teach at your center for a percentage of their income (rent out the room)

Buy a house in a resort town, and have a bed and breakfast as well as a Yoga center.

Run a small Ashram, with specific Gurus teaching. People live in (room and board). Have regular Satsangs etc. Also have a bookstore and gift shop.

I had the most unique center. I had a regular 9 to 5 job. My brother and I bought a house in town. We formed a nonprofit organization, rented the 2nd and 3rd floors and made a Sivananda Yoga Center on the first floor.

I was initiated by my Guru H. H. Swami Vishnu-Devananda. I also gave initiations into the Yoga path to those sincerely interested. Every Sunday we had a free Hatha Yoga class from 4 p.m. to 5:45 p.m. and Satsang, from 6 p.m. to 8:30 p.m. On our altar are pictures of Swami Sivananda, Swami Vishnu Devananda, and Mother Durga. After my wife died in 1984, we added her picture on the altar. My students and I taught Yoga on weeknights.

We started our center in 1965. In our center we do not pay anyone, including myself. All the money we collect is used to print books and make cassettes and distribute them. We also use the money to run a weekly TV show on public access television. We give money to an eye hospital in India for free cataract and eye operations for the poor. Now we hope to start a one-room school in India in a village where there is presently no school.

Once I tried to run free Yoga classes for the public. But only a few people joined and almost all of them dropped out after a while. One time I offered free Yoga classes for college students. Some enrolled, but after a couple of classes they also dropped out. I am reminded of a story from The Reader's Digest, about a man who walked dogs for money. He used to advertise his business in a newspaper. He charged $1 an hour to walk people's dogs. And he had two clients. Then one day, the newspaper wrongly printed the rate as $10 an hour. All of a sudden the man had 10 clients. The moral: if it costs more it must be better. So I suggest that you do not give free Yoga classes unless you are doing volunteer work.

How to Advertise

If one is teaching at an institute like the YMCA or J.C.C., and does not advertise, it is good to print business cards and pass them out to friends and others who show some interest in Yoga.

If one is teaching at a rented place, an advertisement in a local newspaper or Yoga or New Age magazine will boost income. One can put Yoga flyers on local grocery store bulletin boards or in your church or temple. The best advertisement, however, is word of mouth. Tell your students publicize the message.

First Class Is Free

Say this in your advertisement that the first class in the course is free. This will attract those who are not sure about trying out your class, and if they like it, they will sign up. You could print a coupon, which will entitle the holder to one class free. This will help you introduce your classes.

It works this way. Suppose you offer seven classes for $60. Since the first class is free, you actually will be charging $60 six classes. If someone joins in the second class, you charge $50 for the remaining five classes.

What to Do on the First Day

Take the students' names, addresses, telephone numbers, fax and/or email addresses.

Give out a handout which has your address, telephone number, and information about your classes and when they are held. Include:

1. The Yoga routine recommended by you or your Guru etc.

2. Pictures of the Asanas you will be teaching,

3. The book or books you recommend, etc.

4. On the first day, ask them to come to the next class even if they do not feel well (mentally); tell them that they will feel great after the class.

5. Tell them not to worry if they miss one or two classes, but just come back to class.

How to End the Class

It is important to start a class properly; it is important to end the class properly to be successful in teaching. In India, we call it "Yagna," which is more than effort, it is sacrifice.

Usually relaxation is the last thing done. After the second or third class, ask your students how their relaxation was. Have them give their brief comments. This will help you evaluate the effectiveness of your teaching of Yoga and relaxation. If they have difficulty in relaxing, guide them on how to relax better next time.

On the last day of the class, before adjourning, give them an evaluation form. There can be many types of evaluation forms. I like the simple one below.

Evaluation Form

Teacher's Name_____ Date_____
Class Held at_____
   I. Rate the class 1 to 10 (1 = Very Poor 5 = Borderline 10 = Excellent)
RATING
   II. Three strong points
      1.
      2.
      3.
   III. Three weak points
      1.
      2.
      3.
   IV. Your Additional Comments

May God and the Practice of Yoga Make You Healthy, Happy & Free

The above evaluation form will help improve your teaching.

Who Is a Successful Teacher?
The following is a yardstick for a successful Yoga teacher.
   1. The teacher inspires students to come regularly and ensures there are few or no dropouts.
   2. Gives a routine or structure that students can practice at home without any trouble.

3. Inspires students to start practicing at home and start reading about Yoga.

4. Students take the Yoga class again and bring a friend with them.

5. Students feel good and relaxed after each class.

6. Students feel good about all religions.

7. Inspires students to go from Hatha Yoga to Jnana, Raja, Mantra, Karma and/or Bhakti Yoga

8. Inspire the students to take the Yoga teachers training course and become a Yoga teacher.

Authentic Yoga

Many people think Yoga means stretching exercises or Hatha Yoga. But Hatha Yoga is more than just stretching postures. Hatha Yoga includes Pranayama or Yogic breathing, Mudras, Bandhas, Siddhis, Tantras, Nindra, diet, fasting, etc. To me this is what Hatha Yoga is.

To teach one has to know the authentic or "Complete Yoga." You may doubt whether students will like authentic Yoga or not, but my experience over the last 35 years assures me that most people like complete Yoga, and come back repeatedly to learn more.

A Few Recommendations

1. Always keep a notebook and write down when and where you gave the Yoga class, besides the name, address and phone number of each person who attended.

2. To teach Yoga you do not need any special or fancy clothing, but it is good to wear something white, for example, white pants and T-shirt. White clothing gives a professional look.

3. During the first class, one could test the following things on their students.

a. Sit in an Easy Posture, keep both hands in the air and then stand up. Every person should have enough strength to carry his or her own body.

b. Have them close their eyes and connect the index fingers.

c. Tell the students to lie down on their backs, put one hand on their chests and the other on their stomachs. Then tell them to take a breath and exhale. Make them do this about six times. Then ask them what went up. Their chests should not go up and down. Only their stomachs should.

4. Tell the students that they are not competing against anyone. They should not force themselves to stretch more than they are able to. Tell them, "Do your best, but know your limits."

5. Tell the students to wait for about 1 ½ hours after a meal before doing Hatha Yoga

6. Those with high blood pressure may need to refrain from doing the Headstand or Shoulder Stand.

7. Happy Hatha Yoga

Chapter 34

Yoga at Delaware Prisons

Yoga at the Women's Correctional Institution

An Indian friend asked me, "How did you get involved with teaching at the Women's Prison?" I replied that if you take one step toward something, the next step comes to you, and then the third step and more are waiting for you. The first step I took when I was 10 years old, in Ambavad, India, and I told my father about a debate in my school.

He said to me, "Son, there are Shepherds and there are sheep. A Shepherd guides the sheep. He or she decides what has to be done and tells the sheep to do it. If you want to be a leader, you have to learn public speaking. To do this, you have to take risks." So, he advised that I participate in the schools debate. I agreed.

When the teacher asked who would like to participate, I raised my hand, although secretly hoping that he would not notice. But he did, and put down my name for the debate. I prepared my talk.

The evening I had participated in the debate, my father sat waiting for me at the door. As I slowly walked up to him, he asked me if I had been a "Tiger or a Goat?" I said "Goat," because I got up to speak and I got frozen, and I sat down faster than I had taken to get to the stage, and without saying anything. I was really hurt. I went to my mother and sat down next to her. I said to her "some people are born leaders." She said, "you are OK, at least you got up and that is a good start." I never forgot that.

In 1952, I came to the US to study. In my third year at the Philadelphia College of Textile and Sciences, there was an International Club Election. I put my name for the President and gathered all my courage to get up and tell the students and faculty: "If you elect me as the President, I will start a cricket team in the College." They elected me and I started the team. I remember the next year, after my graduation, the Dean saw me at the College and told me that the Philadelphia College of Textile and Sciences beat Harvard University at cricket. The Dean was very proud of that accomplishment and thanked me for starting the team.

After graduating from the College, which is now known as Philadelphia University, I was lucky to get a job at the E. I. DuPont DeNeumors and Co. Textiles Fibers Research Department as an engineer. Every week, we had to give a speech to our group on the status of our projects. As I was a very poor speaker, and all of the others in the group were PhDs, I decided to join Toastmasters International, a public speaking group, which met once a week. In the group, you must prepare a speech and they critically evaluate it. And a Toastmaster of the week is elected. I was the worst speaker in the group and in six months never won even once. One day, while coming home, I was really depressed. Tears were running down my face. I made a decision to win at least once in the club. I thought it would be great if I could win the city contest, and the state contest as well. So I joined an English class for a year at the University of Delaware, and a lady teacher helped me improve my pronunciation as well as organizing my speeches.

The hard work, won me my first Toastmasters club award. I then won the City contest, and followed it up with the State of Delaware contest and the Tri-State contest. Eventually I became the District 18 Toastmaster Governor with 1,000 members. This illustrates the hard work involved to achieve the goals you set. I was a member of Toastmasters International for 40 years before I retired (1957—1997).

I realized that Toastmastering had helped me a great deal and believed it could be a tool for better communication and for helping people understand themselves better. It also builds self-confidence.

I realized that the men's correctional institution would benefit greatly from this knowledge. So I started the first Toastmaster's International Club at the Smyrna Correctional Institution. I volunteered there for only a year, but I was heartened to see a tremendous difference in those who participated in this program.

Gopal (Gregg Hill), one of my Yoga students and member of the Sivananda Yoga Center of Delaware, was so inspired by the story above that he decided to volunteer to teach Yoga at the same prison. There was a story he told about his classes that I really liked. His students in the prison used to complain that they couldn't get Yoga pants to practice their Asanas. So he used to wear two pairs of Yoga pants to his class and give away one pair. So Gopal is the first one I know of in Delaware to volunteer to teach Yoga in a correctional institution.

This training also helped me teach Yoga. In 1990 I started a TV Show called "Yoga for Health, Happiness, and Liberation." This led me to volunteer at the Vishwa Hindu Parishad summer camp for two weeks each year to teach Mantra Yoga and Yoga from 1983 to 2005. In India, I have attended the RSS Children's Program. I started the HSS Shaka in Delaware and one time I was director at the HSS Summer camp in Pennsylvania.

One day I got a phone call from a physician friend who worked at a mental hospital "Delaware Hospital." He felt that Yoga would help the patients a great deal and asked if I would consider volunteering at the hospital. Thus began a new phase of my life, which continued for two years. My classes held up to 40 or 50 patients at a time, which was quite huge for a Yoga class. There, I met one of my Toastmaster colleagues Dr. Mel Rosenthal, who had learned Yoga from me. He also began teaching Yoga at the Delaware Hospital. Then came a new director and he discontinued the program. From there Dr. Rosenthal went on to teach Yoga at the Baylor Women's Correctional Institution. He would often come with his wife to attend my Satsang at the Sivananda Yoga Center.

Once he expressed his love for Hindu philosophy. So I introduced him to Swami Dayananda, and his wife and he began attending Swami Dayananda's programs on weekends until they decided to move there on his retirement.

Before leaving Wilmington Dr. Rosenthal asked me if I would take his place for teaching Yoga to the girls at Baylor. Interestingly, the director had seen my Yoga TV show and so already knew who I was. The rest is history.

The Baylor Women's Correctional Institution in New Castle, Delaware, 19720, has 400 women, 300 in the general population and 100 in the Village, with which is mostly for drug and alcohol related issues. The village is divided into four groups or "Pods." Each pod has about 10 rooms, with 25 women and girls per pod. The Village is loosely structured and allows the inmates to obtain their GED, and offers training in computers and other related subjects. I have permission to teach the girls Yoga once a week (one hour class) in the Village. I have been teaching there for the last six years. I distribute treats for most Holidays to brighten them and show them some support through their most difficult time. I have found through the years that my efforts mean a great deal to the well-being of these girls. They have shown unbelievable appreciation and love. One girl told me that I am the only one who comes to see her.

I am allowed to teach Yoga to these 100 women and girls who are part of the drug addiction program. The first three years I went on Wednesdays for an hour. The girls sat on the floor while I taught them Yoga. Then at my request, my session was shifted to Friday mornings, when the Catholic and Protestant Ministers also have sessions, so that the girls have a choice to go to any of the three sessions or do not have to go to any of the sessions. This way the girls interested in Yoga are in my sessions. In 2000, about 20% of the attendees were white women; now it is about 40%. In addition, the girls now have the choice to sit in chairs or to sit in the middle of the floor and do Yoga.

I always start my class by asking all of the girls to sit erect, close their eyes, and hold their hands straight with Dhyana Mudra and chant Om three times and say Shanti three times. Then I teach Asana (postures) for 15 minutes and breathing for 10 minutes or Meditation, sometimes I do relaxation techniques, sometimes I read from my book, "Spiritual Clouds" (locally printed for the Women's Prison; I give two copies as incentives at each class), and sometimes I give a spiritual talk. I have also tried Laughing Yoga. Sometimes I ask their names and ask them to tell an inspiring sentence.

The Women's Prison Authority usually asks me to give a seminar on Yoga twice a year, at which all the 100 girls are together. At that time I take my daughter, Meeta, who demonstrates the postures and gives a relaxation session. They also use in their group meetings, a tape Meeta made for relaxation. I teach Pranayama (Yogic breathing).

One time, during Thanksgiving, I asked the girls what kind of special food they would be having—were they going to have cake? They said "No, we are not going to have cake!" So then I asked the director if I could bring cake or something for the girls for Thanksgiving. She approved, as she is a very kind and loving person. I asked the girls, "Would you like to have cake or something else?" They all unanimously said, "We would like to have Chocolate!" So, I told my daughter to buy 100 chocolate bars. After that, I realized that I had become very popular. We now do the same thing at Christmas as well. One time we gave all of the girls a t-shirt that said Yoga and Om on the T-shirt. And at Diwali (A Holiday similar to Christmas) we distributed Indian sweets.

Author's Experiences at the Women's Prison

You Are a Spirit Soul

I had arrived a little early for one of my Yoga classes, and before everyone got there, one girl came up and sat down next to me on the floor. She was almost in tears as she told me that she felt terrible, because everyone tells her that she is evil, ugly and bad. Those words hurt her a great deal. She wanted to know how to overcome all these bad feelings. I told her that Hindus believe there is no devil and no one is evil, but people do wrong things because of their ignorance. I told her to tell these people that "God has made me and God likes me the way I look and the way I am." I taught this to 25 girls in my class, but because the words could not fully convey the message, I decided to have them use body language:

Step 1: Put both hands on your hips and say, "I am not this body."
Step 2: Put both hands on your forehead and say, "I am not this mind."
Step 3: Put your left hand on your heart and your right hand straight up towards the sky and say, "I am spirit soul."

Step 4: Put your right hand on your heart and your left hand straight up towards the sky and say, "I am part of God."

Step 5: Put both hands in front of you with your palms facing each other but not touching and say, "I am divine bliss."

Step 6: Then put both hands out to the sides and say, "I am joy forever."

Step 7: Then put both hands down and say, "But I feel like hell because I forgot who I am."

This brought tears to the girls' eyes from laughing, and they said they all felt much better about themselves. When I teach the above message in my children's class with hand gestures I change the 7th step to "But I don't feel good, because I forgot who I am."

Hanging the Red Rose

Every morning I spend some time in Meditation and sometimes I get a message from my Guru's Guru Swami Sivananda. About two years ago I got a message, to go with flowers on Mother's Day to the Village. I disregarded the message, because it didn't seem very practical, but the message persisted.

So I decided, hesitatingly, to go to out on the morning of Mother's Day to buy some roses. At first I intended to give each girl one rose, but that would have been very expensive. So I decided to buy four bunches of roses—one for each pod.

That morning I went to the Women's Prison with the roses. To my surprise, the women guards were very excited and happy and watched me enter the building. When the girls saw that I had come with the roses, they too, were very excited. They put each of the four bunches in a cup of water—one for each pod.

Two weeks went by and I returned to the Women's Prison. The girls told me that the roses looked as fresh as when I brought them. I told them that because of their love the roses, remain fresh.

A month went by and I returned to the Women's Prison. I asked the girls if they liked the flowers I had brought them on Mothers Day. One of the girls asked me to wait for a minute, ran to her room and then came back with two of the roses that were dried and tied with a string. I asked her why she had dried the roses. Then she told me that no one had ever given her a rose before. So she hung them above her bed to remind herself that someone loves her and how special they made her feel. I get tears in my eyes whenever I think of how much such a little thing meant to her. This little thing wouldn't mean much to an average person. But for these girls, it is something they never had nor been given. Since that first Mother's Day, I have been taking roses to the girls every year.

Mantra and Japa Yoga
When I went to India, I bought 500 malas (rosaries) for teaching Mantra and Japa Yoga to the girls at the Women's Prison. At first, I explained to the girls what Mantra Yoga is, and I told them that one of the greatest Mantras is Om. There are also many traditional Mantras in Yoga.

An important Mantra for Divine Mother is "Shakti Ma," and for Father and Mother is Om Namah Shivaya. I made the group sing with me. Every time I went, I took 10 malas with me and gave one to whoever wanted to do Japa Yoga. Then I taught them how to do Mala traditionally. This was a very popular session each time I taught Mantra Yoga. Some of the girls asked why didn't I bring a drum. I said I didn't, because that could jeopardize the entire program. The girls make arts and crafts. I told them about Mother Durga. One of them saw the picture of Mother Durga in my prayer book, made a beautiful painting of Mother Durga and gave it to me.

Holidays
Every Easter, Meeta gave bags of candy to the girls. Quite a few girls came and thanked me for the candy, because when their children visited them on this holiday, they had nothing to give them, except this candy. It really made them feel good, they said, "God bless you."

Favorite Story
One girl at the Prison asked me to tell them my favorite story. I told them I had received a story by email, that I thought everyone should know. A young man learns what's most important in life from the guy next door. It had been some time since Jack had seen the old man. College, girls, career, and life had

got in the way. In fact, Jack moved clear across the country in pursuit of his dreams. In the rush of his busy life, Jack had little time to think about the past, often had no time to spend with his wife and son. He was working for his future, and nothing could stop him.

Over the phone, his mother told him, "Mr. Belser died last night. The funeral is Wednesday." Memories flashed through Jack's mind like an old newsreel as he sat quietly remembering his childhood days. "Jack, did you hear me?" "Oh, sorry, Mom. Yes, I heard you. It's been so long since I thought of him. I'm sorry, but I honestly thought he died years ago," Jack said. "Well, he didn't forget you. Every time I saw him he'd ask how you were doing. He'd reminisce about the many days you spent over 'his side of the fence' as he put it," Mom told him. "I loved that old house he lived in," Jack said. "You know, Jack, after your father died, Mr. Belser stepped in to make sure you had a man's influence in your life," she said. "He's the one who taught me carpentry," he said. "I wouldn't be in this business if it weren't for him. He spent a lot of time teaching me things he thought were important...Mom, I'll be there for the funeral," Jack said. As busy as he was, he kept his word. Jack caught the next flight to his hometown. Mr. Belser's funeral was small and uneventful. He had no children of his own, and most of his relatives had passed away. The night before he had to return home, Jack and his Mom stopped by to see the old house next door one more time. Standing in the doorway, Jack paused for a moment. It was like crossing over into another dimension. The house was exactly as he remembered. Every step held memories. Every picture, every piece of furniture.... Jack stopped suddenly. "What's wrong, Jack?" his Mom asked. "The box is gone," he said. "What box?" Mom asked. "There was a small gold box that he kept locked on top of his desk. I must have asked him a thousand times what was inside. All he'd ever tell me was 'the thing I value most,'" Jack said. It was gone. Everything about the house was exactly how Jack remembered it, except for the box. He figured someone from the Belser family had taken it. "Now I'll never know what was so valuable to him," Jack said. "I better get some sleep. I have an early flight home, Mom." It had been about two weeks since Mr. Belser died Returning home from work one day Jack discovered a note in his mailbox. "Signature required on a package. No one at home. Please stop by the main post office within the next three days," the note read. Early the next day Jack retrieved the package. The small box was old and looked like it had been mailed a hundred years ago. The handwriting was difficult to read, but the return address caught his attention. "Mr. Harold Belser" it read. Jack took the box out to his car and ripped open the package. There inside was the gold box and an envelope. Jack's hands shook as he read the note inside.

"Upon my death, please forward this box and its contents to Jack Bennett. It's the thing I valued most in my life." A small key was taped to the letter. His heart racing, as tears filling his eyes, Jack carefully unlocked the box. There inside he found a beautiful gold pocket watch. Running his fingers slowly over the finely etched casing, he unlatched the cover. Inside he found these words engraved: "Jack, Thanks for your time! -Harold Belser."

"The thing he valued most was...my time." Jack held the watch for a few minutes, then called his office and cleared his appointments for the next two days. "Why?" Janet, his assistant asked. "I need some time to spend with my son," he said. "Oh, by the way, Janet, thanks for your time!"

Think about these things. You may not realize it but they are true.

1. At least two people in this world love you so much they would die for you.

2. At least 15 people in this world love you in some way.

3. A smile from you can bring happiness to anyone, even if they don't like you.

4. Every night, SOMEONE thinks about you before they go to sleep.

Source Unknown

Laughing Yoga

In India a new kind of Yoga has been started, they call it "Laughing Yoga." I was in India in 2002 and I went to my hometown, Amadavad (Karnavati) and a friend of mine told me about it. He goes to the park every Sunday morning where they have a group meeting where they conduct Laughing Yoga. I told him I'd really like to attend one of these meetings. He took me with him and I really enjoyed it. When I came back to America I introduced it to my Yoga class as well as to the girls in the Women's prison. Everyone really enjoyed it. Once you start laughing you can't stop.

I guess Laughing Yoga started because in this modern life there is too much mental tension and stress. People need a release, especially in big cities with so much traffic, pressure, and pollution. This is also the reason why Hatha Yoga is so popular around the world.

Wall Street Journal also had an article in the 9/13/96 issue about Laughing Yoga in which it says that Dr. Madan Kataria popularized ancient Yoga breathing and laughing posture. Dr. Kataria organized a group of five people to share jokes outside his home last October. Within a week the jokes were stale, but 50 people had joined in to laugh their cares away. Now enthusiasts estimate there are more than 100 laughing clubs across India.

This is how it is done. Just before sunrise, in the Park, the laughing club members line up in a row or a semi circle. They begin by doing a few Yoga stretches, such as touching their toes and raising their arms while deep breathing, then they start with a warm up laugh, building slowly to "ha ha ha's" and "ho ho ho's" to stimulate deep breathing. Slowly serious laughing begins. They laugh hard enough to break a sweat, slapping hands with the person on the left and right at the same time. Sometimes they bend down, touch their toes, and then come up laughing. The meeting lasts about one hour.

Wall Street Says, "Experts can master special laughs: the silent 'joker laugh' (make a funny face, laugh with open mouth but no sound); the low-pitched 'etiquette laugh' (lips closed) or the classic 'Bombay laugh' (fill chest with air and roar).

Chhaganbhai Sheth, 72 years old, says his grandchildren find him less irritable since he started laughing regularly four months ago. He says he laughs with his teeth clenched to prevent his dentures from falling out.

'Earlier I used to look down upon these people as crazy,' says Ajit Kamlani, a gasoline dealer. Now he's dedicated to his regimen. 'No other activity exercises the 32 muscles of your face," he notes."

After I came home from the laughing club in India I was light hearted all day. I really got a kick out of it. The girls in the women's prison were laughing even after the class was over.

Some of the Women's Experiences at the Women's Prison:

May 2006
Dear Mr. Bharat,

We first met you around the end of 2005 at the Village, and it's safe to say we'd reached the lowest point in our lives and were spiritually disconnected. We started attending your groups on Fridays and started practicing Yoga. Your visits are our highlights of the week. You always bring with you such a sense of peace. Your presence is so heartwarming and your humor is great. Audrey is so inspired that she reads your book over and over and now dreams of becoming a Yogi and opening her own Yoga Center. Anyway, we just wanted you to know what a wonderful man you are and how much we appreciate and look forward to your visits. Thank you for helping us to heal and grow into more spiritually whole women. We couldn't forget you if we tried. You've left a mark on our hearts and we love you so very much.

The girls presented me with a large knitted blanket that they made for Father's Day and my Birthday. One of the girls wrote this letter to accompany the blanket.

6/18/06
Dear Mr. Bharat,

This blanket is made with tender love and care. We made this blanket in gratitude for all the wonderful things you do for us.

Each square represents the hope and love you have shown each one of us by all the stories you shared and by the way you teach us Yoga, and the spiritual aspect of Meditation.

You always say something to lift our spirits especially mine. It's a joy to see you come walking through those doors on Friday mornings. You have inspired me to change my habits and be a better person.

Thank you for your time and inspirational words.

Love, Karen Coleman

Dear Mr. Bharat,

My first Yoga class with you was on January 13th, 2006—and the energy I left with was beyond words. It was a monumental experience I will never forget. Soon after as luck would have it, my roommate gave me your book

"Spiritual Clouds," and I fell in love with Yoga. Yoga has opened up my heart, mind and spirituality. I am now a committed Yogi. I am teaching my fellow inmate sisters breathing techniques and postures. I have the utmost respect for you and I consider you my Guru. I am truly blessed to have you in my life. Thank you Mr. Bharat. You are a true inspiration and I will always remember you.

Your Spiritual Follower,
Audrey Becker

One of the girls wrote this poem and gave it to me. I present it here:

Spread Sunshine Wherever You Go

Try to spread sunshine
    Wherever you go,
Grow a lush garden
    from seeds that you sow.
The fragrance will linger
    In each grateful heart,
Where life's a bit brighter
    Than it was at the start.
Try to give comfort
    To each troubled soul,
That longs for a friend
    When trials take their toll.
When you spread sunshine,
    Wherever you go
You will find flowers
    That bloom in the snow.

By Pamela Richardson
Thank you Bharat for everything you do.

5/11/2001

Dear Mr. Bharat,

Words could never express the change and growth you have helped me to accomplish at the very turning point of my life. You teach very valuable valid lessons. I opened my mind and you touched my spirit-soul. You have so many great things instilled in your heart and mind that you could be very close to perfect (Divine Bliss). You have a lot of compassion that only comes from practicing love.

Love is....
Love is a bond never broken;
Love is often unspoken;
Love is unconditional and strong;
Love will last a life long.

The more I've gotten to know you the more I've gotten to know myself. I have learned that....

I am forty-one years old.
My hair he has lined with silver and gold,
He gave me eyes more beautiful than emeralds.
Rubies are my lips and pearls are my smile
I am a diamond in his light I shine
And my value is worth,
more than anything on earth.
Sincerely, Patricia Trusty

My student Gregg Hill (Gopal), whom I mentioned early, taught Yoga at the men's prison. During his classes he told his students about me my teachings and Swami Sivananda's messages. The word spread and some prisoners started writing to me.

Prisoner Seeking Hindu Philosophy

A man in the Smyrna, Delaware Prison, wrote to the President of the Mahalakshami Hindu Temple of Delaware to seek deeper knowledge of Hindu Philosophy. The President of the Temple asked me to correspond with and help this man in his spiritual quest. The following is a summary of his experiences as well as my experiences from corresponding with him.

This man wrote about his struggles and asked how to control the deep emotions that were influencing his life so much. He also wanted greater peace and love, and wanted to give that of himself.

His interest in spirituality told me that he is a spiritual person seeking higher consciousness. I felt great compassion for his situation and struggles to overcome his negative environment. I told him I would pray for his health, happiness and inner peace.

I sent him a Sivananda Yoga Center Prayer Book and told him it would help him experience love and peace. He was happy with the prayer book. He started reading it regularly and requested 2 more copies to spread Swami Sivananda's messages within the prison. He wanted to leave a book on display so that hopefully others will find the secrets within. He wanted to read and practice gradually with the prayer book. After corresponding for some time, he told me, 'It felt so good after reading the prayer book for the first time. I have been here four years now, and I felt as if I was not here, so good like it must feel when enlightened!'"

In his letters, he is not very confident about his abilities. But I told him that we work on improving ourselves every day, that introspection is an important part of our growth as human beings. Then he disclosed he has noticed improvement, is happy in recent months after reading and starting to apply the prayer book and other Hindu truths.

Recently he told me, "I am so glad that I found you. I find myself more flooded in love as I write you. It is so great. (tears)"

Chapter 35

Students' Experiences with Yogi Bharat

Since 1967 a lot of people came through the doors of the Sivananda Yoga Center of Delaware and participated in Yoga classes, seminars, workshops and various other activities. People continue to come to our Satsang and vegetarian potluck dinners.

The Sivananda Yoga Center of Delaware, that was on Baynard Boulevard in Wilmington Delaware, held a Satsang every Sunday evening, and on Sunday mornings a children's Yoga class. I gave Yoga classes twice a week. We also held Yoga, Marriage, and Meditation Seminars once a year. Once a year Rupal (Anandi Narayani Ma) and I had a Yoga retreat at Ocean City, MD. from Friday to Sunday. We rented a few condos, did Yoga and Meditation at sunrise on the beach. We also brought a vegetarian potluck dish to share. This was a very special get-together for many of our Yoga students and they have fond memories of these occasions. All proceeds from all events went directly to the Sivananda Yoga Center and no one was paid for these events. From time to time we had lectures by visiting Yogis and Swamis including Swami Vishnu Devananda Maharaj who is my Guru.

Below are letters and stories about the Yoga Center and experiences my students had while participating in the Yoga Center activities and what it meant to them.

Hi Bharat,

It was so wonderful to hear your voice again and to feel your Presence today at my Yoga class.

I was teaching the students about one of the two basic Yogic breathing techniques you share in your Yoga book, about the cleansing breath, Kapalabhati. One of the students felt a presence around me while her eyes were closed and she opened them to see what was happening. She described you and told the class what you wore and how you held your two hands together in front of you in prayer. She said you were whispering something to me. Before the breathing experience took place, I was reading to the students your writing on Pranayama, and about the Yoga Sutra information from Patanjali. I could not continue to read because your presence and love came in so strongly for me that tears started filling my eyes. I had to stop reading and asked another student to continue where I left, off which she did.

Earlier, I had shown them your photo and Rupal's photo on the cover of another book you had put together with Swami Sivananda's photo on it.

You asked me to write to you about my experiences. I have been teaching Yoga ever since I left Wilmington, DE, in 1978. I have taught in gyms, martial arts centers, community schools for Volusia County here in FL, churches, and had my own television show for thirteen weeks, 3 times a week where I taught Yoga and how to be beautiful inside as well as out (modeling classes). I co-founded my own healing sanctuary with my husband Chris in 1989 in Enterprise, FL. We moved to Deltona, FL and at our center, The Doolin Healing Sanctuary, I teach Hatha Yoga for beginners and intermediates and offer Yoga workshops for the community at libraries. I offer Rebirthing sessions, Reiki classes (First—Third Degree), Reiki Sessions, teach Power of Visualization Techniques for healing, offer spiritual counseling for adults, children, squirrels and pets. I am an author, and you wrote an endorsement for my latest book, The Only Way Out Is In, which should be published between Dec 2005—Jan 2006.

I love teaching Yoga and I am now Registered with the Yoga Alliance who does a thorough interview and use of references so they can endorse your being a worthy teacher with their reputation behind you. I am a singer/songwriter with my husband and our first CD, "Level Seven" has just been released. We both play guitar, write and sing.

I have had a wonderful life with Yoga and Reiki. Yoga led me to Reiki. I am 65 years old as of Jan 3, 2006 and I feel like I did when I was 35 years. I am so very thankful that I kept persisting in finding the Sivananda Center open one day. Every day I came by the Center it was always closed back in 1970-

71 or so. I was determined to find out what did Sivananda mean and why was no one was ever there to answer my question of what the building was all about. I persisted until one day I found you there, came to Satsang (didn't know what that was either), and I have been hooked ever since meeting you and your family.

My life has been blessed with two sons, a beautiful partner who loves music, and many, many things I love. My partner attends my Yoga classes every moment he can and he says it keeps him supple and keeps his back flexible. I see that I affect the lives of others in the same beautiful way you affected my life because Spirit is behind our intentions in everything we say, how we live, what we do, and what we think. I have you, Swami Sivananda, and Swami Vishnu Devananda to thank, Shantanandaji (though I don't know where he is now or how to find him) and all the Spiritual help and guidance I have been given from those I cannot see and all the people I have met in my life who have been teachers to me.

I am now an Ordained Unity Minister with World Federation of Practical Christianity and give workshops/seminars and talks on radio and TV as well as in churches.

I'd love to have a copy of your book when your ten chapters are done and it's complete. I'll send you my copy of The Only Way Out Is In when it's ready.

Om Shanti, Shanti, Shanti,

Love,

Daya (Devi-Doolin)

Comments by Bharat: *When you pray to Guru, and experience his/her presence it is always God who comes but as you love your Guru you see his presence except when it is a saint like Swami Sivananda.*

Jan. 4, 2004

I want to tell you a story about one of my disciples and member of the Sivananda Yoga Center named Haridas (Geesung). He is from South Korea. A few years ago, a man living in Fort Meyers, Florida telephoned and asked me if I'm Yogi Bharat. When I said, "Yes," he told me his name and said he had heard that I give Mantra initiations and that he wanted to be initiated. He also told me that he wanted to become a Hindu. I told him that would not be a problem. He went on to ask me if I could make him a Hindu Brahman. I asked him if he were qualified. He felt he was since he had studied the Vedas and the Upanishads, that he knew and understood Hindu Philosophy and that he was a vegetarian. He felt that he was a Hindu Brahman.

So I asked him to come. He drove from Florida to Wilmington and I gave him the Mantra initiation, as I have to so many others in Delaware and I prayed to Swami Sivananda for his name to be joined to the lineage of Sivananda. In my Meditation the name Haridas came to me. So I called Geesung and told him that he was Haridas.

I have never seen or heard anyone as happy as he to have his new spiritual name. He said, "I will wear a Bindi and a yellow cape or shawl with Hindu Mantras on it. He asked me how to perform Hindu wedding ceremonies. I have done many weddings, so I taught him how to do weddings. In Fort Meyers he gave Mantra initiations to many people and spread the word of Swami Sivananda. He taught karate, Yoga, and Indian Astrology, in which he was an expert. He used to go to Hindu Bhajans, prayer meetings and helped the Hindu community build a temple. After he was initiated, he called me every week. He was the only one who called me Guruji. He would ask what message I gave on my television show that week. Twice a year he would come to see me. He would bring along a bunch of flowers and Korean tea, though I would tell him not to do. But he wanted to. I used to sit on a chair and he would sit near my feet, touch my feet and say, "Guruji, please bless me." I would always say, "I bless you." He taught me devotion. He called me one day and told me that he had four beautiful tapes by Bhagawan Rajaneesh that he wanted me to listen to. I asked him to send them to me at my cost. He insisted that he wanted to give them to me and I consented when he agreed to let me send him 20 Om pendants that I had got from India".

Soon after he called to tell me that his father had just died and left him some money and he desired to go to India with his two children. He wanted to visit the Sivananda Yoga Ashram there and take a bath in the Ganges. I told him that I would talk to my niece and get some information on how to do that economically. Then, on September 13, 2004, I received a phone call from the President of the Hindu Temple of Fort Meyers whom I visited with Haridas. She gave me sad news. Haridas died in a car accident. A drunk driver came into his lane and had a head on collision. Fortunately, Haridas's mother had gone to Fort Meyers and taken charge of the children, who were 13 and 16 at the time. On September 14,[th] 2004, I received the four tapes that Haridas had sent me. I cried. At the Sivananda Yoga Satsang we prayed for his soul and did a yagna ceremony for his soul. May God bless his soul.

(Karen Foley was in college when I gave her a Mantra initiation with the spiritual name of Gayatri. After she graduated, she served our Guru, Swami Vishnu Devananda for several years in India when his health was deteriorating. Everyone at the Sivananda organization headquarters had great respect for her. When I went to teach the Bhagavad Gita in the Bahamas for the teacher's training course, I met Swami Saroopananda for the first time. He told me that he didn't know me, but that he knew my student Gayatri, and because of her he had respect for me. I felt very proud of her.)

Dear Bharat

I first started taking Yoga classes at the University of Delaware in 1981 through the East West Yoga Club founded by Gregg Hill (Gopal). The classes were free and I attended once a week. One day Gopal asked the class if we would like to attend a satsang with Bharat at the Sivananda Center in Wilmington. The class was quite big about 60 or so students per week, but of those, I was the only one who wished to go.

Gopal drove and as soon as I entered the Sivananda Yoga Center, I had an inexplicable, immediate sense of coming home. I had never met Bharat until then, never been to the Center before, yet felt I had found something that I didn't even know was missing. I was not familiar with the program or with what was going on, but my heart was happy. After that initial introduction, I continued to attend satsangs and became a regular member of the Center.

Then one day in the Spring of 1985, Bharat told us that Swami Vishnu Devananda would be visiting the Center as part of a National tour. We had heard about Swami Vishnu Devananda through Bharat and even though most of us did not know Swamiji personally, Bharat's sincere love and devotion passed onto us. The night Swami Vishnu came, we were all very excited to meet him. We all wore white clothes and tried to behave in a way that was most honorable and respectful.

I remember Swami Vishnu's lecture was about Subject vs. Object. He spent a lot of time explaining this to us and used various examples and different ways to help us distinguish between the two. Swamiji told us that Subject never changes and is our Self. Object always has the quality of change inherent in it and has limiting adjuncts—it is everything else but the Self.

After Swamiji's lecture we performed Arati, and then sat and shared Prasad. I was sitting quietly when Swamiji looked at me, pointed to me and said

"Visit me in Canada." I just simply said "Yes, Swamiji" and didn't think much more about it.

A few months later I was talking to Gopal and he said he had booked a trip to go to the Ashram in Canada, but he had to cancel his plans. He asked if I would like to go in his place, since he already has the plane ticket, the room etc. I accepted his kind offer and that summer much to my surprise, I found myself at the Sivananda Ashram in Val Morin, Canada.

Since that time much has happened. Swami Vishnu Devananda has entered Samadhi, and after 30 years the Sivananda Yoga Center on Baynard Blvd has closed. I moved from Delaware and presently am not formally part of a Center, but what I learned and what I experienced through Yoga is an enormous part of my life. Sometimes it's in a quiet, solitary way, sometimes it's through a mini satsang with Bharat by phone, sometimes it's by going to the Ashram in Val Morin or sometimes just by simple association with other Yogis.

Even though things continue to change on the material plane, to me Yoga qualifies as the Subject—the same topic I heard Swami Vishnu Devananda talk about the first time I met him. Everything else has changed and continues to change, everything else has limiting adjuncts, and everything else is temporary. Everything but Yoga. Yoga has been the one constant. Unchanging and Eternal.

Subject vs. Object....

Gayatri (Karen Foley)

One of my other students Chris Miller (Anandi Ma) read about this in our Sivananda news letter and wrote the following:

Hari Om Bharat,

"So sad about Haridas—sad for you. You helped him so much. He was happy because of the things you told him and the things he wanted to learn from a great guru like you. You touched his life and he touched yours. May you find peace and acceptance in his passing.

With much love and concern for you, and thank you for being my Guru too. You have touched the heart of many. Your words and your love for others have been stamped on this earth.

This is a girl who took the children's Yoga classes from Rupal and I, over 20 years ago. Today 2/1/06, she wrote this letter.

Dear Bharat,

I don't know if you remember this or not. I am Anna Matthew's daughter—Jennifer Matthews. I used to take Yoga classes with you in Wilmington with your wife Rupal. I then saw you again in 1995 for a weekend seminar. It's been a long time, but I wanted to get in contact with you because I would like to talk to you.

I remember being in class with Rupal and she showed/taught me to move the energy around my body. I have never lost sight of her teachings; they have always been there. She taught me how to relax and Meditate. Making the energy move in and out of my body is something that I have always cherished. In 2001 I had a bad experience, and I shut myself down to the energy work. Now, five years later I am ready to allow myself to experience that type of energy work again.

Rupal comes into my thoughts often and I feel her around me. My memories of her are very special to me. When she comes to me, she is always wrapped in blue. I then feel her wrapping me in a blue cascade of light.

I remember you talking with us, and I was wondering, do you still teach? Do you still have classes? I am all the way in California in San Francisco.

I hope that you are doing well.
Sincerely, Jennifer Matthews

Hi Bharat,

Here is a story that is most memorable to me.

In October of 2002 my father was gravely ill and we made the decision to take him off life support and let him die naturally. I sat by his bedside to be with him while he died. He was a very strong willed man and it occurred to me that he might linger for a day or two while his spirit was leaving his body. After a few hours of my vigil, I got a strong message to pray to Swami Sivananda. I asked him to grant my father peace and comfort as he was leaving this life. I felt a great sense of relief after that prayer. Within 15 minutes my father had died. Right before he died he opened his eyes and tears were streaming down his face. I do believe that at the end he saw the wonder of eternal life. I believe that Swami Sivananda intervened to give my father a peaceful death.

I hope you can use this story. I thank you for your continued prayers for my Mom and our family. We will keep you posted.

Blessings,

Cindy Krahn (Shivani)

I'm Bharat's daughter Meeta, and my Mother passed away in 1984 when I was 19 years old. She was a Yoga teacher also and when I was a little girl I used to watch her teaching Yoga in the basement of our house in Green Acres. I remember how happy she looked when she was teaching. I learned Yoga from my parents and have been practicing Yoga since I was 4 years old. In 1997 I started teaching Yoga and during my classes I would sometimes become overwhelmed with the sensation that my mother (Anandi Narayani Ma) Rupal was around me almost as if she was experiencing the joy of practicing the Asanas with me and through me. It would bring tears to my eyes. I could feel my own Yogic lineage of teacher to student in my spiritual connection to my mother and her to her Guru Swami Vishnu Devananda and so on. This has only happened a few times during the 8 years I've been teaching Yoga.

Meeta Gajjar Parker

Red Rose

I met my wife Anandi Narayani Ma (Rupal) on Valentines Day Feb. 14th, and after we met a few times she gave me a rose bud, which had not bloomed. This became a symbol throughout our marriage. So when we bought our first home, I planted her a rose climber in the front of the house. We loved that rose bush, and it happened to blossom an over abundance of roses every year. We lived in that Green Acres house for 12 years. When I sold the house and bought another house, I forgot to tell the new owner that I wanted to take the rose bush to my new house. It was too late; I had already sold the house so I had to leave that rose bush behind. I apologized to that rose bush for that mistake. Three or four months after I sold that house, I drove back to see how the rose bush was doing and to my surprise it died.

In 1984, after 25 years of marriage my wife died in her sleep. One year after her death, on Valentines Day, a package came to my house with a note from Washington, DC. I opened the package to see a red rose with a note that said, "I took your Yoga seminar in Washington, and I'm a physic, I communicate with spirits and I'm sending this rose because your wife asked me to send you a red rose today." Nobody but my wife new about the Red Rose and I knew that she must have spoken to this woman. I don't remember who she was, but I was very touched that she had taken the time to reach out to me on behalf of my wife's request from the other side.

Yogi Bharat J. Gajjar

Mantras Are Powerful

In my Yoga classes I always taught my students the "Gaya Ganesha" Mantra. You can see the Chapter on Mantras. I have a few stories about that. I had a student who was pregnant who used to come to class and she really liked the Mantra "Shakti Ma." I told her to "Think about your baby in the womb when you Chant that Mantra," and later she told me that when the baby was delivered, the Doctor turned her upside down and she was smiling. The Doctor said, "I've never seen a baby come out smiling." Then she told me that whenever the baby cries, I Chant Shakti Ma, my Mantra, and the baby stops crying.

Another student told me that she has a horse that she rides regularly, and one time after learning to chant Mantras she decided to chant it out loud while she was riding her horse. The horse stopped trotting and started dancing when it heard the Mantra being Chanted.

Here is another story I remember from one of my students. She told me that she didn't see any purpose to Chanting the Mantras, so I asked her if she had any problems in her life at this time? She told me she had a boyfriend and that lately he doesn't call her anymore. I told her that after she leaves class, while driving home, think about your boyfriend and chant this Mantra, "Saravanabhava, Saravanabhava, Saravanabhava Pahimam, Subramanya, Subramanya, Subramanya, Rakshamam." The next week, when she came to class, she told me that when she reached home her boyfriend had called her, and she became a believer of Mantras.

There was another girl who told me that she also did not see any purpose in Mantras. I told her that Mantras are the word of God, so when you are chanting you are loving God. I told her at 3:00 in the afternoon I would think about her and be Chanting a Mantra, was that ok? She said, "yes." The next week when I saw her in class, she said, "at 3:00 I felt incredible power and love around me. I felt energized at that time, it's unbelievable that Mantras work."

One day, I had gone to the Pocono Mountains and decided to take a walk by myself in the woods. I thought entered my mind, "if Mantra has a power to love, and if all these trees around me have living souls within them, then if I Chant my Mantra it should affect both of us. So I started Chanting the "Jaya Ganesha" Mantra out loud. To my surprise, I experienced a surge of love coming from the trees at me. I'd like to ask you, if you believe what I'm saying to chant to the trees? Try it sometime.

At one time in my life, I lived in a townhouse that didn't have much space for a garden, so I planted one tomato plant and every time I passed that plant coming or going from my house I would chant my Mantra and send love to the plant. That tomato plant grew so big and had so many tomatoes I had to give them away. One of my friends stopped over my house and couldn't believe that it was only one plant because it was so big with so many tomatoes. I never had a green thumb, but a green thumb must really mean a person who loves their plants.

Hi Bharat Bhai,

Hi to all from the Sunshine land of South Africa—(rainbow nation). I will always treasure and remember the fond memories of attending the Sunday Satsangs in Wilmington at the Sivananda Yoga Center of Delaware.

I worked for the State of Delaware from 1990—1994. I had no family or friends in USA, apart from the work colleagues. I always thought when I was at Satsang and chanting that this was a home away from home for me and looked forward to seeing all the people at Satsang. I met some amazing people there who always had a smile on their face and encouraged me. I always looked forward to going to Satsang, which kept me going for the 4 years I worked in Delaware. I attended the Yoga teachers training program in Montreal in 1994. I returned to South Africa after that. I still miss the Sunday Satsangs and chanting.

Love Anita / Laxshmi

BE GOOD DO GOOD

2/24/06

Dear Bharatji,

Yoga has helped me so much because of Chanting and Meditating. I was doing my Meditation on wanting goodness to come to me. I had given up the need to have a relationship. Well after getting my initiation (which by the way was such a wonderful feeling), things started to turn around for me. My guru Bharatji told me that Master Sivananda would be watching over me. Soon after, I told a non-Yoga friend of mine that I was not interested in meeting anyone because I was happy being by myself and with my cat Herbie. My friend insisted on my meeting a certain gentleman. She introduced me to my husband-to-be in a Wawa of all places. She had never tried to do this before. I told Bharatji about this and told him about this man I had just met. It turned out that Bharatji had worked with this man for 35 years at DuPont, and he said that I was in good hands. Bharatji's opinion meant a lot to me. Soon I realized how wonderful a man my husband-to-be was, and the fact that Bharatji new him was awesome. Bharatji married us a year later at the Sivananda Yoga Center with a Hindu wedding ceremony. This was a blessing I had never expected since I used to always seem to pick the wrong kind of man for me. I'm so thankful for this wonderful gift I received from Meditation because of Yoga. I've never been happier. The blessings keep coming too. My husband also has an open mind towards Yoga because of his friend Bharatji. He loves to go to Satsang where we have developed some wonderful friendships. Meditating on my Mantra brings me peace and a feeling of safety too.

Bharatji, thanks for writing your book. We would love a copy. Thank you for giving me my initiation and helping me to change my life.

Thank you for sharing the other member's stories with all of us. It made me remember just how lucky I was to have Yoga in my life. To have met you again after 30 years when I first met you. Thanks to my sister who read about you celebrating Yoga's 30-year anniversary in Arden at Gild Hall. I followed you ever since. You showed all of your students love and acceptance where I never felt that anywhere else. Until I met my husband who knew him from working with him at DuPont.

I am so happy to have been part of this wonderful spiritual family. My Mantra has brought me peace too, also now I can Meditate easier. I have met some very good people some of who I still see today. I remember when one of the members taught me some of the things she learned from V. Devananda. She would get groups together to chant, I loved that so much and miss it even to this day. I remember chanting on New Year's eve-how calming it was. The love energy was there always to fill the room even when we left to return home I needed this oh so badly. Times where rough for me outside of the center so when I saw your face and your smile I felt comforted. Yoga is a deep part of who I am now. And, so it is.

Om Sri Ram,

Love,

Anandima (Chris Miller)

Hi Bharat,

February 25, 2006

My name is Shiva (Bob Krahn) and I've been involved with the Sivananda Yoga Group since 1983. A close friend had begged me to attend Satsang for over a year—when I came, I immediately knew this was for me, attended classes and took initiation very quickly. Among my earliest memories are going to Satsang led by you and Rupal, and seeing Swami Vishnudevananda that year at our center.

Yoga has given me many life-long friendships, starting with a special depth of spiritual experience at Satsang, classes and many cherished retreats at Ocean City, MD and camp in NJ. A real peak experience was the 'Thirty Years of Yoga' Reunion in 1995 when all of us put real energy and creativity into a very special get-together of so many of your students.

Yoga has become so integral to my life that it is hard to pick out specific events. I regularly Meditate, chant Kirtan on my daily walks, read daily readings from Swami Sivananda and the Bhagavad Gita. I try to apply the principles of Vedanta Yoga to my life and share that understanding with others as a practicing spiritual healer and counselor. These teachings have never failed to inspire me and keep me on a Yogic path.

A recent highlight was my marriage to Shivani performed by you at our Sunday Satsang 3 years ago. Shivani has often commented about the 'old-time' Yogis and the specialness they all seem to share from a very committed association.

I give eternal gratitude to you for helping me and hundreds of others learn to live by spiritual principles as taught so clearly by our Guru, Swami Sivananda.

Dear Bharat,

I remember so well those early days of the Sivananda Yoga center when I was attending. My children were little at the time, and they attended Rupal's Yoga classes for children. They are all involved in Yoga in their own ways now and think back on those times with love. Rupal gave Jennifer Matthews an Om pendant when she was little and I kept it for her all these years. Last month Jennifer was visiting me in Florida where I make my home and as we were reminiscing, she remembered the pendant. I pulled it out and gave it to her. She cried with joy and we felt Rupal's presence and blessings all over again. To me, Bharat, you and Rupal made the biggest impact on my life to this day I never forget your Satsangs.

I am so blessed to be a part of this family.

Anna Matthews (Radha)

Dear Bharat

My first experience with Bharat and the Delaware Sivananda Yoga Center was a weekend retreat in Ocean City, Maryland. I found out about the retreat from a man who was teaching a Hatha Yoga class in Newark (Gregg Hill (Gopal). During the weekend retreat, we went for a silent walk on the beach at sunrise. I had a spiritual experience that was beautiful, profound, and quite amazing. God touched my soul. By the end of the weekend I knew that I would be initiated and that my initiate name would be Shakti. Many years later, I continue to read the Bhagavad Gita Daily Readings every day and I try to live by the words of Swami Sivananda, "Be Good, Do Good." I feel blessed that I found the Sivananda Yoga Center when I did. I had been searching for a long time and when I found it, I felt like I was home.

Terri Lee (Shakti)

Guruji,

Dearest Bharat,

It was a delight to receive your email. So many memories flood into my head as I read through it. Tears welled up in my eyes and trickled down my face. You and the Sivananda Yoga Center were so special to me at a very tough time in my life. As I am sure Peter mentioned, I have been living in New Zealand for the past 14 years now and I love it. I have kept a photo from Oct. 1984 of you on my little table (attached) along side. I also now have one of my mother Bobbe too. My Guru's.

I want to share a poem by George Eliot I have over the past years come to treasure—"Oh the comfort, the inexpressible comfort of feeling, Safe with a person; Having neither to weigh thoughts nor measure words, But to pour them out. Just as they are—chaff and grain together,

Knowing. That a faithful hand will take and sift them, Keep What is worth keeping and then with the breath of the kindness, Blow the rest away."

It is as if I have these deep spiritual ties, which have been there my entire life, different segments very strong at times and others somewhat fragile but always there.

I remember two times at the center very clearly at the Sivananda Yoga Center -

Once we were all sitting in a circle meditating and a greenish line glowed from the top of my head across the room to the top of Shakti's. It's as if we were connected in some kind of magical way. I'll never forget it, so strong and clear.

A few times I brought my very young son along, "Jason." He would sit quietly beside me but preferred to sit in my crossed legs. This particular Sunday evening you were not there and Gopal was leading the Satsang and we were chanting. At the end of the chanting, my young son looked up into my eyes and asked "Mom where is God?" I looked at him quizzically and he then said, "You know 'God,' he sits over there." He wanted to know where you were Bharat (As you might recall we the Free's were all raised with a very strong Catholic background).

I also cherish the sunrises of the retreat I attended at Ocean City, MD as well as Rupal's ashes being sprinkled to the sea…although I cannot remember if I was physically there, it is set in my being.

It makes me very happy that you remember me by my maiden name. It is a name I treasure, but felt unable to go back to after my divorce because of the confusion it might have had on my 2 boys at the time.

I am so blessed having had your presence in that time in my life.
Much Love,
Natalie—Rama

Dear Bharatji,
At our Gita Path, you took a ½ an hour before we started reading the Gita to teach and practice Meditation with us at our monthly meeting. At that time, you always chanted the Jaya Ganesha Mantra. About 5 years ago, I moved to Washington, DC and a very interesting thing happened the other day. One of our friends invited my wife and I to dinner and they said that before dinner, we usually chant this Mantra and we sing along. They played the tape and to my surprise it was your Jaya Ganesha Mantra tape. My wife and I looked at each other in recognition. I just thought you would enjoy hearing about this.
Ravi Mathur

I met Bharat in Feb. 1980 after 4 years in the 82nd Airborne Division (Infantry). I wanted an exercise class that had women in it and I heard Bharat talking about reincarnation, being vegetarian, etc. I disagreed with just about everything but I kept listening. My first time in Wilmington was pretty wild, totally different. I once asked Bharat why we couldn't sing in English. I think it was the only time he said, NO...There were maybe 6 of us in Satsang. Rupal was the best, a class act.

One weekend in 1984 when Rupal died, a group of 20 people took Rupal's ashes to Ocean City, MD. (Half of Rupal's ashes were send to India to her sister to put into the Gangis) Ram and I went into the ocean to place Rupal's ashes in the Sea. The sunrise was beautiful, the people were very nice and tuned in. Princess Diana with all her "pomp" never had it that good! I have Rupal's smile locked into my thoughts. (Rupal treated Gopal and Ram as her own children.)

I always have remembered Rupal and Bharat. Meeta & Ajay (their children) were such a treat to the center. Rupal could say a few words and everyone would understand. I took my brothers to the University class Bharat had at the University of Delaware. There he told one of them to look at what he, my brother, was doing in his Asana and not to look around the room. We howled all night over that!

380

I just gave the LA Center most of my Yoga collection of books (2 full book cases). For 11 years I have had www.japanesemassage.net, a massage business. I have done almost 6,000 sessions in honor of my parents, Bharat / Rupal, Master Sivananda, and Swami Vishnu Devananda. The whole world has come in there. I remember Swami Vishnu Devananda was walking by himself to his house and I was pulling weeds. He asked me how I liked it. I told him, " I like it very much." He was standing there and I told him I was going back to work because I wanted the flowerbed to look right. He had a big smile and shook his head in approval. I promised to myself I would live and help out in the Ashram. I plan to go to the Ashram in Trivandrum where they have a health clinic and offer my skills, etc. In 1980, Swami Sahajananda, in South Africa, invited me to South Africa as I had bought so many books from their Ashram. Once his people were planning an event and they said to Swami Sahajananda something about me being an American. He said Gopal has been a devotee of Master Sivananda for many, many, lifetimes. That was neat to hear. Everything Swami Vishnu Devananda & Bharat have said has come true since 1980. I heard 27,000,000 are now doing some form of Yoga in the U.S. How fortunate to be one of the 6 or 7 people who heard it first at the Sivananda Yoga Center in Wilmington Delaware. I have always felt protected and been given life's homework to do. It's been a hell of a ride, but it's the only game in town. Thanks, Rupal & Bharat and Meeta & Ajay for having the best Yoga Center in the world. It's stands by itself, second to none. I'm trying to live what I have learned for all of you.

Jai Sivananda. Jai Vishnu Devananda. Jai Bharat & Rupal.

Gopal (Gregg Hill)

Gopal wrote the following message about the Yoga center. Swami Vishnu Devananda was recorded live on audio tape at the Sivananda Yoga Center in Wilmington, DE on April 24, 1986. Gregg was transferring it to CD. He sent this message regarding its completion.

Wild Day…The best part was the CD and everybody we know was laughing, Swamiji, Bharat, Meeta, Gayatri, Bob Krahn etc. My ears heard that. Wow. Swamiji & everyone laughing, a small group, God as the teacher, God as the listener, God as the vegetable & fruit cutter. Even the 2 tapes together in my hand, those 2 tapes are literally heavier than any other 2 out of 150. I'll have all the other tapes by next week. Bharat, I can only put this into words that all the years you put into the Center. These CD's reflect that in every way. These CD's will jump right out and stay with all of you. It's as if everything about the Center is trying to do or the reason it was there is in those CD'S. To all of you, I'll send these CD's to every town & village. You will have everything I have, all these CD's each has a personality of it's own. We'll have these the rest of our lives always use them. They are alive. Funny, dramatic, crazy, interesting, serious. Every human emotion is there. Ruby Blue (with affection) calls Swamiji " a flawed saint " He says " I have faults, I have weaknesses. " he told us in New York, Gayatrima, (I think you were there), Not to look to him but go to Master Sivananda, we have found that in our own lives. With a tear (of profound joy) in my eye I can play these CD'S to someone and say, " This is My Yoga Center where I got started…" When you hear these CD'S and feel the love etc. This is proof that what we have is second to none. Run to the mailbox everyday. It is on it's way. These CD's are a reflection Of Master Sivananda in all his glory. Swamiji, once said, " Hundreds & Hundreds of thousands of people went to Rishikesh maybe 40—50 people could figure it out." These CD'S will validate we are protected and guided and everything is all right. My first Sunday night at the Center, I remember signing the guest book after Rupal gave me some noisemakers! She was chanting and such a big smile, Pearl Fertell, Charlie, Russ Apple now Ram, no more than 6 people one crazier than the next. I kept going back to Rupal in eye contact and she would just smile and then I remember Bharat speaking and thought I need to look at this place in another way as this was very different than anything I had ever seen. I also disagreed with everything Bharat said. Reincarnation, meat eating etc. "Anything you don't like just leave here, he would say. Harry would sit next to me and Bharat would tell him to clean his feet! I went to a Hare Krishna temple in Berkley Calif. where all the hippies of 40 years know to show up for the Sunday night feast and the head devotee trained the hippies (in 2005) to at least wash their feet. And they would stick out their feet to show him they had washed their feet! I was rolling in laughter. Somebody's feet did stink and the devotee asked him if he washed his feet. He said, he didn't, but he took a swim in the Ocean the day before in the morning (36 hours ago) is that okay! I had a flood of memories from Baynard Blvd when I heard that. Enjoy your prasad from Texas, it's pretty good.

Gregg Hill

Gopal

Thanks Bharat & Thanks Rupal from which all good things come…
Bharat, Swamiji calls you Brother Bharat. That why Swami Swaroopananda asked you in the Bahamas maybe if you were his brother.

Guruji,

I met Yogi Bharat Gajjar in 2001 through a friend. I had been practicing and teaching Yoga for several years and wanted to have a spiritual name. I e-mailed Bharat and he was very kind in explaining the process. After some time he arranged for me to come visit so we could get to know each other. My wife and I met with him for dinner and we got to know each other. Bharat arranged a time for my initiation and a fire ceremony at the Sivananda Yoga Center.

Bharat's kindness and sincerity have left a lasting impression on me. I remember during the fire ceremony he took a yellow Meditation shawl and as he put it around me and said, "I'll make you a preacher." And he did. Since then we've moved to Kansas City and have conducted Satsangs and Yoga classes. Bharat is my inspiration. I treasure the memory of my short time with him. More than any teacher I've had, he deserves to be called guru. He shows the way by example in his kind and gentle way. I owe much to him.

Blessings,
Ramji Goodman
Kansas City MO

Commentary by Bharat: Every Summer I used to go with my family to spend a week, at the Sivananda Yoga Camp in Canada, to be with my Guruji, H.H. Swami Vishnu Devananda and learn Yoga. One time, I showed him my Sivananda Yoga Center of Delaware Prayer book. He browsed through it and told me that Master Sivananda wanted all his students to publish and spread the message of Yoga. He was very happy that I was doing that and teaching Yoga. My message to all my students is to learn Yoga, practice it and continue learning Yoga and at one point teach Yoga, and spread the word. I'm very happy that Yogi Ramji Goodman and his wife Stephanie are doing just that by teaching Yoga. In addition, they give seminars on Yoga. He has a blog (http://www.eternalself.blogspot.com/) and writes about Advaita philosophy and Meditation through articles and poetry. He also has the blessings of Divine Mother.

Hello Bharat,

It is truly amazing how positively meeting you and your family has influenced my life and how much of a blessing being initiated into the Sivananda Yoga Center has been. I was 21 when I met your family, and was also initiated that year. I have never felt alone since and have been able to draw strength from the Mantra I received and the Satsang that I have enjoyed over the years. I am now 52 and look forward to Satsang as ever. Rupal's presence is always there and Swami Sivananda too. We have always had speakers at Satsang, but you are always are best and most inspiring. My husband Barry was very open to our Yoga Center after I explained to him how important our center was to me when we first met in 1994. Again, I am blessed as he thinks the world of you and loves the chanting and the wonderful friendships he has made at the Center. We are truly blessed!! Thank you!! Hari Om!!

Parvati (Kathy Levin)

Dear Bharat

When I moved here in 1983 I was in the midst of taking philosophy, Meditation, and also Hatha Yoga classes in England. I was very homesick and wanted to connect somehow. I searched and searched. I even contacted the same group for philosophy classes, but they were only in NY on the East coast. (They are now in Philadelphia too). I telephoned around—no Internet, just the yellow pages. I finally spoke to someone who had a karate studio. He mentioned a man named Bharat Gajjar who had a Yoga Center in Wilmington. I was so excited. I called Bharat and he told me to go to the Yoga Center for an evening class that week. I turned up, and when Bharat arrived, we went in. I was not at all skeptical. Being English, I have roots in India and everything was familiar to me. We lay on the floor for Meditation and I was shaking. I knew I was home.

There has been no turning back. I was initiated. My new name is Ganga, which translates to River Ganges. I met my husband-to-be Ram, there. And Bharat married us 18 years ago. It is a wonderful way of life. Non-violence is deep-rooted in me. I am a true vegetarian—for compassionate and spiritual reasons. Bharat changed my life. Swami Vishnu Devananda changed my life. Swami Sivananda changed my life. I am whole now.

Hari Om Tat Sat!

Ganga (Trudy Apple)

Dear Bharat,

I remember very well as a teenager attending Satsang at the Sivananda Yoga Center and Meeta as a little beautiful girl. Bharat and Rupal were so generous and loving. We would have Satsangs on Sunday nights, and I would play the harmonium and Bharat would play the murdanga (Indian drum). We would chant, Bharat would give a talk about spiritual topics, we would have prasadam, and then Bharat would say, "Okay, who wants ice cream?" Bharat's family and I would all jump into our cars and go for ice cream and have a great time.

I was fortunate to also have gone to Val Morin (Sivananda Headquarters in Canada), which was incredible. I remember meeting Swami Vishnu Devananda there and I also became involved with the Sivananda organization in Los Angeles in the early 1980's.

Bharat's Yoga classes were fantastic. He was an incredible teacher. Bharat and Rupal were great cooks as well, and I was fortunate to attend dinners at their home. Also Bharat was so gracious in giving me rides to Satsangs and classes. I also think he gave me my first Bhagavad Gita.

Another example of Bharat's incredible generosity of allowing Scott Davison (another member of the Sivananda Yoga Center) to stay at his parents home in India free, for an entire year to study Tabla (Indian drums).

I remember us all renting a bus to take a field trip to New York City and attending the Sivananda temple service there.

It was a very special, magical inspiring time in my life. I have gone on to become a professional clown/puppeteer and teacher in Los Angeles. I still have my altar and chant, and am greatly blessed to have met and married a wonderful, spiritual man. We have a beautiful home high up in the hills. I want to thank Bharat and Rupal for helping me along on my spiritual journey.

Hari Om Tat Sat
Radha, "Debbie" Alice Jones

At Bharat's Sivananda Yoga Center, I learned how to surrender to life's events through the ancient science of Mantras. Mantras can be chanted, written on paper or used in Meditation. The use of Mantras creates a Web of Godly Vibrations. I think that we, all of Bharat's students, are connected to one another through this Vibration Web. Therefore, our friendships are deep.

Spontaneously or intuitively we call or visit each other at times when this exchange is very necessary, when one needs help and the other understands what kind of help is needed.

Master Sivananda is in charge of this Networking Web. Thank you, Bharat, for all your efforts to run and maintain the Delaware Sivananda Yoga Center. Thank you for your love to each one of us, your students.

Love from your student,

Maya (Elly)

The Gift Of Yoga

In the Indian tradition, presents are not exchanged. But my parents gave me the biggest gift. I was born into a family of Yogis. My Mother and Father are Yogis. When I was four years old I began practicing Yoga every evening before dinner. I practiced Yoga, because that's what my family did. When I was little, Yoga came so easily.

Children are close to God. Spirituality is a big part of their soul, and their bodies are new, they function the best they ever will. A child who is given the gift of Yoga cannot fully appreciate this gift until it grows up. The gift is most appreciated between 30 and 40, when stiffness and back pain begin to be felt.

As an adult when I practice Yoga, my blood flows into areas which need it; deep breathing relaxes me, and my energy blocks are released, I realize how blessed I am to have received this gift of Yoga from my parents. I am a professional singer, a Hatha, Bhakti, and a Naada Yogini. Which means that I connect with God and my audience through sound and music. I started teaching Yoga 10 years ago, and I use my voice to relax my students as well as teach Hatha Yoga.

I grew up as an unconscious vegetarian until I was 20. Yogis do not eat meat, especially red meat, because it stiffens your arteries. It is also preferred (not) to eat lower forms of life out of compassion to animals. Then I became a conscious vegetarian. In college, I did a report on vegetarianism and learned a lot. I learned that meat from a live animal is Grade A meat, while meat from a dead animal becomes dog food. Animals are kept free of disease and illness by giving them antibiotics. But then they became immune to diseases and illnesses, and law only requires that the diseased part be cut off.

I also learned that three-fourths of the world could be fed with the grains used to fatten animals. Why get your food second hand and make your stomach a graveyard? I read about how the animals are killed and how the trauma of the death experience leaves the animals' bodies in the stressed state. When people eat the animal they almost take on the animals' karma, the energy of their trauma. In my heart, soul, I have no desire to eat animals. After marriage, my husband became a vegetarian too.

Your spirituality grows with practice of Yoga. Something happens inside you. A calmness grows inside of you, your heart becomes bigger, you begin to feel, know and understand the word compassion in a whole new way. Your eyes shine with clarity and the word love is understood.

Meeta Gajjar Parker

Dear Bharat,

I moved to Delaware in 1982 and soon after, went through a divorce I didn't want. As I was putting the pieces together, I met Cyndi Dombrowski (Sita), who took me to a hatha Yoga class at the Sivananda Center on Baynard Boulevard. It was several years before my next visit; a cousin and I went to a hatha class and stayed on for Satsang. To my surprise I found myself humming the "Arati" melody all the next week! I began going regularly to the hatha Yoga classes and to satsang, and found a whole new community of loving and kind individuals. Bharat initiated me in the late 1980's. 1991 I went to Val Morin to be certified to teach Yoga. Because of Yogi Bharat's teaching, I knew the bhajans, I knew how to Meditate and to chant, and much of the philosophy even before going. My weeks there were the last summer of Swami Vishnu Devananda's life.

After that I taught every Sunday at the Yoga Center for several years. It is because of Bharat and the community he created that I have made my dearest friends and found peace with my new life in Delaware. Satsang, though its venue has changed, always reunites me with this kind community, and—even more importantly—with myself and with God.

Linda Letson (Gita)

5/7/06

Dear Bharat

In 1964, Rupal Gajjar gave birth to Meeta, and I went to Wilmington to see my brother's family. At that time he was living in an Apartment and wanted to buy a house. I asked him where he would like to buy it. He said, "Green Acres, but I don't think I can afford it." I called a realtor, who showed him a house. Bharat liked it and bought it. At that time Bharat told me that when the children get a little older, he'll send them to India for proper education. I asked him, "Why do Indians always have to run to India? Why can't we make India here?" He said, "Sounds good to me." During that same visit, we had that same realtor show us a house in the city. We bought that house together, as a Hindu Center and that building eventually became the Sivananda Yoga Center. After 35 years, when he wanted to retire and he couldn't find anyone to take over, he sold that building for $100,000, which he gave to me to open schools in India.

Here is an account of how we have used the proceeds from the sale of the Sivananda Yoga Center (HC Inc.) and the donation of the revenue. In August 2003, we started 60 new schools, 30 with Vishva Hindu Parishad (VHP) and 30 with Rastriya Seva Sangh (RSS) in interior Gujarat, India. Both these groups are non-profit organizations and are run by volunteers.

These 60 schools were started in villages where no schools existed, where children had no opportunity to get any education. On the average each school has one room and 30 to 35 children.

Because of our involvement and contributions, about 1,800 children are getting an education, which they would not have had without our assistance.

Every month we continue to contribute to these schools. We have received overwhelming positive feedback and gratitude from the villagers where our schools are located. You and I believe that providing education is one of the best kinds of charity as it gives people dignity and means to help themselves.

Love, Navin J. Gajjar

VHP Summer Youth Camp

In 1983, I decided to volunteer at the Vishwa Hindu Parishad (VHP) and my goal was to teach the children and the parents Yoga and Mantra Yoga. I used to go for two weeks and there were 100 boy and girls and 50 parents in each of two camps. I went to the camps every year until 2005.

The following is a letter to me from one of the mothers who attended the camp with her children.

Aadarniya Bharat ji:

Namaste.

I am fine and we all are trying to adjust to life after camp. I wish there were more such camps so that we could go to them year round. Then we will not feel the deep vacuum of missing India so much.

The children came home and sang the Aarti on Saturday evening to their father. They have been talking about the camp to all their friends. That is the great fruit of all the efforts of the whole organizing committee.

Waiting for 51 weeks is really too much.

Other Indian groups should know how VHP camps are serving the Hindu community and doing such a great job.

I thank you from the bottom of my heart for doing all that you do for Hindus of the next generation, as well as the present one. You are a role model to us.

With regards—

Sucheta Maheshwari

This is a young man who received his Mantra initiation and spiritual name from me and he is teaching Yoga in Russia.

10/2/92

Dearest Guruji!

How are you? How are things? How is your Yoga? What News? At last I am staying at home and writing this letter to you. I haven't written to you for almost a year. It was due to my intensive work and frequent long business trips. Now I will be devoting more of my time to teaching Yoga.

So many changes have happened since my last letter and the main one is that I live in a newly independent country. Unfortunately I couldn't come and visit you as I had planned, but it would be splendid to restore our contact again. May God bless you and your children!

Om Shanti

Shiva (Alex Loubenski)

8/16/06

Dear Mr., Gajjar,

I recently saw a copy of your prayer book. I think it is a beautiful work of devotion. I am wondering if you would happen to have a scanned, digital version of the prayer book or if you would be willing to send me a physical copy via the post. I am willing to pay for any expenses incurred.

Thank you and again Congratulations on such a lifework of devotion.

Best Regards,

Tomás Fonseca

São Paulo, Brasil

Dear Ones,

On September 14,1997 I was initiated by Bharat starting at his home and continuing the ceremony at The Sivananda Yoga Center. My spiritual name of Shri Devi, it was given to me that day by Bharat. This name means Love Goddess in the most spiritual sense to me. The image brought to Bharat as he gave me this name sparkled in his eyes and the magnitude of knowledge that was imparted to me over numerous years with Bharat were imparted at that moment. I learned and grew with the Hindu teachings of Bharat my Guru. I have the BE GOOD—DO GOOD bench on our front porch now and everyone sits there as they come to get Acupuncture from my husband of whom I met through my interactions with Ma Devi at The Sivananda Yoga center!!! That is the most incredible event besides my Mantra initiation, the birth of my son, and prior experience as an RN for a Hindu family for 3 years caring for a child raised in the Hindu beliefs and rituals on a day-to-day basis. This is my 20th year as a nurse. The last important event (thus far in my physical life) that occurred from my time being taught self-acceptance at The Sivananda Yoga Center on Baynard Blvd. in Wilmington, DE, was knowing that my son Kyle B. Wawrzenski (12.6yrs.young-2006/9) had in fact been a Yogi when he was born and demonstrated 10 years later (or so) that fact; when his gym teacher asked if anyone new Yoga (asked in Medford, NJ), all the kids said no!! EXCEPT KYLE!!! He was then asked to demonstrate what he knew:

1. Lotus Pose-with prayerful hands
2. Fish Pose
3. Bridge Pose
4. Shoulder Stand

He had resisted doing this with Michael E. Moore, L. Ac., M. Ac.(my husband) and I Sheri L. Moore, R. N., B.S.N. The fact is that Yoga is always with us at all ages through the postures, Mantras, masters—BHARAT GAJJAR, and the realization of Maya. HARI OM TAT SAT!!!

Chapter 36

Your Life-Altering Wisdom

One day Meeta came to me and suggested this idea for a chapter. It would provide everyone with an opportunity to give their personal life altering wisdom to others. It should be something that you use to guide your life. So please read the following and reach inside yourself, Meditate and find a life-changing sentence to share. If it comes from someone else, tell us where it came from. We need your name along with your 1 or 2 quotations.

1)   Meeta Gajjar Parker (Parvati Devi)
"You only get love by giving love." My Mother
"Tomorrow never comes, because when it comes, it comes in the form of Today." Bhagawan Rajneesh

2)   Frank Parker
"Everyone determines their own fate."
"The most important thing in life is how you treat other people."

3)   Kathy Levin (Parvati)
"All paths lead to the same river" Swami Sivananda

4) Bharat J. Gajjar
"If you do anything three times or more it is a habit"
"When a bride enters the house and the child is in the cradle, they show their colors and it never changes." Gujrati Proverb

5)   Cindy Kerr
"Treat people like it is the last time you are going to see them."
"Slow down and enjoy life and don't let life pass you by."

6)   Agatha Fuller
"You are the creator of your destiny"

7)   Gregg Hill (Gopal)
"If you give mercy, you get mercy." Tamal Krishna Goswami
"The world to me is a ball of fire." Swami Vishnudevanada

8) Marie Allen
"Accept and enjoy the positive opportunities that are presented to you; you may not have another chance at what is being offered."
"The unselfish effort to bring cheer to others will be the beginning of a happier life for ourselves" Helen Keller

9)   Theresa Danberg
"If you don't wind, you don't have to unwind." Bharat J. Gajjar

10)   Alice Jones (Scott)
"Hold fast to dreams for when dreams die, life is like a broken winged bird that cannot fly." Langston Hughes
"Life is not a dress rehearsal."

11) Lee Scott
"Time is relative, but no relative of mine." Donald Gauthier
"Be here now." Ram Dass

12) Jeanne Poggi Kraszewski
"We shall never know all the good that a simple smile can do." Mother Teresa

13)   Chris Miller (Anandi Ma)
"Meditation gives you the opportunity to come to know your invisible self. It shatters the illusion of your separateness."
"A mind at peace, a mind focused on not harming others, is stronger than the universe."

14)   Karen Foley (Gayatri)
"Man Proposes, God Disposes."
"Rejection is Protection."

15) Andy Ednir
"Don't sweat the small stuff."
"You're born, you die, and in between you watch birds."

16) *Judi A. Herring*
"You cannot be more than your nature allows"

17) Marc Weisburg (Arjun)
"Be a friend to all." Swami Sivananda
"Lead a life of continuous improvement. For every problem there is a solution." Bharat Gajjar

18) Kathleen Taylor and Mayra   This is an American proverb.
"There is no free lunch." Bharat Gajjar

19) Ajay B. Gajjar
"Prana is the life force (shakti) which runs the body. Your body is also made of Shakti. If you recognize this, your body can be healed or cured in an instant."
"Those who play in school work hard later and those who work hard in school play later." Bharat's School Teacher

20) Yogi Vitaldas
"A Yogi not only knows how to live, but knows how to die."
"A true Yogi knows when he will be leaving this material world and die consciously."

21) Patricia Trusty
"The shadow of my past leans on an invisible path guiding me directly to my future."

22) Rosemary Lort
"When you change the way you look at things, the things you look at change." Dr. Wayne W. Dyer
"A belief is only a thought you keep thinking." The Teachings of Abraham

23) Jennifer Dize

"An ounce of practice is worth more than a ton of theory." Swami Sivananda

"Use things and love people. Don't use people and love things" Unknown

24) Pamela Randall

"To love myself, is the greatest gift to myself."

"Life is a precious gift. Be careful when handling."

25) Danielle Farmer

"A person can only do what you allow them to do to you."

26) Shelly Hack

"If a small thing has the power to make you angry, does that indicate something about your size?" Sydney Harris

"Forgiveness is the final form of love." Reinold Niebuhr

27) Tracy Marvel

"It's better to deserve honors and not to have them, than to have them and not deserve them." Mark Twain

"Mistakes are often garments of miracles." Unknown

28) Natasha Davis

"Life isn't about finding yourself it's about creating yourself." George Shaw

29) Michele Pennington

"Life is not measured by how many breath's we take, but by the moments that take our breath away." Unknown

"Today is a gift; Tomorrow is a promise of hope, and yesterday is the wind at your back."

30) Audry Becker (Yogini)

"Worse than blindness is sight without vision." Helen Keller

"Dance like no one is watching. Love like you've never been hurt, and live each day like it's your last." Unknown

31) Tom Lundy
"Trust in God; but tie your camel up first." Ancient Arab wisdom

32) Bob Krahn (Shiva)
"There is nothing either good or bad, but thinking makes it so."
Shakespeare—Hamlet, Act II, Scene II:
"Shave the Mind, not your head"—Swami Sivananda

33) Leo Waters
"When I was young, I could eat a horse and my wife was a lousy cook. Now, I'm old, can't eat anything, and she's become a great cook. That's the way life is."

34) Jaybhadhra G. Gajjar
"Get ahead by working hard not by sweet talking."
"It has no meaning to say 'I wish I had done that.'"

35) Robert A. Kasey
"When public speaking, Summarize the message you want them to take with them, explain it, say it again, then sit down."

36) I. E. DuPont de Nemours and Company
"Do it right the first time."
"Don't say it, write it."

37) Cindy Krahn (Shivani)
"Believe nothing, no matter where you read it, or who said it—even if I have said it—unless it agrees with your own reason and your own common sense." Buddha

38) Mary Britt
"Every little bit counts, no matter how small no matter how insignificant it may seem."